SOFTWARE SINGLE-USER LICENSE AGREEMENT

D1278034

1. NOTICE. WE ARE WILLING TO LICENSE THE PRODUCT *Potter: Software to accompany Medical Office Administration: A Worktext* ("SOFTWARE PRODUCT") TO YOU ONLY ON THE CONDITION THAT YOU ACCEPT ALL OF THE TERMS CONTAINED IN THIS LICENSE AGREEMENT. PLEASE READ THIS LICENSE AGREEMENT CAREFULLY BEFORE OPENING THE SEALED DISK PACKAGE. BY OPENING THAT PACKAGE YOU AGREE TO BE BOUND BY THE TERMS OF THIS AGREEMENT. IF YOU DO NOT AGREE TO THESE TERMS WE ARE UNWILLING TO LICENSE THE SOFTWARE PRODUCT TO YOU, AND YOU SHOULD NOT OPEN THE DISK PACKAGE. IN SUCH CASE, PROMPTLY RETURN THE UNOPENED DISK PACKAGE AND ALL OTHER MATERIAL IN THIS PACKAGE, ALONG WITH PROOF OF PAYMENT, TO THE AUTHORIZED DEALER FROM WHOM YOU OBTAINED IT FOR A FULL REFUND OF THE PRICE YOU PAID.

2. Ownership and License. This is a license agreement and NOT an agreement for sale. It permits you to use the Software Product on a computer network only on the terms set forth in this Agreement. The Software Product and its contents are owned by us or our licensors, and are protected by U.S. and international copyright laws. Your rights to use the Software Product are specified in this Agreement, and we retain all rights not expressly granted to you in this Agreement.

- You may use one copy of the Software Product on a single computer.
- After you have installed the Software Product on your computer, you may use the Software Product on a different computer only if you first delete the files installed by the installation program from the first computer.
- You may not copy any portion of the Software Product to your computer hard disk or any other media other than printing out or downloading nonsubstantial portions of the text and images in the Software Product for your own internal information use.
- You may not copy any of the documentation or other printed materials accompanying the Software Product.

3. Transfer and Other Restrictions. You may not rent, lend, or lease this Software Product. You may not and you may not permit others to (a) disassemble, decompile, or otherwise derive source code from the software included in the Software Product (the "Software"), (b) reverse engineer the Software, (c) modify or prepare derivative works of the Software Product, (d) use the Software in an on-line system or (e) use the Software Product in any manner that infringes on the intellectual property or other rights of another party.

However, you may transfer this license to use the Software Product, to another party on a permanent basis by transferring this copy of the License Agreement, the Software Product, and all documentation. Such transfer of possession terminates your license from us. Such other party shall be licensed under the terms of this Agreement upon its acceptance of this Agreement by its initial use of the Software Product. If you transfer the Software Product, you must remove the installation files from your hard disk and you may not retain any copies of those files for your own use.

4. Limited Warranty and Limitation of Liability. For a period of sixty (60) days from the date you acquired the Software Product from us or our authorized dealer, we warrant that the media containing the Software Product will be free from defects that prevent you from installing the Software Product on your computer. If the disk fails to conform to this warranty, you may, as your sole and exclusive remedy, obtain a replacement free of charge if you return the defective disk to us with a dated proof of purchase. Otherwise the Software Product is licensed to you on an "AS IS" basis without any warranty of any nature.

WE DO NOT WARRANT THAT THE SOFTWARE PRODUCT WILL MEET YOUR REQUIREMENTS OR THAT ITS OPERATION WILL BE UNINTERRUPTED OR ERROR-FREE. WE EXCLUDE AND EXPRESSLY DISCLAIM ALL EXPRESS AND IMPLIED WARRANTIES NOT STATED HEREIN, INCLUDING THE IMPLIED WARRANTIES OF MERCHANTABILITY AND FITNESS FOR A PARTICULAR PURPOSE.

WE SHALL NOT BE LIABLE FOR ANY DAMAGE OR LOSS OF ANY KIND ARISING OUT OF OR RESULTING FROM YOUR POSSESSION OR USE OF THE SOFTWARE PRODUCT (INCLUDING DATA LOSS OR CORRUPTION), REGARDLESS OF WHETHER SUCH LIABILITY IS BASED IN TORT, CONTRACT OR OTHERWISE AND INCLUDING, BUT NOT LIMITED TO, ACTUAL, SPECIAL, INDIRECT, INCIDENTAL OR CONSEQUENTIAL DAMAGES. IF THE FOREGOING LIMITATION IS HELD TO BE UNENFORCEABLE, OUR MAXIMUM LIABILITY TO YOU SHALL NOT EXCEED THE AMOUNT OF THE LICENSE FEE PAID BY YOU FOR THE SOFTWARE PRODUCT. THE REMEDIES AVAILABLE TO YOU AGAINST US AND THE LICENSORS OF MATERIALS INCLUDED IN THE SOFTWARE PRODUCT ARE EXCLUSIVE.

Some states do not allow the limitation or exclusion of implied warranties or liability for incidental or consequential damages, so the above limitations or exclusions may not apply to you.

5. United States Government Restricted Rights. The Software Product and documentation are provided with Restricted Rights. Use, duplication, or disclosure by the U.S. Government or any agency or instrumentality thereof is subject to restrictions as set forth in subdivision (c)(1)(ii) of the Rights in Technical Data and Computer Software clause at 48 C.F.R. 252.227-7013, or in subdivision (c)(1) and (2) of the Commercial Computer Software-Restricted Rights Clause at 48 C.F.R. 52.277-19, as applicable. The manufacturer is Elsevier Science, the Curtis Center, Suite 300, Independence Square West, Philadelphia, PA 19106.

6. Termination. This license and your right to use this Software Product automatically terminate if you fail to comply with any provision of this Agreement, destroy the copy of the Software Product in your possession, or voluntarily return the Software Product to us. Upon termination you will destroy all copies of the Software Product and documentation.

7. Miscellaneous Provisions. This Agreement will be governed by and construed in accordance with the substantive laws of the Commonwealth of Pennsylvania. This is the entire agreement between us relating to the Software Product, and supersedes any prior purchase order, communications, advertising or representations concerning the contents of this package. No change or modification of this Agreement will be valid unless it is in writing and is signed by us.

Medical Office Administration:
A Worktext

Brenda A. Potter, BS
Instructor
Northwest Technical College
Moorhead, Minnesota

SAUNDERS
An Imprint of Elsevier Science
Philadelphia   London   New York   St. Louis   Sydney   Toronto

SAUNDERS

An Imprint of Elsevier Science

The Curtis Center
Independence Square West
Philadelphia, PA 19106

MEDICAL OFFICE ADMINISTRATION: A WORKTEXT

ISBN 0-7216-8746-6

Library of Congress Cataloging-in-Publication Data

Potter, Brenda A.
    Medical office administration: a worktext / Brenda A. Potter. — 1st ed.
      p. ;   cm.
    Includes index.
    ISBN 0-7216-8746-6
      1. Medical offices — Management — Problems, exercises, etc. 2. Medical
secretaries — Problems, exercises, etc. 3. Medical records — Problems, exercises, etc.
I. Title.
      [DNLM: 1. Office Management — Problems and Exercises. 2. Medical
Receptionists — Problems and Exercises. 3. Medical Record Administrators — Problems
and Exercises. 4. Medical Records — Problems and Exercises. W 18.2 P866m 2002]
    R728.8 .P665 2002
651′.961 — dc21   2001031150

Publishing Director: Andrew Allen
Senior Acquisitions Editor: Adrianne Cochran
Senior Developmental Editor: Rae L. Robertson
Project Managers: Linda Lewis Grigg and Natalie Ware
Designer: Steven Stave

PI/QWK

Printed in the United States of America.

Last digit is the print number: 9   8   7   6   5   4   3   2   1

To my husband and my children, who provided enduring support whenever and wherever I needed it, and for their love, patience, and understanding while I pursued this dream; to Mom and Dad, who taught me to dream big and to strive for the best in everything; to my sisters and entire family, who are my shelter and foundation; to my friends, who were a constant source of encouragement; to all of my students, past, present, and future, who are the inspiration and motivation for this work. I have been truly blessed.

PREFACE

The best interest of the patient is the only interest to be considered. — *Mayo Clinic founders, late 1800s*

No better words than these can describe the focus of and purpose for Medical Office Administration. The patient is, indeed, the very purpose of anyone's work in heath care—whether a student is preparing for employment in the business aspect of the medical office or in direct patient care. Each patient is the very reason for our presence in the office.

Over the last 20 to 25 years, the health care industry has undergone a tremendous metamorphosis. Health care is increasingly similar to the marketplace. Outpatient clinics have gone from 9–5 Monday through Friday hours to evening and weekend availability. Physicians now *advertise* their services to potential patients. The industry is extremely patient-focused and customer-sensitive, and it treats the patient as any thriving business treats a customer.

Medical Office Administration explores the career of a medical administrative assistant, beginning with the examination of the profession and the health care industry and continuing on to the daily responsibilities of a medical administrative assistant. The text is organized into five units and 15 chapters that are designed to prepare the student for employment as a medical administrative assistant.

Medical Office Administration is designed to meet the medical administrative competencies as developed by the American Association of Medical Assistants and the American Medical Technologists. Procedures checklists provide a detailed outline to help students meet administrative competencies and to assist instructors in evaluating those competencies. The text can be used by anyone desiring to understand the day-to-day business activities of a medical office.

In writing *Medical Office Administration,* my basic philosophy included developing exercises that encouraged problem solving, team building, and critical thinking. Although memorization of some facts is necessary, I strove to encourage higher level thinking skills in the majority of exercises and projects within the text. It is not just enough to know the facts, but students must be able to apply their knowledge of these facts to various situations that may occur in the medical office. The worktext focus of this text encourages that application.

This text uses several features to present the complexities of the medical office environment:

- Everything needed for primary instruction in medical office administration is included in the text.
- The text is an *all-in-one worktext,* which consists of a textbook and workbook along with a medical office software program component that takes the learning process to a higher level.
- The workbook feature of the text includes exercises, activities, and discussions related to topics presented within each chapter.
- *Lytec Medical 2001* is a medical office management program featuring computerized appointment scheduling, registration, billing, and insurance activities. The text includes many practical scenarios that involve operation of the program.

CHECKPOINT

Features included in each chapter give students the opportunity to apply knowledge gained in the chapter to a critical-thinking situation.

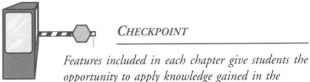

YOU ARE THE MEDICAL ADMINISTRATIVE ASSISTANT

is a feature that allows the reader to apply knowledge learned in the chapter to realistic medical office scenarios.

Procedure boxes offer step-by-step instructions on how to perform specific administrative tasks.

- Competency checklists, based on the AAMA curriculum components, spell out the individual steps required to complete a full range of administrative procedures and allow the instructor or student to evaluate performance.
- A comprehensive Instructor's Curriculum Resource includes lesson plans, numerous resources, information on how to set up a curriculum, and additional ideas for classroom instruction as well as answers to worktext exercises and tests for each chapter.

Throughout my various career experiences in health care and in the business world, I have lived and breathed what students will experience in the workplace. Quality customer service is essential to the success of a health care organization today and is a common thread woven throughout this text. How we interact with others is crucial to the success of any organization. In my career as an instructor at Northwest Technical College in Moorhead, Minnesota, I have assisted numerous students with gaining employment in the medical administrative assisting, medical transcription, and medical coding professions. It is with that understanding that I am pleased to present this publication for your use.

BRENDA A. POTTER

EDITORIAL REVIEW BOARD

ACKNOWLEDGMENTS

I would like to offer sincere and profound thanks to everyone involved with this project, especially:

- To Rae Robertson, my Senior Developmental Editor, who kept me on track with this project. Her sheer persistence has made this textbook a reality;
- To Adrianne Cochran, Senior Acquisitions Editor, who saw with me the vision for this work and gave me the chance to realize this accomplishment;
- To the Production and Art & Design staff for all their support in seeing this project to its fruition: Natalie Ware, Linda Grigg, and Steven Stave;

- To the staff at Lytec Medical for providing the software and technical support for this project;
- To the many reviewers whose valuable input provided the needed guidance to make this text a reality;
- To my colleagues at Northwest Technical College for their enthusiasm, advice, and encouragement to pursue this project;
- And to medical administrative assisting instructors everywhere who find inspiration and merit in this work.

I am eternally grateful to all of you.

BRENDA A. POTTER

CONTENTS

Working in the Health Care Environment

CHAPTER OUTLINE

LEARNING OUTCOMES

On successful completion of this chapter, the student will be able to

1. Recognize various titles for office positions usually filled by medical administrative assistants and recognize the places where an assistant might find related employment.
2. Relate typical job duties of a medical administrative assistant.
3. Explain desired personal qualities of a medical administrative assistant.
4. Demonstrate appropriate professional appearance for a medical administrative assistant.
5. Identify professional skills needed by a medical administrative assistant.
6. Identify employment information (e.g., earnings, employment trends, and forecasts related to the medical administrative assistant profession).
7. Examine professional organizations and related certifications for medical administrative assistants.
8. Describe the importance of a student portfolio and begin a portfolio.

RMA COMPETENCIES

1. Employ appropriate interpersonal skills in the work place.
2. Know terminology associated with medical secretarial and receptionist duties.

VOCABULARY

Certified Coding Specialist
Certified Coding Specialist–Physician Based
Certified Medical Assistant
Certified Professional Secretary
compassion
confidentiality
empathy
medical administrative assistant
medical assistant
medical transcriptionist
Registered Medical Assistant
student portfolio

THE CAREER OF A MEDICAL ADMINISTRATIVE ASSISTANT

Two important things are to have a genuine interest in people and to be kind to them. Kindness, I've discovered, is everything.

—*Isaac Bashevis Singer*

Wanted: Enthusiastic, caring, empathetic individual with an interest in health care to work in a large or small office with few or many coworkers. Must be able to handle the stress of a heavy workload one day and a light workload the next.

This is quite an interesting job description, isn't it? Although such an advertisement would probably never appear in a newspaper, it is very descriptive of what many employers expect of a medical administrative assistant.

Students electing to pursue a career in the medical office may or may not already have an idea of what a medical administrative assistant does.

Students select this job for a variety of reasons. For example, they may have an interest in health care, they may enjoy working with people, or they may be looking for a rewarding career.

What can be expected of an assistant on the job? Let's take a look at the career of a medical administrative assistant.

CAREER DESCRIPTION

When seeking employment as an administrative assistant in health care, one of the first things to note is that there are many different titles for this type of administrative support position.

In this text, the title **medical administrative assistant** has been chosen to identify an individual who serves patient and organizational needs by performing a huge variety of office support functions in a health care organization. The position is identified with a variety of titles, a few of which are listed in Box 1–1. The title *medical administrative assistant* is used because *administrative assistant* is a commonly used and accepted term for an individual performing office support functions and *medical administrative assistant* identifies an individual who performs these activities in a health care setting (Fig. 1–1).

Job Duties

Although a variety of job titles exist for the position of medical administrative assistant, the essential duties remain the same. What might those duties include?

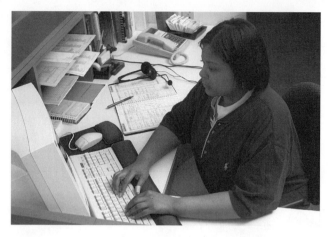

Figure 1–1. A medical administrative assistant performs a wide variety of a medical office's administrative support functions.

A typical job description for a medical administrative assistant can vary widely depending on the specific duties of the position in a particular office. Each office has its own unique needs that depend on the structure and purpose of the organization. An assistant's job description may include *any* or possibly *all* of the common administrative duties listed in Box 1–2, and, depending on the employer, the job description could include additional duties.

It is a medical administrative assistant's job to provide office support for the efficient operation of the medical office. Administrative responsibilities are also part of another multi-skilled position known as **medical assistant.** The term *medical assistant* is used to describe an individual who is qualified to perform both *administrative* and *clinical* duties in a medical office. The clinical responsibilities of a medical assistant will also vary with the needs of the office and can include some or all of the clinical duties listed in Box 1–3.

It is important for a student in a medical office–related program to clearly understand the differences in the job responsibilities of a medical administrative assistant and a medical assistant. A medical administrative assistant performs administrative duties, and a medical assistant may perform administrative duties, clinical duties, or both,

Box 1–1 Possible Titles for a Medical Administrative Assistant

- Medical secretary
- Medical office assistant
- Medical office specialist
- Patient services representative
- Patient services specialist
- Patient services assistant

Box 1–2 Administrative Duties of a Medical Administrative Assistant

- Schedule appointments.
- Screen and make telephone calls.
- Obtain and verify patient registration information.
- Transcribe medical dictation.
- Maintain medical records.
- Prepare correspondence.
- Prepare patient billing.
- Prepare insurance claims.
- Perform financial and bookkeeping procedures.
- Arrange outside appointments and admissions.
- Manage office activities.

Box 1–3 Clinical Duties of a Medical Assistant

- Use precautions necessary in a health care environment.
- Obtain patient's medical history.
- Obtain patient's vital signs.
- Perform routine laboratory and diagnostic tests.
- Prepare patient for examination.
- Prepare the office for patient examinations and treatments.
- Assist with examinations and procedures.
- Prepare and administer medications.
- Apply sterilization procedures.

depending on the needs of the health care organization in which she or he works. The terms *medical administrative assistant* and *assistant* are used interchangeably to represent the same position, but the terms *medical administrative assistant* and *medical assistant* cannot be used interchangeably because of the scope of their responsibilities. The medical administrative assistant and the medical assistant do perform the administrative skills of the office, however, and those skills are presented within this text.

A Typical Day at the Office

What is it really like to work in a medical office? Job descriptions highlight the major job responsibilities, but many other things happen as part of everyday activities. From one day to the next, the job can be quite surprising and challenging. Each day, by providing patients with the best possible service, a medical administrative assistant has the opportunity to make a difference in someone's life.

The responsibilities of an assistant will be greatly influenced by the size of the organization. In a large organization, an assistant sometimes specializes in a specific area of responsibility or a combination of specific areas, such as billing, insurance, registration, appointments, transcription, or medical records. In a small organization, an assistant often has a variety of different responsibilities and may even be responsible for all of the administrative responsibilities listed previously.

In addition to the administrative duties, an assistant may be asked to assume other office-specific duties, such as arming and disarming alarm systems used for office security; providing after-hours instructions using voice messaging systems for patients who need care after the office is closed; or devising, reorganizing, and implementing procedures to improve patient services. At the same time, an assistant needs to be ready for any possible medical emergency that could present in the office. All of these things may be required to be done *in addition to* the administrative skills previously mentioned. There are days that can go by in the blink of an eye and other days that give an assistant an opportunity to

catch up on office tasks that were postponed because of a heavy patient load. An assistant must be prepared for almost anything while at work.

Personal Qualities

If the ability to perform the office duties were all that a medical administrative assistant had to bring to the job, it might be easy for many individuals to simply learn the steps of a procedure and repeat them on the job. But there are other attributes that are important for a medical administrative assistant to possess. Granted, a medical administrative assistant's ability to perform the tasks necessary for the position is important, but equally important are the personal qualities and characteristics that a medical administrative assistant possesses and refines while receiving training in the profession. And that is what this position should be considered—a profession.

An assistant should always keep in mind the qualities and characteristics that are necessary to provide patients with the best possible service. Exceptional service for patients is extremely important. Patients are the reason for the work of medical professionals.

What are some of the personal qualities and characteristics that employers look for in potential employees?

Empathy. Empathy is probably one of the most highly desired qualities of a medical administrative assistant and of many other health care professionals. Empathy means that an individual has a deep understanding of what another individual is experiencing. For example, the parents of a child who is ill may be waiting for the results of some diagnostic tests. A medical administrative assistant might offer a quiet place for the parents to sit with their child. An assistant, knowing the parents may be experiencing some stress, would try to make their office visit as comfortable as possible. An empathetic assistant reacts to a situation with an understanding of what a patient and family must be experiencing.

Compassion. Working in a medical office can, at times, be hectic, but it is also very rewarding. Every day, a medical administrative assistant has an opportunity to make a difference in people's lives by providing assistance to patients with varying medical concerns. Compassionate individuals display a genuine caring and concern for people. They are kind and considerate and often put one another's feelings ahead of their own. Assistants are usually very friendly individuals and enjoy working with people.

Sometimes a patient's or family's experience with a family member who is ill can be very difficult emotionally. An assistant, while interacting with a patient, needs to be careful to not become so personally and emotionally involved with the situation that it prevents him or her from performing assigned job duties. Some situations can be very challenging, and an assistant will need to remember the boundaries of professional behavior.

Dependability. A physician expects the front office staff to provide office support when and where needed and to manage the activities of the office with as little intervention as possible from the physician. Staff members must be punctual by reporting to work on time, taking only the specified amount of time for coffee and lunch breaks, and covering the front desk at all times. If a staff member is ill, he or she may need to secure a replacement or notify the supervisor early enough to find a substitute for the day. To provide the best possible patient service, all office staff members must work as a team, and staff members must be able to depend on one another to accomplish the work of the office.

Confidentiality. All health care personnel are expected to hold confidential all that they hear, see, or do in regard to patients and the care that patients receive. A patient's reason for care and medical history are often very sensitive issues, and all health care personnel must take the utmost care that such issues remain secret.

Attention to Details. A medical administrative assistance must be well organized and thorough in performing the daily activities of the office. Because of the serious nature of many patients' health care needs, an assistant must be precise and accurate when performing office duties.

Other Desirable Personality Traits. When interviewing new employees, employers may look for a variety of personal attributes. An assistant who, in addition to the traits mentioned, is honest, courteous, sincere, and conscientious will have a greatly increased chance of being hired.

Professional Appearance

Another highly desired personal quality is a professional appearance. The type of clothing worn and other things a person does regarding his or her outward appearance create a lasting impression. That impression must be a good one. When working in a medical office, it is extremely important for a medical administrative assistant to possess a professional appearance and be well-groomed. A professional appearance will help create the impression that an assistant will do everything he or she can for a patient and that the assistant will serve a patient in an appropriate manner. A professional appearance adds to a patient's confidence in the medical staff.

A very important thing to remember when choosing clothing and preparing for work in a medical office is that **health care is very conservative.** Outrageous fads, outlandish clothing, and the like have no place in a health care setting. An extreme or peculiar appearance could destroy patient confidence in the office staff. Conservative clothing does not mean that clothing must be fancy, lavish, or expensive—it means that clothing should be modest or traditional. Even casual clothing can be conservative—for example, a pair of khaki pants and a coordinating polo shirt would be tasteful and very appropriate for some offices.

Office Attire

Depending on the facility in which they work, medical administrative assistants wear a variety of apparel. The types

---

Box 1–4 Do's and Don'ts for Professional Appearance

Do

Dress like the people in the position above yours. At promotion time, you'll already look as though you'll fit in.

Be mindful of the colors you wear. In a high-pressure situation, some colors create more excitement than others do. Navy is a traditional business color.

Wear some type of hosiery at all times, even in the hot summer months. Bare legs are not acceptable in a business environment.

Don't

Wear clothing that is outlandish or very unusual.

Wear fads. Wait until the fad becomes the style.

Wear seductive, provocative clothing. For women, short skirts, see-through blouses, and bare midriffs are an absolute no! For men, open shirts without an undershirt are not appropriate.

---

of clothing worn at a medical office range all the way from casual dress and uniforms to business dress. The trend lately has been for quite a few places of business to allow staff members to dress in a casual way: pants, sweaters, knits, and so forth. Some medical employers prefer to select a uniform or variations of a basic uniform for their employees to ensure that all staff members are dressed appropriately for the environment. Some guidelines for selecting clothing for work are listed in Box 1–4.

Uniforms

Uniforms are popular in some medical offices (Fig. 1–2). A uniform may be either casual in style or have a "business" look. Casual uniforms generally consist of a comfortable pair of pants (usually white in color), a colorful smock-type top that allows the wearer to wear a shirt of some kind underneath, and a pair of white tennis shoes. This type of uniform is extremely comfortable and wears well. The tennis shoes are an added bonus to the uniform in that assistants can expect to spend long hours on their feet, and tennis shoes help minimize the chance of foot injuries that can arise with these types of work demands. A disadvantage to wearing a casual uniform is that if the front desk staff and nursing or other staff members wear the same type of uniform, patients may confuse the front desk staff with others in the office.

A business uniform consists of a collection of business apparel in a few color choices. The basic pieces of the uniform are available to purchase in colors that coordinate with one another. For example, the uniform pieces might be available

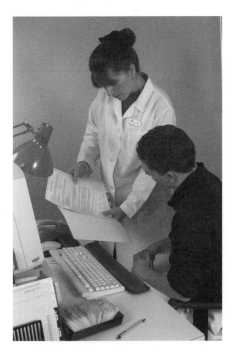

Figure 1–2. A uniform helps identify the office staff.

in navy, khaki, and burgundy. Employees could then choose from uniform components in one or more of the selected colors. The basic pieces of the uniform would include blazers, pants, and skirts for women and jackets and pants for men. An assistant may then be allowed to wear any shirt or accessory that fits within the color scheme. A disadvantage to business uniforms is that the uniform can be costly. Also, as personnel come and go from the facility, the uniform must be available in open stock to ensure that all assistants look the same.

Other Office Apparel

For those facilities not requiring uniforms for their office staff, some type of business dress will be expected to be worn to work (Fig. 1–3). The office may allow casual dress as mentioned previously or may require the staff to wear more formal business clothing. A good rule of thumb is that if you are not sure what to wear to work, observe what *most* of the rest of the staff members are wearing. Ask your supervisor specifically if there is a dress code to follow for work.

Personal Appearance

Medical administrative assistants should have impeccable grooming habits. They should pay attention to every detail.

Fingernails should be kept clean and trimmed because hands are often in view while an assistant is helping patients. Women choosing to wear nail polish should be careful to wear subdued colors and should avoid shockingly bright or neon colors. Polished nails should be maintained and should not be allowed to chip.

Hair. In addition to being neat and well kept, it is often wise to choose a hairstyle that is easy to maintain. Hairstyles that require a lot of "fuss" to look just right might not hold up in a busy office.

Scents. Use perfumes, after-shaves, and other fragrances with caution in a medical office. If they are used to excess, they can wreak havoc for patients and coworkers who may be allergic to fragrances. Make sure a fragrance is not overpowering.

Jewelry. Try to limit jewelry to three or four pieces. There is no need to decorate every appendage of the body with a piece of jewelry. If ears are pierced, avoid several earrings on one ear.

Trends. From time to time, unusual trends related to appearance circulate around the country. Unusual hair color, body piercing, and tattoos are usually frowned on for employees in a health care setting. Remember, the health care environment is very conservative. Employers are not likely to look with favor on employees who come to work with an unusual appearance.

Professional Skills

Career preparation for medical administrative assistants is available at many public and private educational institutions throughout the United States. Curriculum for this profession provides training for necessary job skills and usually consists of courses in the following:

Medical Terminology, Anatomy and Physiology, and Disease Processes. Medical terminology training provides an understanding of medical terms and abbreviations. Training in anatomy, physiology, and disease conditions covers the structure and function of the human body as well as disease and disorders that affect humans. An understanding of these subjects is essential for serving patients and conducting the business of health care. The medical administrative assistant is a vital communications link among the patient, the physician, and the rest of the office staff. Whether transcribing medical reports, processing a patient's bill, taking a message, or scheduling an appointment, an assistant must possess an exceptional command of medical language to serve as that communications link.

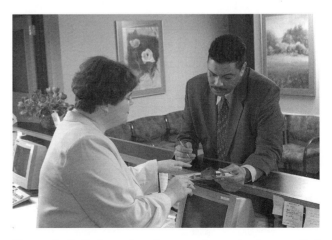

Figure 1–3. Business dress is appropriate attire in a medical office.

Medical Office Procedures and Practices. Telephone reception, appointment scheduling, medical record maintenance, and other office activities are part of the everyday activities of a medical administrative assistant. Knowledge of what, why, when, and how things are done in the medical office is expected of graduates entering the workforce.

Medical Transcription. The documentation of a patient's encounter with the health care provider is an important part of the activities of the medical office. A physician must keep accurate, complete, and legible documentation of each patient's visit. Medical transcription involves the production of medical reports that provide a record of a patient's visit with a health care provider. These reports are a vital component of the medical record. Medical records are used to provide documentation of patient care, to supply information for billing purposes and statistical purposes, and furnish medical information in a legal case.

Medical Billing, Coding, and Insurance. Preparing monthly statements and insurance claims for patients is an important function performed by a medical administrative assistant. Billing, coding, and insurance are interconnected, and an understanding of each of these processes is essential for a well-trained assistant in the medical office. Proper billing practices help ensure that the medical office stays financially stable.

Communications Skills. A medical administrative assistant should possess proper oral and written communication skills. During a large part of the workday, an assistant communicates with patients and coworkers, and the ability to communicate in a professional manner is a public and employer expectation.

Computer Technology. Today, most medical offices conduct many patient-related activities by means of a computer system. Computers are used for scheduling appointments, retaining patient registration information, billing patients, processing insurance claims, and transcribing medical reports and correspondence. Industry trends indicate that soon even patients' medical records will be kept electronically. Offices today need medical administrative assistants with strong computer skills and keyboarding ability to maintain information in a computer system.

Internship. Many educational programs provide the opportunity for students to experience the activities of a medical office through an internship or through practical experience. During an internship, a student works in a medical office and performs many office activities under the supervision of an employee of that office. This experience allows the student to practice skills learned in school and gain on-the-job experience.

Student Portfolio

After enrollment in a medical office program, students should begin to collect samples of projects and course work that they complete while enrolled in the program. Students should also keep track of accomplishments and special activities in which they participate. This information is gathered to create a **student portfolio** that can later be presented to a prospective employer. Examples of information that might be kept in this portfolio include—but are not limited to—a bookkeeping project for a medical billing course; samples of medical transcription, letters, and other medical office documents produced by the student; and even certificates of achievement for participation in school activities. The portfolio helps a student keep track of important items from the student's educational experience and serves as documentation to an employer of the student's abilities.

Places of Employment

Medical administrative assistants work in a variety of organizations. Of course, a private practice, clinic, or hospital are probably the first locations that come to mind, but there are many other employment possibilities if a student has interests elsewhere. Assistants may find employment in such places as nursing homes, home health agencies, pharmaceutical businesses, dental offices, independent laboratory and radiologic facilities, and even legal firms that handle medical-related cases.

CHECKPOINT

Explain why education as a medical administrative assistant would be beneficial for employment in a dental office.

Earnings

Information on the earnings of a medical administrative assistant in a specific area can usually be obtained through state government agencies that provide employment services. Information is also available from the Bureau of Labor Statistics of the federal government; however, this information is a national average.

Several factors affect potential earnings. Supply and demand for medical administrative assistants affect regional earnings. Earnings also vary regionally according to economic conditions, with salaries possibly being higher in metropolitan areas. In addition, employees who obtain certification that is applicable to their field may expect to earn more than employees who do not have a certification.

Employment Trends and Forecasts

Although individuals find employment in a medical office under an assortment of job titles, the employment statistics kept by the federal government are usually tracked under the occupation titles of *medical secretary* or *medical assistant*.

The future of employment in these areas looks promising. The U.S. Bureau of Labor Statistics forecasts that many jobs in health care will have tremendous growth through the year 2006. This increase in jobs will be due in large part to the overall growth of the health care industry because of rapid technologic advances in medicine and the aging of the population. If the health care industry continues to grow as expected, this increase will require businesses to hire additional office support staff. Because of this anticipated growth, medical administrative assistants should expect many opportunities when seeking employment.

PROFESSIONAL ORGANIZATIONS

There are a few professional organizations to which individuals working in a medical office may wish to belong. Membership in a professional organization is voluntary and is a very practical way to keep current with changes in the profession. Organizations hold conferences and conventions to communicate the latest news about the profession and to give the members a chance to network with others in the field. Several organizations have professional publications that contain articles related to the profession. Many employers encourage membership in a professional organization by paying a portion or all of membership costs and sometimes by paying expenses for attending conferences or conventions.

Professional organizations have one or more certification examinations that a student may be eligible to take, depending on the qualifications required to take the examination. Specific information regarding these organizations, the certifications they sponsor, professional publications available, and other information is available by using the information in Table 1–1 to contact the organization desired.

American Association of Medical Assistants

The American Association of Medical Assistants (AAMA) is a professional organization serving members of the medical assisting profession. The organization is responsible for promoting the profession of medical assisting. The AAMA has identified competencies necessary for medical assistants and conducts a certification examination that assesses an applicant's knowledge of those competencies. The examination covers both administrative and clinical competencies required for employment in the profession. An individual passing the certification examination is known as a **Certified Medical Assistant** (**CMA**). A list of applicable CMA competencies is available at the beginning of each chapter of this text.

The members of the AAMA, in upholding the standards of the profession, have established a code of ethics (Fig. 1–4) to guide medical assistants in the expected ethical behaviors of a medical assistant. The AAMA code of ethics should serve as a guide for all medical office staff when performing the responsibilities of their position.

American Medical Technologists

The American Medical Technologists (AMT) is a national group for medical assistants that conducts a certification examination different from the one conducted by the AAMA. The certification examination sponsored by the AMT is the **Registered Medical Assistant** (**RMA**) examination. The AMT has established a group of administrative and clinical competencies that is assessed on the RMA examination. Depending on the requirements of the state in which he or she wishes to practice, a medical assisting student would take either the CMA or the RMA examination. Competencies for RMAs are listed at the beginning of each chapter of this text.

International Association of Administrative Professionals

The International Association of Administrative Professionals (IAAP) is an organization dedicated to advancing the profession of administrative support professionals. The organization was formed in 1942 and currently has more than 40,000 members throughout the world.

Table 1–1. Professional Organizations of Interest to Medical Administrative Assistants

Organization Name	Address	Phone	Internet Address
American Association of Medical Assistants	20 North Wacker Drive, Suite 1575 Chicago, Ill 60606-2903	312-899-1500	www.aama-ntl.org
American Medical Technologists	710 Higgins Road Park Ridge, Ill 60068-57655	847-823-5169	www.amtl.com
American Association for Medical Transcription	PO Box 5761875 Modesto, Calif 95355	800-982-2182	www.aamt.org
International Association of Administrative Professionals	10502 NW Ambassador Drive PO Box 20404 Kansas City, Mo 64195-0404	816-891-6600	www.iaap-hq.org
American Health Information Management Association	233 North Michigan Avenue Suite 2150 Chicago, Ill 60601-5519	312-233-1100	www.ahima.org

---

AAMA Code of Ethics

The Code of Ethics of AAMA shall set forth principles for ethical and moral conduct as they relate to the medical profession and the particular practice of medical assisting.

Members of AAMA dedicated to the conscientious pursuit of their profession, and thus desiring to merit the high regard of the entire medical profession and the respect of the general public which they serve, do pledge themselves to strive always to:

A.   render service with full respect for the dignity of humanity;

B.   respect confidential information obtained through employment unless legally authorized or required by responsible performance of duty to divulge such information;

C.   uphold the honor and high principles of the profession and accept its disciplines;

D.   seek to continually improve the knowledge and skills of medical assistants for the benefit of patients and professional colleagues;

E.   participate in additional service activities aimed toward improving the health and well-being of the community.

Figure 1–4. The AAMA code of ethics serves as a guide for all medical office staff. (Courtesy American Association of Medical Assistants, Chicago.)

For its members, the organization provides
- Education in the form of workshops, seminars, and conferences,
- Networking opportunities for its members who attend meetings,
- A publication, *The OfficePRO,* which provides current information related to the administrative support field, and
- A certification examination known as the **Certified Professional Secretary** (**CPS**) examination for members wishing to demonstrate excellence in their field through the certification process.

The IAAP was formerly known as Professional Secretaries International (PSI). The organization recently instituted a name change to reflect "the broader range of job titles and expanded responsibilities held by today's administrative support staff."

American Association for Medical Transcription

The American Association for Medical Transcription (AAMT) is a professional group organized to support the members of the medical transcription profession. Each year,

the AAMT holds a national meeting somewhere in the United States, and several states have their own chapters that hold regional meetings. The AAMT's publication, entitled *The Journal of the American Association for Medical Transcription,* is published six times yearly and provides information that transcriptionists will find invaluable in keeping up with their profession.

One of the functions of the AAMT is to establish the guidelines for the **Certified Medical Transcriptionist** (**CMT**) examination. To obtain employment as a medical transcriptionist, it is not required that a transcriptionist be certified. Attainment of the certification, however, demonstrates the high level of proficiency that a transcriptionist has achieved. The designation of CMT can make a difference to an employer interested in hiring a transcriptionist.

American Health Information Management Association

Medical office staff members may be familiar with this professional organization for health information, or medical records, personnel. The American Health Information Management Association (AHIMA) also sponsors two certification examinations known as the **Certified Coding Specialist** (**CCS**) and **Certified Coding Specialist–Physician-based** (**CCS-P**) examinations. These help maintain professional standards in the field of medical coding, an important component related to billing and insurance in the medical office.

Additional Certifications

There are other professional organizations that sponsor their own certification examinations. Even worldwide companies—Microsoft, for example—sponsor certification examinations that assess an individual's ability to utilize their product. Although some examinations are not as widely known as others, they still may be highly regarded by a health care employer. When considering a certification examination, an individual may wish to consult employers in the area about their preference for hiring certified individuals.

Continuing Education

Once assistants finish their formal education, take any certification desired, and secure employment in their field, their education is still far from over. Health care is a dynamic field and is changing constantly. Workshops, seminars, and college courses are often available to keep medical administrative assistants informed of the latest changes and trends. Conferences sponsored by professional organizations often allow members and nonmembers to attend and upgrade their skills and knowledge about their field. A genuine interest in learning new things is a very desirable trait in an employee, and employers often encourage staff members to attend these conferences to keep current with health industry trends.

SUMMARY

The health care field offers numerous employment opportunities for medical administrative assistants. Employers look for individuals with the right training and qualities who will provide exceptional service to the patients of the office. An individual wishing to be hired as a medical administrative assistant will need to have appropriate educational preparation to perform many duties in the medical office. Even after an assistant is employed, he or she will need to pay particular attention to keeping current in the career. Professional organizations related to medical office responsibilities provide a wealth of information and support to enhance the career of the medical administrative assistant.

Bibliography

Internet Resources

American Association for Medical Transcription
American Association of Medical Assistants
American Medical Technologists
International Association of Administrative Professionals
Mayo Clinic
U.S. Department of Labor, Bureau of Labor Statistics, Occupational Employment Statistics

YOU ARE THE MEDICAL ADMINISTRATIVE ASSISTANT

Picture yourself as a medical administrative assistant in a medical practice. What would you do in the following situations?

1. Parents of a 2-year-old patient with cancer are bringing the boy to the office because he has taken a turn for the worse. The parents come in carrying the child, who is obviously very weak and has lost all of his hair. As the assistant, what will you do?
2. The clinic manager wants to hire an additional staff person to help cover the front desk in the office. The labor market is tight, and the manager thinks that a person with no office experience or medical background would be all right for the position. Do you agree? Why?
3. On a coffee break, a coworker mentions that she would like to get a tattoo on her ankle. How do you reply?

Suggested Readings

There are many *Chicken Soup for the Soul* books on the market today. These books provide wonderful stories that eloquently portray empathy, compassion, kindness, and other desirable human virtues.

Exercise 1–1 TRUE OR FALSE

Read the following statements and determine whether the statements are true or false. Record the answer in the blank provided. T = true; F = false.

_____ 1. It is common in large health care organizations for a medical administrative assistant to specialize in a specific administrative area of the organization.

_____ 2. CCS means certified corporate secretary.

_____ 3. *Patient services specialist*, *medical office specialist*, *medical secretary*, and *medical administrative assistant* are job titles that could be used to describe the same position.

_____ 4. Composing a letter to a patient may be part of an assistant's responsibility.

_____ 5. Continuing education is necessary to remain a valued employee.

_____ 6. Handling telephone calls is part of a medical administrative assistant's responsibility.

_____ 7. Wearing the latest styles is important for the medical administrative assistant to create a professional appearance.

_____ 8. Casual clothing is not appropriate in any medical office.

_____ 9. A medical administrative assistant's appearance may influence a patient's perception of an assistant.

_____ 10. Uniforms are the only type of clothing appropriate for a medical administrative assistant on the job.

_____ 11. If the office staff and the nursing staff wear the same uniform, a patient may confuse the office staff and the nursing staff.

_____ 12. To become a medical transcriptionist, an assistant must be certified.

_____ 13. To transcribe medical reports, knowledge of medical terminology is necessary.

_____ 14. The study of human anatomy and physiology covers the structure and function of the human body.

_____ 15. Because most patient contact is in person in the medical office, it is not necessary for a medical administrative assistant to have proper written communication skills.

_____ 16. Computer skills are not widely used in the medical office today.

_____ 17. Membership in a professional organization is mandatory for all medical administrative assistants.

Exercise 1–2 ADMINISTRATIVE AND CLINICAL DUTIES IN THE MEDICAL OFFICE

Identify whether the following duties in the medical office are administrative or clinical. Record the answer in the blank provided. A = administrative; C = clinical.

1. Prepare insurance claim. _____

2. Take and record patient's blood pressure. _____

3. Sterilize instruments. _____

4. File medical records. _____

5. Provide assistance to physician during a procedure. _____

6. Obtain patient's medical history. _____

7. Perform routine laboratory test. _____

8. Prepare treatment room for patient. _____

9. Schedule appointments. _____

10. Record patient's payment on account. _____

11. Prepare statement of patient's account. _____

12. Remove patient's bandage. _____

13. Take and record patient's temperature. _____

14. Make daily bank deposit. _____

15. Record patient's change of address. _____

Exercise 1-3 DESIRABLE PERSONALITY TRAITS OF A MEDICAL ADMINISTRATIVE ASSISTANT

Desirable personality traits of a medical administrative assistant are listed here. Match the characteristics on the left with their meanings on the right. Record the answer in the blank provided. Each answer is used only once.

_____ 1. Compassionate   (a) Keeps information secret

_____ 2. Dependable   (b) Thorough

_____ 3. Conscientious   (c) Envisions things from the patient's perspective

_____ 4. Honest   (d) Appropriately dressed

_____ 5. Confidential   (e) Caring

_____ 6. Personable   (f) Works well in a group

_____ 7. Team player   (g) Friendly

_____ 8. Punctual   (h) Reliable

_____ 9. Empathetic   (i) Truthful

_____ 10. Well-groomed   (j) Arrives on time

Exercise 1-4 PROFESSIONAL ORGANIZATIONS

Match the statements below with its associated organization. Choose the best answer. Some answers may be used more than once. Record the answer in the blank provided.

    (a) American Association of Medical Assistants
    (b) American Medical Technologists
    (c) International Association of Administrative Professionals
    (d) American Association for Medical Transcription
    (e) American Health Information Management Association

_____ 1. Conducts CMA certification examination.

_____ 2. Professional organization for health information personnel.

_____ 3. Professional group for medical transcriptionists.

_____ 4. Conducts CPS examination.

_____ 5. Publishes *The Journal of the American Association for Medical Transcription*.

_____ 6. Conducts RMA examination.

_____ 7. Conducts CCS and CCS-P coding certification examinations.

_____ 8. Publishes *The OfficePRO*.

_____ 9. Conducts the CMT examination.

_____ 10. Formerly known as Professional Secretaries International (PSI).

Exercise 1–5 PROFESSIONAL APPEARANCE

Read each statement regarding personal appearance and determine whether or not the appearance is professional. Record the answer in the blank provided. Y = yes, this is professional; N = No, this is not professional.

1. Bright red nail polish _____

2. Navy blazer and pants _____

3. Pierced lip and tongue _____

4. Shorts _____

5. Conservative hairstyle _____

6. Purple-streaked hair _____

7. Khaki pants and coordinating shirt _____

8. Miniskirt _____

9. Tennis shoes with white uniform _____

10. Lightly worn cologne _____

1
ACTIVITIES

ACTIVITY 1–1 Research employment opportunities in the medical administrative assistant field using the Internet, newspapers, or any other source. Find at least three openings for which a medical administrative assistant would be qualified. Find at least one opening outside your state. Take note of the titles of the positions advertised. On each of the listings, highlight the information that identifies educational requirements, personal qualities, and other information regarding medical administrative assistants that is found in Chapter 1.

ACTIVITY 1–2 Research the professional organizations identified in this chapter. You might be interested in the following:
- How much are dues?
- Does the organization have a local chapter in your area?
- Where and when is the next annual convention or national meeting?
- Is the organization sponsoring any workshops in your area in the near future?

ACTIVITY 1–3 Interview a person who is currently working as a medical administrative assistant. Prepare a list of interview questions to be approved by your instructor.

ACTIVITY 1–4 Chapter 1 gives examples of professional and unprofessional appearance for the medical office. Using magazines, newspapers, the Internet, or any other sources available, find two pictures of professional business dress appropriate for the medical office, one picture of an appropriate uniform for the medical office, and two pictures of unprofessional appearance.

Cut out each picture and secure each to a separate sheet of $8\frac{1}{2} \times 11"$ paper.

On each sheet, describe how each picture portrays professional or unprofessional appearance.

ACTIVITY 1–5 Start a portfolio to be used to gather samples of your work while in school. An accordion-style paper folder can be used to hold many items. Discuss with your instructor what items should be included in the portfolio. Periodically review your portfolio, placing like items together.

ACTIVITY 1–6 Research computer software certifications such as the MOUS certification from Microsoft. Find answers to such questions as
(a) What are the types of certifications?
(b) What are the requirements to take a certification examination?
(c) How much does a certification examination cost?

ACTIVITY 1–7 Research certifications from the organizations mentioned in the chapter. Find answers to the questions listed in Activity 1–6 for those organizations.

ACTIVITY 1–8 Consider the following role-playing situations. What are the appropriate responses to the situations given?

    (a) A coworker named Nancy, on a whim, wanted something new for her hair. She decides a really "funky" thing to do would be to color her hair (temporarily) green. She tells you about this idea during your lunch break. What do you say?

    (b) Another coworker, David, and a few of his buddies have decided it would be fun to pierce their lips and noses. David reports to work one day with a silver stud through his lower lip and another through his nose. What do you say?

1

DISCUSSION

The following topics can be used for class discussion or for individual student essay.

DISCUSSION 1–1 Read the quotation at the beginning of the chapter. How does this quotation apply to a medical administrative assistant's career?

DISCUSSION 1–2 What is the importance of the statement "Patients are the reason for the work of medical professionals"?

DISCUSSION 1–3 Discuss the application of the medical assistant's code of ethics to the position of medical administrative assistant.

DISCUSSION 1–4 Several employees want to wear jeans to work. Are jeans appropriate for the medical office?

DISCUSSION 1–5 You want to work in a medical office and have decided to become a medical administrative assistant. Why do you want to work in health care?

CHAPTER OUTLINE

HEALTH CARE PROVIDERS
Physician
Physician Assistant
Nurse Practitioner
Certified Nurse Midwife
Podiatrist
Chiropractor
Optometrist
NURSING PROFESSIONALS
Registered Nurse
Licensed Practical Nurse
Certified Nursing Assistant
ALLIED HEALTH PROFESSIONALS
Medical Assistant
Medical Transcriptionist
Health Information Professional
Physical Therapist
Physical Therapy Assistant
Occupational Therapist
Occupational Therapy Assistant
Respiratory Therapist
Radiology Technologist
Medical Laboratory Technologist and
    Technician
Pharmacist
CONTINUING EDUCATION
PROFESSIONAL ORGANIZATIONS
HEALTH CARE FACILITIES
Clinic
Private Practice
Hospital
Urgent Care Center
Outpatient Surgery Center
Home Health
Nursing Home, Assisted Living
Public Health
SUMMARY

LEARNING OUTCOMES

On successful completion of this chapter, the student will be able to
1. Describe the members of the health care team and their area of responsibility in the health care environment.
2. Identify the common settings for delivery of health care.

CMA COMPETENCIES
1. Perform within legal and ethical boundaries.

RMA COMPETENCIES
1. Know credentialing requirements of medical professionals.
2. Know terminology associated with medical secretarial and receptionist duties.

VOCABULARY
ambulatory care
assisted living facility
board certified
clinic
emergency room
home health
hospital
inpatient
managed care
nursing home
outpatient
outpatient surgery center
primary care
private practice
provider
public health agency
reciprocity
residency
urgent care center

2

THE HEALTH CARE TEAM

Use what talents you possess: the woods would be very silent if no birds sang except those that sang best.

—*Henry Van Dyke, American educator*

Who are the significant players on the health care team? What do they do for the patient? What is required of these professionals?

It is important that a medical administrative assistant know the answers to these questions so that the assistant understands (1) how these professionals interact with patients and one another and (2) what their responsibilities are in a health care setting.

In addition, this chapter introduces the common types of facilities in which health care is provided to supply a frame of reference for the places in which a medical administrative assistant may work. Although a medical administrative assistant may work in a variety of locations, the most common location is a clinic, whether a private practice or group practice, which is the focus of the chapters in this text.

Many different employment opportunities are available for people with an interest in health care. No matter where a health care professional may work, however, anyone entering a health care profession should do so with one focus in mind: patient service. Patients are the reason that a health care facility and its staff members provide services, and optimal service can be provided only with continuous and heartfelt consideration for all patients.

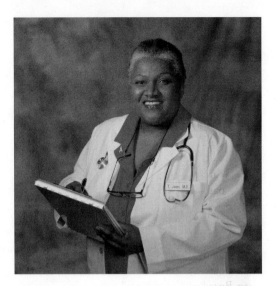

Figure 2–1. A physician is chiefly responsible for developing and overseeing the treatment plans for her patients.

HEALTH CARE PROVIDERS

The term **provider** is used in health care to describe the individuals who are chiefly responsible for coordinating and delivering health care services. Providers examine patients; order laboratory or radiologic testing; and may prescribe medications, treatments, or therapies for illness or injury. They also provide preventive health care. Physicians, nurse practitioners, and physician assistants, to name a few, are examples of providers. A provider relies on many other health care professionals to supply many other necessary services related to a patient's visit to a health care facility.

Physician

A physician's practice of medicine involves providing preventive care or providing or coordinating treatment of patients' illnesses or injuries. A physician also relies on other health care professionals to provide additional services for patients. For example, a physician treating a patient with a suspected fracture will order an x-ray, but a radiology technologist will take the actual x-ray. Although physicians may not actually conduct all treatments or therapies, they are chiefly responsible for developing and overseeing the treatment plans for their patients.

A physician (Fig. 2–1) is usually the leading health care professional in most of today's medical offices. Although many offices do employ other providers—such as physician assistants, nurse practitioners, and certified nurse midwives—a physician or group of physicians must supervise

the activities of those health professionals and is responsible for the actions of those professionals.

Physician Education

The road to becoming a physician is long and difficult. A student wishing to become a physician usually completes a 4-year bachelor's degree program in a science, such as biology or chemistry, or completes a program designated as "premed." Such a program provides the student with a base of knowledge necessary to continue in medical school.

After the student completes 4 years of college and is accepted into medical school, he or she spends the next 4 years in the medical school program. A few colleges offer a combination bachelor's degree program and medical school curriculum that can be completed in 6 years. After graduation from medical school, the student holds the degree of Doctor of Medicine (MD) or Doctor of Osteopathy (DO). Of 142 medical schools in the United States, 125 prepare MDs and 17 prepare DOs, with a total of approximately 15,000 medical students graduating each year.

Both MDs and DOs are physicians and are required to be licensed to practice medicine. Each type of physician is trained to treat illness and injury and to offer preventive health care. Each type is allowed to prescribe medications and perform surgery. One of the key differences between these two types of physicians is the osteopath's approach to medicine: osteopaths believe that a healthy musculoskeletal system is essential for good health.

Licensure

Before a medical school graduate is allowed to practice medicine, the graduate must be licensed by the state in

Box 2–1 American Board of Medical Specialties Member Boards

American Board of Allergy & Immunology
American Board of Anesthesiology
American Board of Colon & Rectal Surgery
American Board of Dermatology
American Board of Emergency Medicine
American Board of Family Practice
American Board of Internal Medicine
American Board of Medical Genetics
American Board of Neurological Surgery
American Board of Nuclear Medicine
American Board of Obstetrics & Gynecology
American Board of Ophthalmology
American Board of Orthopaedic Surgery
American Board of Otolaryngology
American Board of Pathology
American Board of Pediatrics
American Board of Physical Medicine & Rehabilitation
American Board of Plastic Surgery
American Board of Preventative Medicine
American Board of Psychiatry & Neurology
American Board of Radiology
American Board of Surgery
American Board of Thoracic Surgery
American Board of Urology

apply to perform a residency in a specialty of his or her choice. These graduates are known as **residents,** and this period of education is known as a **residency.** Residents are physicians and must be licensed to practice medicine but are also students, continuing their education in a chosen specialty. Residency training programs for medical specialties vary in length from 3 to 7 years depending on the specialty.

Because health care is so complex and the amount of medical knowledge is so extensive, many doctors usually choose to specialize or concentrate their further studies in a specific area of medicine. The American Board of Medical Specialists has 24 boards that set the standards for physicians choosing to pursue further training in a specialty area (Box 2–1). Each board identified in Box 2–1 sets the standards for its specialty. In some specialties, there are also subspecialties that allow a physician to further specialize his or her practice of medicine. For example, a physician specializing in surgery may wish to further specialize in pediatric surgery, or an obstetrician may wish to further specialize in reproductive endocrinology. Table 2–1 describes the focus of care of many of the more common medical specialties.

Once a resident has completed a residency in a specialty area, the resident may choose to take an examination related

which he or she wishes to work. Each state, the District of Columbia, and all U.S. territories has its own licensing board that oversees the practice of medicine in the region. This board is called the State Board of Medical Examiners. The Board of Medical Examiners is responsible for regulating the practice of medicine within each state or jurisdiction.

Application for licensure requires that a doctor be a graduate of an accredited medical school and that he or she has passed a licensing examination known as the United States Medical Licensing Examination (USMLE). Applicants for licensure must also disclose their medical history and any record of arrests or convictions. Many states allow a physician who is licensed in another state to obtain a license in that state through an agreement called **reciprocity.** Reciprocity allows the physician who has met the requirements in one state to obtain a license in another state without retaking the USMLE.

Once licensed, the physician must then renew his or her license as required by the state in which the physician works. Many states require that the physician take part in a specified amount of continuing education in order to renew his or her license to practice.

Residency and Board Certification

After graduation from medical school and licensure by the state in which the physician works, the physician may

Table 2–1. Common Physician Specialists Found in Health Care Facilities

Specialist	Provides Care For
Allergist	Individuals with abnormal hypersensitivity to a substance
Anesthesiologist	Patients requiring the administration of an anesthetic for surgical purposes or pain management
Cardiologist	Heart disorders
Dermatologist	Integumentary system (hair, skin, nails) disorders
Endocrinologist	Endocrine system disorders
Family practice physician	Primary care for patients of all ages (infant to elderly)
Gastroenterologist	Gastrointestinal disorders
Nephrologist	Disorders of the kidney
Neurologist	Nervous system disorders
Obstetrician/gynecologist	Female reproductive system disorders; also provides prenatal and postnatal care
Ophthalmologist	Eye disorders
Orthopedist	Musculoskeletal disorders
Otolaryngologist	Disorders of the ear, nose, and throat; allergic disorders
Pathologist	Laboratory examination of patient specimens
Pediatrician	Children up to age 18
Psychiatrist	Patients with psychological disorders; can prescribe medications
Pulmonologist	Respiratory disorders
Radiologist	Patients requiring radiologic examinations or treatments
Rheumatologist	Disorders of the joints
Surgeon	Patients requiring surgical treatment of a condition
Urologist	Disorders of the urinary system

to his or her specialty to become **board certified.** The resident also may practice for a few years before taking the board-certification examination. If the physician successfully completes the board-certification examination, the physician is then known as a Diplomate and is said to be board certified. The achievement of the designation *board certified* indicates that the physician is recognized as an expert in his or her chosen field.

Current Trends

Many years ago, it was common for a physician to practice independently in a small office located either within his or her own home or, perhaps, in a small storefront on the main street in town. Physicians were on call almost every day of the week and had little support from fellow physicians, owing to the geographic distances among them. Since the 1950s, increasing specialization in medicine has led many physicians to group together in multispecialty clinics.

In today's health care industry, physicians are much more likely than they were in years past to work as part of a group practice. A group practice helps provide some relief for physicians in providing emergency coverage for patients. A group practice allows physicians to communicate more readily with one another and allows the physicians in the group access to one anothers' expertise. This arrangement also allows the practice to pool resources to buy more state-of-the art equipment to diagnose and treat patients and to provide more health care services.

Currently, the health care industry is undergoing a shift in the types of physicians that will be needed to fill jobs in the future. The growing number of **managed care** plans today means that more **primary care** physicians will be needed to serve the U.S. population.

Primary care physicians are physicians who treat disorders of all parts of the body. Physicians in specialties such as family practice, pediatrics, and internal medicine are examples of primary care physicians. They provide care for patients' routine health needs on a regular basis and refer patients to other physicians when necessary for more specialized care.

Managed care plans normally require that a patient see a primary care physician, who acts as a "gatekeeper," when seeking help with a medical problem or for preventive care. The gatekeeper role means that the primary care physician always sees the patient first (except in emergency cases) and refers the patient to a specialist only when necessary. The use of primary care physicians results in an overall reduction in health care costs for the consumer. More information on managed care is included in Chapter 11.

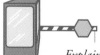

CHECKPOINT

Explain why a group practice may want to employ more primary care physicians than specialists.

Physician Assistant

Physician assistants (PAs) provide routine health care under the supervision of a physician. They examine patients, may order and interpret laboratory tests, and make diagnoses. They can treat injuries that require sutures, splints, or casts. In most states, PAs may prescribe medications. Depending on the requirements of the state, the extent of the PA's duties may be decided by the state regulating agency or by the supervising physician.

Admittance to many PA training programs requires a minimum of at least 2 years of undergraduate education and some work experience in health care. PA programs last about 2 years. The PA curriculum involves health-related courses and clinical experiences in areas such as obstetrics and gynecology (OB-GYN), emergency medicine, pediatrics, and surgery.

Almost all states and the District of Columbia require that PAs pass the Physician Assistants National Certifying Examination in order to practice in their state. Once a PA has passed the examination, he or she is allowed to use the credential PA-C (Physician Assistant—Certified). PAs must complete 100 continuing education hours every 2 years to keep their certification.

Nurse Practitioner

A nurse practitioner is an advanced practice nurse who diagnoses and treats patients in a chosen field. Many nurse practitioners choose to specialize in fields such as family medicine, pediatrics, or women's health. Nurse practitioners are allowed to prescribe medications in most states, but the types of medications that they are allowed to prescribe may vary among states.

Like PAs, nurse practitioners usually work under the supervision of a physician. The extent of the supervision required is determined by the state in which they work.

As mentioned previously, a nurse practitioner is an advanced practice nurse and has met additional educational and clinical requirements beyond that of a master's degree in nursing. A nurse practitioner course of study usually lasts 1 to 2 years.

Like other health care providers mentioned previously, certification and licensure requirements for nurse practitioners vary from state to state. Some states require that nurse practitioners pass a certification examination before they are eligible for licensure. A nurse passing the certification examination is known as a Certified Nurse Practitioner (CNP).

Certified Nurse Midwife

Somewhat similar in practice to that of a nurse practitioner, a certified nurse midwife (CNM) is an advanced practice nurse who conducts routine yearly physical examinations for women, delivers babies, prescribes medications, and provides prenatal and postnatal care for routine (i.e., without serious complications) obstetrics patients. Certification requirements for nurse midwives vary from state to state.

Podiatrist

A Doctor of Podiatric Medicine (DPM), also known as a podiatrist, treats disorders of the foot and lower leg. Podiatrists treat a variety of foot disorders, from corns, calluses, and bunions, to foot disorders caused by diabetes. Podiatrists are allowed to prescribe drugs, perform surgery, treat fractures, and order tests to diagnose foot problems. They make customized inserts, known as orthotics, to correct foot abnormalities and even custom design shoes.

Most applicants to a college of podiatric medicine have a bachelor's degree before admission. Podiatric colleges offer a 4-year curriculum that includes courses in a variety of sciences as well as clinical rotations in clinics and hospitals. A graduate of a college of podiatric medicine is known as a DPM.

After becoming a DPM, podiatrists usually complete a residency training of 1 to 3 years. Residents receive advanced education in anesthesiology, surgery, and other related areas.

To practice podiatric medicine, podiatrists must be licensed by the state in which they work. Each state outlines the requirements for licensure to practice in their state. Many states have reciprocity agreements that allow podiatrists to easily obtain licensure in more than one state.

Chiropractor

A Doctor of Chiropractic (DC), also known as a chiropractor, treats patients with disorders associated with the musculoskeletal or nervous system. Chiropractors believe that musculoskeletal problems can cause problems throughout the body and may obstruct the body's ability to fight disease.

Chiropractors do not prescribe drugs or perform surgery; instead, they treat patients, when appropriate, by manipulating or adjusting the spine. They may also treat patients with ultrasound, massage, or heat therapy.

A person wishing to become a chiropractor must have a minimum of 60 semester hours of undergraduate education in order to apply to a chiropractic college. Some colleges now require a bachelor's degree for admission.

Chiropractic programs consist of 4 years of study: a student takes science courses during the first 2 years and clinical experiences and related courses during the last 2 years.

Chiropractors, like other health care providers, must be licensed by the state in which they work. All states and the District of Columbia regulate the practice of chiropractic within their boundaries. Some states have reciprocity agreements allowing a chiropractor with a license in another state to easily apply for a license to practice in their state.

Optometrist

Optometrists (also known as Doctors of Optometry, ODs) perform eye examinations and prescribe corrective lenses to correct vision problems. Optometrists provide a large portion of the primary eye care in the United States.

Both optometrists and ophthalmologists perform eye examinations and can prescribe corrective lenses for patients. The difference between the two is that the ophthalmologist is an MD who performs eye surgery, prescribes medication, and diagnoses and treats all eye diseases.

Most optometry students have a bachelor's degree on entrance to an optometry school. Optometry curriculum consists of courses in health and visual sciences and is usually 4 years in length.

All states and the District of Columbia require licensure of optometrists who wish to practice within their boundaries. Optometrists are required to be a graduate of an accredited college of optometry and must pass a licensure examination. Continuing education credits are required for license renewal.

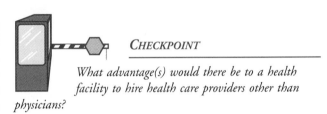

CHECKPOINT

What advantage(s) would there be to a health facility to hire health care providers other than physicians?

NURSING PROFESSIONALS

Registered Nurse

Registered nurses (RNs) comprise the largest health care occupation in the United States. RNs work in many different settings, from clinics and hospitals to nursing homes, home health, public health, and health-related administrative positions.

The chief focus of the nursing profession is the caring process. Nurses help patients recover from or live with illness or injury, observe patient progress, administer medications, and assist physicians. Nurses are also a key component in providing health education.

Depending on the location in which they work, job conditions can vary greatly. Nurses in administration may spend many hours behind a desk or computer. Nurses involved in direct patient care may spend long hours on their feet. Some nursing positions require work at all hours of the day or night every day of the week; work hours for other positions may be from 8 AM to 5 PM, Monday through Friday.

Depending on the state in which a nurse chooses to work, educational requirements for an RN can vary. An associate degree in nursing (2 years) or a bachelor of science degree in nursing (BSN) (4 years) may be required to obtain licensure. Over the years, some states have attempted to raise the requirements for licensure as a registered nurse. This can have an impact on RNs who may wish to work in a state in which the requirements are greater than what they have achieved. BSNs have many more career opportunities because of their advanced educational preparation.

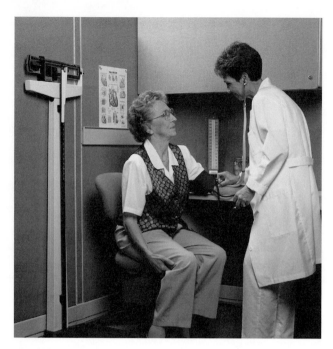

Figure 2–2. Licensed practical nurses perform many of the nursing duties in a medical office.

All RNs must take a national certification examination. Successful completion of the certification examination is a standard requirement for licensure. Each state establishes specific requirements for licensure as a registered nurse in their state.

Licensed Practical Nurse

Licensed practical nurses (LPNs) or licensed vocational nurses (LVNs in Texas and California) (Fig. 2–2) provide basic patient care, such as taking vital signs, performing laboratory tests, providing patients with hygiene care, and reporting patient progress. In some states, they are allowed to start intravenous lines and administer prescribed medications. LPNs usually work under the supervision of a physician or an RN. As RNs have moved into more supervisory positions, LPNs have become more directly involved in patient care, with LPNs performing many of the nursing duties in a medical office.

Educational requirements for LPNs vary from state to state. Most programs are 1 year in length; a few programs are 2 years in length. Education includes health-related classroom courses as well as clinical experience. To work as an LPN or LVN, all states require that LPNs and LVNs be graduates of an approved program and have passed an examination for licensure.

Certified Nursing Assistant

Certified nursing assistants (CNAs) provide personal care for patients in hospitals and nursing homes. CNAs assist patients with eating and personal hygiene. The nature of CNA work is physically demanding, with CNAs often having to lift and transfer patients. Nursing assistants must be careful to avoid injury while at work. All nursing professionals, including RNs, LPNs, and CNAs, are particularly vulnerable to injury because of the nature of their work.

To work as a CNA, an individual usually takes a short course (approximately 3 weeks in length) that involves classroom study and clinical experience and is then usually required to take a state certification examination.

ALLIED HEALTH PROFESSIONALS

Medical Assistant

As mentioned in Chapter 1, medical assistants (Fig. 2–3) are qualified to perform administrative and clinical duties in the medical office. In smaller offices, medical assistants may actually perform both clinical and administrative duties. In a larger office, the medical assistant may specialize in either administrative or clinical duties. Practices with a larger patient volume are often more "departmentalized" than are practices with a smaller patient volume, and a medical assistant is likely to be assigned specific duties.

In some states, medical assistants who will be performing certain clinical duties are required to pass the national certification examination. Two national organizations, the American Association of Medical Assistants (AAMA) and American Medical Technologists (AMT), provide certification or registration for medical assistants, depending on the requirements of the state in which the assistant wishes to work.

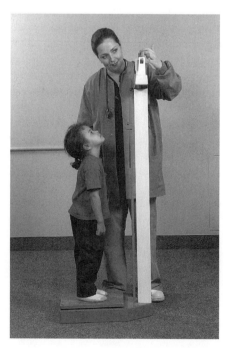

Figure 2–3. A certified medical assistant is qualified to provide clinical, as well as administrative, duties in the medical office.

The assistant may also be required to be a graduate of an accredited medical assistant program before becoming certified or registered. Chapter 1 gives additional information about the organizations mentioned here, (see Table 1–1). Examination is not required for assistants who perform office duties only.

Medical Transcriptionist

A medical transcriptionist's chief responsibility is to transcribe physician dictation. Accurate recording of a patient's encounters with health care providers is an essential piece of any medical record.

Medical transcriptionists must possess an extensive knowledge of anatomy and physiology, medical terminology, and disease processes, and they must have a great deal of computer ability and keyboarding skill. These are all necessary for compiling medical reports, office chart notes, and other essential components of the medical record.

Although it is not necessary for employment, the credential Certified Medical Transcriptionist (CMT) is awarded by the American Association of Medical Transcriptionists to individuals who pass both a written and practical portion of the medical transcription certification examination. A medical assistant or medical administrative assistant may also perform the duties of a transcriptionist in the medical office.

Health Information Professional

There are two types of health information professionals: registered health information administrators (RHIAs) and registered health information technicians (RHITs). Individuals working in the health information profession are primarily responsible for reviewing the health information (medical records) of patients treated in health care facilities. Review of the health information is done to ensure that the records are organized appropriately and are complete and accurate.

This health care profession is unusual in that persons working in this profession have little to no contact with patients. They work primarily behind the scenes, maintaining medical records and supplying information for patient billing and insurance claims.

Health Information Technician

Health information technicians are graduates of a 2-year health information program. After graduating from an accredited program, the graduate may then choose to take a credentialing examination to become a registered health information technician (RHIT). The examination is offered by the American Health Information Management Association, a professional organization for health information professionals. Most employers who hire health information professionals often prefer to hire individuals who have obtained the RHIT credential. Health information technicians are responsible for accurate diagnostic and procedural coding of health care services for billing purposes and for day-to-day maintenance of the medical record.

Registered Health Information Administrator

A registered health information administrator (RHIA) is an individual who has successfully completed a bachelor's degree program in health information and has passed a national certification examination.

RHIAs are usually employed as directors of health information (medical records) departments in health care facilities. They are chiefly responsible for coordinating health information department activities, such as medical transcription, records review, coding, and even tumor registry. RHIAs supervise the health information staff and ensure that a facility's health information practices conform to national accreditation standards.

Physical Therapist

A physical therapist (PT) (Fig. 2–4) provides treatment to improve or restore a patient's ability to move when the patient is affected by disease or injury. Therapists develop treatment plans that may involve exercise, ultrasound, or application of heat or cold to alleviate a patient's suffering. PTs often consult with the patient's provider to plan an appropriate mode of treatment. If a PT is not able to bring about full restoration of a patient's mobility, the therapist works to limit the effects of the disability on the patient's overall health.

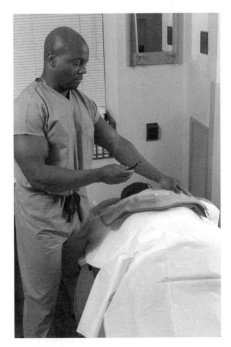

Figure 2–4. A physical therapist provides treatments to help improve or restore a patient's mobility.

To become licensed as a PT, an individual must first be a graduate of an accredited physical therapy program (typically, a master's degree program) and must pass a licensing examination.

Physical Therapy Assistant

A physical therapy assistant (PTA) provides physical therapy treatments as assigned by a supervising PT. Such treatments include exercise, ultrasound, massage, application of heat or cold packs, and, possibly, even traction.

PTA programs generally last 2 years. In 1997, 44 states required that PTAs be regulated. Requirements include certification in cardiopulmonary resuscitation and first aid and a specified minimum number of hours of clinical experience.

Occupational Therapist

Whereas a PT works with patients to help restore or improve the function of the body, an occupational therapist (OT) works with patients to restore skills needed for daily living. These range from personal skills (e.g., dressing, eating, and grooming) to everyday living skills (e.g., homemaking, budgeting, and using transportation). Sometimes, a patient is not able to be restored to a former level of functioning and must adapt to his or her impairment and learn ways to compensate for the loss of function. The OT's objective is to bring the patient to the maximum level of functioning possible.

All states regulate this profession. OTs must graduate from an accredited program with a minimum of a bachelor's degree and must pass a certification examination.

Occupational Therapy Assistant

Just as PTAs provide treatments as planned by PTs, so do occupational therapy assistants (OTAs) provide treatments as planned by OTs. OTAs teach patients how to transfer to a wheelchair properly, cook a meal, or plan recreational activities.

Most states regulate OTAs and require them to be graduates of accredited 2-year programs and to have passed a certification examination. Once the assistant has passed the certification examination, he or she is known as a certified occupational therapy assistant (COTA).

Respiratory Therapist

Respiratory therapists are concerned with treatment and care of patients with respiratory dysfunction. They evaluate the patient's ability to breathe and deliver treatments ordered by the patient's provider. Training for a respiratory therapist generally lasts 2 years, with some programs being 4 years in length. Most states require respiratory therapists to become certified. All graduates of accredited programs may take the examination to become a certified respiratory therapist technician (CRTT). If a CRTT has sufficient education and experience, he or she may then take an examination to become a registered respiratory therapist (RRT). The RRT credential is usually required of persons in a supervisory role.

Radiology Technologist

The field of radiology provides many different services within the health care industry. Radiology involves not only the use of x-rays but also the use of ultrasound, computed tomographic (CT) scans, and magnetic resonance imaging (MRI).

Radiology technologists (RTs) or radiographers (Fig. 2–5) are responsible for taking x-ray images of parts of the body. They can further specialize in the use of contrast material (or dye) that is administered to the patient to allow certain materials in the body to be seen.

Ultrasound technologists (sonographers) utilize ultrasound to create images of a patient's body for interpretation by the physician. Sonographers are RTs who have specialized in ultrasound technique and may even have specialized in taking ultrasound images of specific parts of the body.

Programs training RTs last from 1 to 4 years, with 2 years being the most common length of time. Sometimes, health care professionals from other fields will cross train in a 1-year radiology program.

Most states license RTs, and a voluntary registration of technologists is offered by the American Registry of Radiology

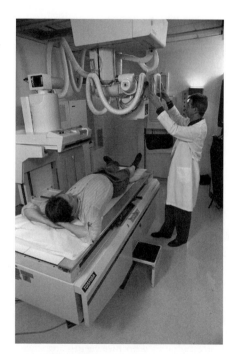

Figure 2–5. The field of radiology involves x-rays, ultrasound, computed tomographic scans, and magnetic resonance imaging.

Technologists. Most employers prefer to hire registered RTs, but in some states, it is not necessary to be registered to perform this occupation.

Medical Laboratory Technologist and Technician

Laboratory testing of a patient's bodily substances is often an integral part of the process of arriving at an accurate diagnosis of the patient's condition. Medical laboratory personnel analyze urine, blood, and other body substances and tissues to establish whether bacteria or foreign substances are present or to determine the level of certain components in the body. Laboratory personnel identify cell characteristics and determine the amount of cells present within the body.

The difference in the training of medical laboratory technologists and technicians is that technologists usually have a bachelor's degree and technicians usually have an associate's degree. Technologists are generally responsible for conducting more sophisticated tests and may be found in supervisory roles. Technicians usually perform more routine or less complicated tests within the medical laboratory. Licensure to work as a medical technologist is required in some but not all states.

Pharmacist

The pharmacist plays an integral part of the health care team. It is the pharmacist's responsibility to dispense medications to patients as prescribed by their physician. The pharmacist also counsels patients about the proper usage of medications the patient is taking. Pharmacists may work in clinics or hospitals, or they may work in outside retail pharmacies. Regardless of where a pharmacist is located, he or she can be in close contact with the physician when necessary for the well-being of the patient.

Pharmacy education consists of either a 5-year bachelor's degree program or a 6-year Doctor of Pharmacy (PharmD) degree program. After graduation, the graduate is eligible to take the state licensing examination. All states require pharmacists to be licensed in order to practice.

CONTINUING EDUCATION

Individuals in health care professions who are certified or licensed are required to regularly update their knowledge of their field by participating in some type of continuing education activity. These activities can include attending conventions, seminars, or workshops; taking college courses; and even reviewing independent study materials.

The purpose of requiring continuing education in order to remain certified or licensed is to ensure that individuals in the profession are keeping current with changes occurring in their profession. Given the advances in medical technol-ogy and technology in general, individuals must constantly be aware of industry advances in order to perform their jobs properly.

PROFESSIONAL ORGANIZATIONS

Nearly every health profession has a professional organization associated with the profession. These organizations often play a large part in establishing and maintaining high standards. Professional organizations are often involved in the development and administration of licensure and certification examinations. Many organizations offer continuing education programs for their membership and are a valuable resource for health information. Continuing education programs help members meet certification or licensure requirements, or both, for continued certification or licensure and provide opportunity for members to stay current in their field.

HEALTH CARE FACILITIES

The public can receive health care in many different types of facilities. The facilities described here are some of the most common types of settings in which health care is provided.

Clinic

In a **clinic** or medical office, a physician or group of physicians and, possibly, other providers (e.g., nurse practitioners, physician assistants, nurse midwives) provide care to patients. This care is referred to as **ambulatory** or **outpatient** care because the patient comes and goes within a 24-hour period and usually is treated within a span of a few hours. A clinic is a chief location of primary care or routine outpatient care delivery. Patients receiving outpatient care usually have routine health concerns and do not have a condition severe enough to warrant an overnight stay in the hospital. Occasionally, ambulatory care patients do arrive at a clinic with a serious medical condition that necessitates admission to a hospital.

Some very large group practices usually have at least one physician in each of the major specialty areas to provide care. Large group practices are prevalent throughout the United States, with physicians from varying specialties practicing together in one clinic location.

One of the largest, and probably most famous, multispecialty groups in the United States is the Mayo Clinic, located in Rochester, Minnesota. This clinic is a prime example of health care availability at its finest, drawing patients from around the globe. In 2002, the Mayo Clinic employed more than 2000 physicians and had an allied health staff of more than 35,000 employees. In addition to providing top-quality patient care, Mayo is also a teaching facility educating physicians and other health professionals. The Mayo

Clinic has greatly influenced the trend toward specialized medicine and group practice.

Some large clinics also provide health care at satellite or branch clinics. Some branch clinics are located in rural areas to provide greater access to health care for rural residents, and some branch clinics are located in suburban areas of a larger city. The branch clinics usually provide primary care on a regular basis and occasionally have specialists in the clinic on a rotating basis. An example of this rotation would be a dermatologist who has office hours at a branch clinic every other Tuesday. A rotation of specialists provides access to specialized health care for individuals who might not otherwise have access. Branch clinics also provide a considerable source of referrals to specialists at a larger clinic.

There are several advantages for physicians who practice in group practices. First, group physicians can "tap into" one another's expertise quickly when faced with a difficult diagnosis. Second, physicians working in a clinic setting usually have reduced responsibility for being available during hours when the clinic is closed. In addition, overhead costs, such as staff, equipment, and buildings, are shared among the entire clinical practice. A large group practice is usually operated by a board of directors that makes decisions on facility operation and management, thereby relieving the group's physicians from having to oversee all aspects of a medical office.

Private Practice

In a **private practice,** a physician provides outpatient medical care from an office in which the physician is the only provider. Some physicians prefer to have their own private practices because they may want the freedom to make decisions about how the practice is run. Physicians who operate a private practice usually maintain an affiliation with at least one hospital so that they may have the right to admit patients when necessary for hospital care. Physicians in private practice may have increased on-call duty and also often shoulder the responsibility of the operation of the medical office.

Hospital

Hospitals vary greatly in the types of services they provide. In general, a **hospital** provides **inpatient** health care—that is, health care that necessitates the patient staying overnight (longer than a 24-hour period) and having the constant attention of the nursing staff at the hospital. Hospitals are designed to provide care for patients with acute conditions, and, therefore, usually all of the services and equipment necessary to serve patients are located within the hospital. Hospitals may also have outpatient services available to provide outpatient care for patients. Hospitals can be operated either for profit or as a nonprofit organization.

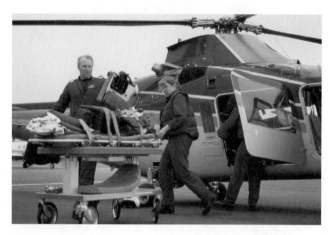

Figure 2–6. Air emergency service is often available at many trauma centers.

Hospitals often differ in the types of services they provide. Some hospitals are trauma centers, meaning they are appropriately equipped to handle emergency cases, such as critically ill or injured patients. Trauma centers may even have helicopter service to bring critically ill or injured patients to the hospital (Fig. 2–6). Not all hospitals are trauma centers. Some hospitals provide only very routine inpatient care and are not equipped or prepared to handle critical cases.

Some hospitals specialize in the type of care they provide. For example, a children's hospital may provide inpatient care only for persons younger than 18 years of age. A rehabilitation hospital may accept only patients needing rehabilitative services because of illness or injury.

Urgent Care Center

An urgent care center might bring to mind thoughts of an emergency room; however, an urgent care center and emergency room are not the same thing.

Most people are familiar with the emergency department in a hospital. The emergency department or **emergency room (ER)** is a place located within a hospital that receives patients who are acutely, seriously, or critically ill or injured. Emergency departments are open 24 hours a day, every day. Sometimes, patients with health concerns such as abdominal pain, severe headache, and musculoskeletal injuries go to the ER because their regular health care provider is unavailable or because the office is closed. Of course, accident victims and patients with critical illnesses such as stroke or heart attack also end up in the ER. The ER provides care to all types of patients with acute conditions, and, if a patient's condition warrants hospitalization, an attending physician will admit the patient.

An urgent care center can be found in various locations. Some urgent care centers are located *within* an ER. Because ERs are open 24 hours a day, urgent care centers located in an ER are usually also open 24 hours a day. (Patients may not even be able to tell where the ER starts and where the urgent care center ends.)

In a combination urgent care center/ER, patients are usually received at a central desk area where a medical administrative assistant takes registration data. The assistant then communicates the patient's arrival to a nurse who interviews the patient, takes vital signs, and assesses the level of care the patient may need. At that point, depending on the type of care needed, the decision is usually made by the nurse about whether the patient will be seen in urgent care or as an emergency patient.

One big difference to the patient will be the amount of money charged for the visit. The cost of urgent care treatment is ordinarily much less than treatment provided in an ER. If at any time the patient requires care greater than that provided in urgent care, the patient will be transferred to the care of the ER.

Urgent care centers provide care for patients who require the attention of a physician but do not have an appointment. These centers are sometimes referred to as *walk-in clinics* because patients can walk in without an appointment and are seen by a health care provider. Patients are usually seen in the order in which they arrive, but acutely ill or injured patients may be given priority over other patients. In addition to hospital settings, urgent care centers are also found in clinic settings. Urgent care centers within a clinic may follow a clinic's regularly scheduled hours or may be open for extended hours.

The tremendous advantage of urgent care centers is that urgent care provides patients with immediate access to health care. No appointment is necessary. The centers provide care for patients' illnesses and injuries ranging from very routine cases such as ear infections, sore throats, and urinary tract infections to more serious cases such as fracture, appendicitis, and severe infection.

Outpatient Surgery Center

As mentioned previously, delivery of health care services has changed drastically since the 1980s. During those years, there was a tremendous shift to outpatient delivery of surgical services. Many surgical procedures that used to require one or more nights in the hospital are now available to patients on an outpatient basis. In an outpatient surgery center (sometimes called *day surgery*), patients are given instructions to prepare for surgery (i.e., no food or water after midnight) and to arrive at the center an hour or two before their scheduled surgery.

Patients are then passed through a series of preoperative steps to ready them for surgery. They sign necessary forms, have vital signs taken, and put on surgical garments. In many instances, patients even walk to the surgical suite (accompanied by a health professional) for their surgery.

After surgery, patients are taken to a recovery area to wait for the effects of any medications to dissipate. In the recovery area, family members are often allowed to visit the patient until the patient is ready to be discharged. At the time of discharge, patients are given postoperative instructions to be followed after they are discharged.

Many different types of surgeries can be performed on an outpatient basis. All patients are not alike, however; in some instances, owing to other preexisting medical conditions, a patient may be a surgical risk and may require inpatient hospitalization. Also, problems may arise during a surgical procedure and a patient may require hospitalization as a result of complications during surgery.

On the whole, outpatient surgery has made an impact in keeping costs down for patients by allowing them to recuperate at home instead of in the hospital.

Home Health

Home health care has become big business. Home health care refers, of course, to care given to a patient in his or her own home. With the rising costs of health care, insurance companies, physicians, and patients have been looking for ways to access health care while sparing some expense. Many insurance companies are willing to pay for home health care services because it is often less costly than having a patient hospitalized.

Home health care agencies make it possible for patients to receive health care in their own home instead of going to a health care facility. Of course, not all health care can be delivered at home, but health care such as physical therapy, occupational therapy, respiratory therapy, and intravenous treatment is sometimes delivered in the patient's home.

Nursing Home, Assisted Living

Nursing homes and assisted living facilities provide continual care to patients (usually called residents). The residents live within the facility and receive the level of health care that they need.

Nursing homes provide round-the-clock care for their residents. Residents may be elderly and feeble with multiple health problems or they may be young individuals who have a serious or life-threatening health problem that does not justify inpatient hospitalization but who are too ill to be cared for at home. RNs, LPNs, and CNAs provide round-the-clock care to residents, with physicians visiting the nursing home when necessary to see patients.

Assisted living facilities may be located with, or separate from, a nursing home. These facilities provide residents with the level of health care required for their particular health situation. Residents live in an apartment-type setting and may require services such as assistance with medication. Meals may be eaten in a central dining area or within the resident's apartment. An assisted living facility can give patients the security of having others around to help when needed, but yet can still leave the resident with a great deal of autonomy.

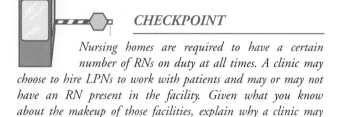

CHECKPOINT

Nursing homes are required to have a certain number of RNs on duty at all times. A clinic may choose to hire LPNs to work with patients and may or may not have an RN present in the facility. Given what you know about the makeup of those facilities, explain why a clinic may not be required to hire RNs.

Public Health

Public health agencies provide an assortment of health care services. The chief focus of most public health agency activities is on keeping the community healthy. Public health programs provide education about healthful living habits, and they work to involve community members in promoting a healthful way of life. Public health agencies also work to prevent or control epidemics and are responsible for tracking and reporting infectious and communicable disease to their respective state health departments. They also provide health care services at little or no cost to low-income individuals.

SUMMARY

After reading this chapter, the medical administrative assistant should recognize the various duties of the health care professionals working in a medical office. No one individual can do everything for a patient, and each member of the health care team is necessary for providing excellent patient service. Whether working in a clinic, hospital, urgent care center, or other health care facility, all members of the health care team contribute to the patient's care experience.

YOU ARE THE MEDICAL ADMINISTRATIVE ASSISTANT

Picture yourself as a medical administrative assistant in a medical practice. What would you do in the following situations?

1. You are working in a group practice with five primary care physicians, one pediatric nurse practitioner, and a physician's assistant. Give a response to the following:
   a. A mother calls with a 3-year-old child who has a possible ear infection. Explain to the mother the role of a nurse practitioner.
   b. A 20-year-old man walks into the clinic with a finger laceration requiring simple closure with approximately four sutures. Is it appropriate to offer the services of another health provider in addition to a physician?

Bibliography

O'Toole M: Miller-Keane Encyclopedia and Dictionary of Medicine, Nursing, and Allied Health, 6th ed. Philadelphia, WB Saunders, 1997.

Internet Resources

American Board of Specialties.
Association of American Medical Colleges, AAMC Medical Education.
U.S. Department of Labor, Bureau of Labor Statistics: 1998–99 Occupational Outlook Handbook.
United States Medical Licensing Examination.

2

REVIEW EXERCISES

Exercise 2–1 TRUE OR FALSE

Read the following statements and determine whether the statements are true or false. Record the answer in the blank provided. T = true; F = false.

_____ 1. A physician's assistant performs the same duties as a medical assistant.

_____ 2. An MD is responsible for coordinating the treatment of a patient's condition.

_____ 3. Wellness education has decreased in recent years.

_____ 4. The most common type of physician in practice in the United States is a Doctor of Osteopathy.

_____ 5. A person entering medical school must have a license to practice medicine in order to be enrolled.

_____ 6. The State Board of Physician Practices regulates the practice of medicine in each state.

_____ 7. A license to practice medicine is granted for life.

_____ 8. Primary care physicians provide care for a wide variety of disorders and diseases.

_____ 9. Some nurse practitioners are allowed to prescribe medication.

_____ 10. Persons living in a nursing home are known as residents.

_____ 11. A psychologist is a medical doctor.

_____ 12. Professional organizations typically provide continuing education opportunities for their members.

_____ 13. Anyone wishing to work as a medical transcriptionist is required to obtain the CMT certification.

_____ 14. Clinics typically provide outpatient care.

_____ 15. A physician working in a clinic setting can expect more on-call duty than can an MD in private practice.

_____ 16. All hospitals are designated trauma centers.

_____ 17. The terms *urgent care center* and *emergency room* are synonymous.

_____ 18. The terms *urgent care center* and *walk-in clinic* are synonymous.

_____ 19. The terms *urgent care center* and *outpatient surgery center* are synonymous.

_____ 20. Home health services often save money for patients and insurance companies.

_____ 21. A typical residency is 1 year in length.

_____ 22. A group practice can help alleviate after-hours responsibility for physicians.

Exercise 2–2 MEDICAL SPECIALTIES

Identify the medical specialties or subspecialties that would treat patients with the following conditions. Some cases are repeated to illustrate the fact that more than one specialty may serve the patient. Refer to Table 2–1 for descriptions of specialties. For further understanding of specialties and disorders, consult a medical dictionary. Choose the specialty that best fits the patient's condition listed. Record your answer in the space provided.

_____ 1. Patient has Graves' disease.
- (a) Neurology
- (b) Endocrinology
- (c) Ophthalmology
- (d) Gastroenterology

_____ 2. Patient has recurrent tonsillitis.
- (a) Plastic surgery
- (b) Thoracic surgery
- (c) Otolaryngology
- (d) Dermatology

_____ 3. Patient is 10 years old; needs a routine checkup.
   (a) Pediatric surgery
   (b) Allergy and immunology
   (c) Ophthalmology
   (d) Pediatrics

_____ 4. Male patient is 10 years old; needs a routine checkup.
   (a) Physical medicine and rehabilitation
   (b) Internal medicine
   (c) Family practice
   (d) Urology

_____ 5. Patient has a seizure disorder.
   (a) Neurology
   (b) Radiology
   (c) Dermatology
   (d) Cardiology

_____ 6. Patient is diagnosed with manic depression.
   (a) Cardiology
   (b) Gastroenterology
   (c) Anesthesiology
   (d) Psychiatry

_____ 7. Patient breaks out in hives repeatedly after eating certain foods.
   (a) Urology
   (b) Allergy and immunology
   (c) Gastroenterology
   (d) Orthopedics

_____ 8. Patient is pregnant.
   (a) Geriatric medicine
   (b) Obstetrics and gynecology
   (c) Hematology
   (d) Rheumatology

_____ 9. Patient has chondromalacia patella.
   (a) Orthopedics
   (b) Dermatology
   (c) Radiology
   (d) Endocrinology

_____ 10. Patient has Parkinson's disease.
   (a) Otolaryngology
   (b) Pathology
   (c) Neurology
   (d) Obstetrics and gynecology

_____ 11. Patient is 35 years old; has influenza.
   (a) Family practice
   (b) Cardiology
   (c) Nephrology
   (d) Ophthalmology

_____ 12. Patient has paronychia.
   (a) Dermatology
   (b) Thoracic surgery
   (c) Plastic surgery
   (d) Allergy and immunology

_____ 13. Patient has congestive heart failure.
   (a) Allergy and immunology
   (b) Hematology
   (c) Nephrology
   (d) Cardiology

_____ 14. Patient is being referred for a CT scan.
   (a) Pediatrics
   (b) Colon and rectal surgery
   (c) Pathology
   (d) Radiology

_____ 15. Patient has brain lesion requiring surgery.
   (a) Psychiatry
   (b) Neurologic surgery
   (c) Plastic surgery
   (d) Nuclear medicine

_____ 16. Patient has a corneal abrasion.
   (a) Ophthalmology
   (b) Hematology
   (c) Gastroenterology
   (d) Otolaryngology

_____ 17. Patient has persistent diarrhea.
   (a) Cardiology
   (b) Neurology
   (c) Gastroenterology
   (d) Nuclear medicine

_____ 18. Patient has a breast lump.
   (a) Urology
   (b) Neurologic surgery
   (c) Obstetrics and gynecology
   (d) Rheumatology

_____ 19. Patient has diabetes mellitus.
   (a) Urology
   (b) Endocrinology
   (c) Gastroenterology
   (d) Cardiology

_____ 20. Patient has recurrent anxiety attacks.
   (a) Psychiatry
   (b) Neurology
   (c) Dermatology
   (d) Radiology

Exercise 2–3 THE HEALTH CARE TEAM

In each group, identify the professional acronym or term given with the **best** description of the profession. Record your answer in the blank provided.

(a) PharmD   (d) DPM
(b) RN   (e) CNP
(c) MD

_____ 1. Observes patient progress, administers medications, and provides health education to patients; this nurse may be found in a supervisory role.

_____ 2. Dispenses medication and counsels patients on the usage of the medication.

_____ 3. Advanced practice nurse; provides health care under the supervision of a physician; may specialize in family medicine, pediatrics, or women's health.

_____ 4. Physician.

_____ 5. Doctor specializing in disorders of the foot.

(a) OD   (d) PA
(b) DO   (e) LPN, LVN
(c) CNM

_____ 6. Provides routine health care under the supervision of a physician.

_____ 7. Physician whose training has the fundamental belief that a healthy musculoskeletal system is essential to good health.

_____ 8. Nurse working under the supervision of a physician or an RN; may be responsible for charting patient progress, taking vital signs, and administering intravenous lines.

_____ 9. Advanced practice nurse who provides routine yearly physical examinations for women and provides prenatal and postnatal care.

_____ 10. Physician who conducts visual examinations.

(a) DC   (d) RHIT
(b) CMA   (e) RHIA
(c) OT

_____ 11. Individual trained in clinical and administrative tasks in the medical office.

_____ 12. Treats patients by manipulating or adjusting the spine.

_____ 13. Generally found as an administrator of a medical records department; supervises activities such as transcription, records review, and coding.

_____ 14. Provides therapy to help patients regain daily living skills.

_____ 15. Technician responsible for maintenance of the medical record.

(a) PT   (d) RT
(b) CMT   (e) CNA
(c) CRTT

_____ 16. Takes x-rays, CT scans, or MRIs.

_____ 17. Provides therapy to patients with respiratory dysfunction.

_____ 18. Transcribes medical reports.

_____ 19. Provides hygiene care for patients; may assist patients in eating or grooming.

_____ 20. Provides therapy to help patients regain bodily function; may use exercise, massage, or ultrasound.

Exercise 2-4 HEALTH CARE FACILITIES

Identify the health care facilities that provide the health care services listed. Choose the answer that most often fits the identified health care service. Record your answer in the space provided.

_____ 1. Chief function is to provide ambulatory care.
   (a) Hospital
   (b) Urgent care center
   (c) Assisted living facility
   (d) Nursing home
   (e) Clinic

_____ 2. Provides operative services not requiring inpatient hospitalization.
   (a) Assisted living facility
   (b) Outpatient surgery center
   (c) Home health
   (d) Urgent care center
   (e) Trauma center

_____ 3. Provides inpatient care for patients with acute conditions.
   (a) Home health
   (b) Urgent care center
   (c) Public health
   (d) Hospital
   (e) Clinic

_____ 4. Takes patients on a walk-in basis.
   (a) Urgent care center
   (b) Public health
   (c) Hospital
   (d) Group clinic practice
   (e) Private practice

_____ 5. Provides health education services and immunizations and reports occurrences of infectious disease.
   (a) Private practice
   (b) Public health
   (c) Clinic
   (d) Home health
   (e) Assisted living

_____ 6. Residents live in an apartment-type setting and may receive assistance in taking medication.
   (a) Public health
   (b) Private practice
   (c) Assisted living
   (d) Group clinic practice
   (e) Trauma center

_____ 7. Provides care for patients in their residence.
   (a) Home health
   (b) Public health
   (c) Nursing home
   (d) Assisted living
   (e) Private practice

_____ 8. Physician providing medical care from an office in which he or she is the only provider.
   (a) Group clinic practice
   (b) Home health
   (c) Urgent care
   (d) Hospital
   (e) Private practice

_____ 9. Place that would receive a patient who is critically injured.
   (a) Clinic
   (b) Emergency room
   (c) Public health
   (d) Home health
   (e) Group clinic practice

_____ 10. Provides care for a patient who may be too ill to be at home but whose health condition does not warrant hospitalization.
   (a) Public health
   (b) Home health
   (c) Private practice
   (d) Nursing home
   (e) Trauma center

Exercise 2–5 VOCABULARY

Read each definition and choose the vocabulary term that best matches the definition. Record your answer in the space provided.

_____ 1. Period of physician training in a specialty.
   (a) Reciprocity
   (b) Ambulatory care
   (c) Managed care
   (d) Residency

_____ 2. Individual chiefly responsible for coordinating and delivering health care services to the patient.
   (a) Primary care physician
   (b) Managed care
   (c) Inpatient care
   (d) Provider

_____ 3. Managed care patient must see this type of physician before seeing a specialist.
   (a) Primary care physician
   (b) Board-certified physician
   (c) Ambulatory care
   (d) Inpatient

_____ 4. Physician licensed in one state is allowed to obtain a license in another state.
   (a) Board-certified physician
   (b) Reciprocity
   (c) Residency
   (d) Group practice

_____ 5. Patient admitted to the hospital.
    (a) Inpatient
    (b) Ambulatory
    (c) Outpatient
    (d) Residency

_____ 6. Physician who has passed an examination in a chosen specialty.
    (a) Private practice
    (b) Managed care
    (c) Board certified
    (d) Primary care

_____ 7. Requires a patient to see a primary care physician/provider before seeing a specialist.
    (a) Primary care
    (b) Managed care
    (c) Ambulatory care
    (d) Public health agency

2
ACTIVITIES

ACTIVITY 2–1 Conduct further research on a health care profession. Choose a profession and identify the chief responsibilities, education, required training, potential earnings, and future expectations for that career. Research can be done with written sources or with personal interviews. Present your findings in report form or to the class.

ACTIVITY 2–2 Using the Internet, locate professional organizations for some of the professions mentioned in this chapter. Obtain answers to the following items or questions:
- Name of organization
- Location of organization's headquarters
- Does the organization provide educational materials or links on their Web site?
- Does the organization have an annual convention or conference? If so, where is the next one held?

ACTIVITY 2–3 Both a psychiatrist and psychologist are involved with helping patients restore good mental health or live with mental disorders. They are both trained in assessing psychiatric disorders and can be involved in counseling and diagnosing patients. Research the differences and similarities in the professions by using the Internet or other reference materials or by interviewing health professionals.

ACTIVITY 2–4 Research the American Board of Medical Specialties on the Internet. Identify subspecialties of the member boards.

ACTIVITY 2–5 Many movies have been made about the healthcare profession. Watch a movie that takes place in a health care setting. Some suggestions: _Patch Adams_ or _The Doctor._

ACTIVITY 2–6 Write a short paragraph relating the quotation at the beginning of the chapter to the variety of professionals who are part of the health care team. Why is this quotation fitting for this chapter?

ACTIVITY 2–7 Examine health care facilities in your local area. Can you find examples of the following types of facilities?
- Clinic
- Hospital
- Nursing home
- Public health agency
- Home health agency
- Urgent care center
- Assisted living facility

ACTIVITY 2–8 Research the State Board of Medical Examiners in your state. Check for information on the following:
- Licensing
- Medical practice guidelines
- Disciplinary actions
- Physician database

CHAPTER OUTLINE

LEARNING OUTCOMES

On successful completion of this chapter, the student will be able to

1. Describe different types of law and their origins.
2. Define and apply legal terminology and concepts.
3. Explain the essential components of a contract and how contract law applies to the physician-patient relationship.
4. Describe medical malpractice and negligence.
5. Explain legal proceedings in a typical medical malpractice suit.
6. Explain confidentiality.
7. Identify requirements for reporting injury, disease, and medical incidents.
8. Explain advance directives.
9. Describe the purpose of the Controlled Substances Act of 1970.
10. Describe the purpose of the Uniform Anatomical Gift Act.
11. Describe the purpose of Good Samaritan Statutes.
12. Identify components of the Health Insurance Portability and Accountability Act of 1996.
13. Explain the concept of risk management.

CMA COMPETENCIES

1. Identify and respond to issues of confidentiality.
2. Perform within legal and ethical boundaries.
3. Perform risk management procedures.

RMA COMPETENCIES

1. Identify the various types of consent and how and when to obtain each.
2. Know disclosure laws, what constitutes confidential information, and what information may be disclosed under certain circumstances.
3. Recognize legal responsibilities of the medical assistant.
4. Know the various medically related laws.
5. Define legal terminology associated with medical law.
6. Use procedures for ensuring the integrity and confidentiality of computer-stored information.
7. Know credentialing requirements of medical professionals.

VOCABULARY

abandonment
administrative law
advance directive
case law
civil law
common law
compensatory damages
confidentiality
consent
consideration
contract
criminal law
damages
defendant
deposition
durable power of attorney for health care
emancipated minor
executive branch
expressed consent
implied consent
informed consent
interrogatories
judicial branch
law

MEDICAL LAW

. . . . 'keeping up' with the law is a never-ending responsibility.

—*Nancy J. Brent, author of* Nurses and the Law

> **VOCABULARY** (*Continued*)
> legislative branch
> legal capacity
> litigation
> living will
> malpractice
> mature minor
> offer and acceptance
> plaintiff
> punitive or exemplary damages
> risk management
> standards of care
> statute of limitations
> statutes
> statutory law
> subpoena
> subpoena duces tecum

A medical administrative assistant needs a broad overview of medical law and how it affects the individuals who work in a health care organization. Legal issues regarding medical practice can affect an assistant directly or indirectly. Knowledge of the law and its concepts as it applies to health care helps a medical administrative assistant understand the complexities of health care delivery, demonstrates how legal and ethical issues have an impact on an assistant when serving patients, and provides an assistant with an understanding of the legal forces at work every day in the health care environment.

LEGAL CONCEPTS AND TERMS

What Is Law?

Laws are written rules established by a society's government. Laws indicate what is acceptable behavior and what is not acceptable behavior. All citizens who belong to a society are obligated to follow that society's laws.

Because change seems to be a constant in today's world, laws are continually updated to reflect society's changes. For example, in the early 1900s, automobiles were owned by an elite few. Now, automobile ownership is commonplace. Because of the proliferation of automobiles today, laws have been developed to govern how they are used. All people who drive automobiles are obligated to follow these laws. If they do not, they are subject to fines or arrest, or both. Likewise, as changes occur elsewhere in society, laws are enacted or changed to reflect those changes.

Origin of Law

Laws can originate at either the federal, state, or local level. The fundamental law at the federal level is the U.S. Constitution. Each state has its own constitution.

The structure of the government is identified in a constitution: at the federal level, the U.S. Constitution; at the state level, each individual state's constitution. At the state level and at the federal level, the structure of the government consists of three parts—legislative, judicial, and executive branch—each with its own authority.

The **legislative branch,** consisting of senators and representatives elected by the people, is responsible for establishing laws. Within state and federal jurisdictions, these enactments are known as **statutes** or **statutory law.** Statutory law is also referred to as legislative law.

The chief function of the judicial system is interpretation of laws. The **judicial branch,** or the court system, establishes **common law,** also known as **case law,** by deciding cases brought before the court. These cases, once decided, establish a precedent, and the court's decision serves as a model for future cases of a similar nature that come before the court. There is an extensive court system at both state and federal levels.

The **executive branch** at both the state level and the federal level is responsible for ensuring that the laws within its jurisdiction are observed. The President of the United States and the governors of each state serve as the executive power within their respective jurisdictions.

To avoid substantial conflict between federal, state, and even local governments, the U.S. Constitution establishes that the Constitution is the primary law of the land and that no state may take away rights that are assured by the Constitution. State law cannot contradict or supersede federal law. No state can take away rights that are guaranteed by federal law.

Administrative Law

Because establishing laws to govern the many facets of society would be overwhelming for elected officials of the legislative branch of government, legislatures give authority to government agencies (either state or federal agencies) to establish regulations and enforce those regulations, or **administrative laws,** within their jurisdiction. For example, the Drug Enforcement Agency (DEA) establishes guidelines for the manufacture and dispensing of potentially addictive prescription drugs. The Environmental Protection Agency (EPA) establishes regulations that safeguard the environment. The Center for Medicare and Medicaid Services (CMS) oversees the administration of Medicare and Medicaid benefits. These federal agencies are then charged with carrying out enforcement of the administrative law within their authority.

Civil and Criminal Law

Legal cases pertaining to health care can be either civil or criminal in nature. **Civil law** involves the relationship between individuals or a group. Civil cases are brought with the contention that the one party did something that adversely affected or injured another party. An individual who alleges that a health care worker was negligent in providing care is making a civil claim. Civil cases usually involve the injured party asking for a sum of money to compensate for the damages he or she has incurred.

Criminal law, on the other hand, involves the relationship between an individual and the government. By enacting laws, legislatures determine what constitutes criminal behavior and what punishment is suitable for a crime. If an individual breaks a law, the government has the responsibility for upholding the law to protect the rest of society. For example, a health care worker who assists a patient in obtaining prescription drugs illegally would face criminal charges. The penalty for violating criminal law can include fine or incarceration, or both.

Standards of Care

In the health care field, health care professionals are required to perform consistent with expectations of their profession. This concept is known as **standards of care.**

In other words, a health care professional is expected to carry out his or her duties as other reasonable health care professionals in their profession would carry our their duties. For example, in a particular situation, a physician is expected to perform as other reasonable and prudent physicians would perform. In turn, a nurse is expected to perform as other reasonable and prudent nurses would perform. Physicians and other health care professionals are held to standards of care for their particular profession and are expected to perform as others in their profession would perform. If they fail to perform up to standards for their profession, they risk being accused of malpractice.

Medical Malpractice and Negligence

According to the *Miller-Keane Encyclopedia & Dictionary of Medicine, Nursing, & Allied Health,* **malpractice** is "any professional misconduct, unreasonable lack of skill or fidelity in professional duties, or illegal or immoral conduct." A widely held view of malpractice is a physician failing to do something a reasonable and prudent person would do or a physician doing something a reasonable and prudent person would not do.

Because of their advanced training, physicians are held to their profession's standards of care when administering medical care. Physicians may be liable if they act or if they do not act. They can be found guilty of malpractice if they make a mistake while administering medical treatment or if they fail to recognize treatment that should be given in a particular situation.

Malpractice is a type of negligence. To prove negligence in a court of law, an individual must be able to demonstrate all of the following:

1. An obligation or duty existed on the part of the physician to provide services for a patient.

2. The physician failed to provide proper care for the patient's medical condition.
3. The physician's failure caused the patient's injury.
4. The patient suffered damage or injury.

Respondeat Superior

Is the employer responsible for the wrongdoings of an employee? The Latin phrase *respondeat superior* means "let the master answer." Essentially, this establishes liability on the part of the employer for the actions of an employee. When an employee performs job duties, the employer (e.g., a physician, clinic, or hospital) may be held responsible for any negligence or wrongdoing of the employee.

Respondeat superior is an important concept of the law because it pertains to many of the activities in the medical office. To protect a health care facility, a physician, and themselves, it is vital for assistants to understand the meaning of this term.

Because it would be virtually impossible for physicians to conduct all business of a practice, physicians hire an office staff to help perform the activities necessary to run a medical office. All employees are deemed to act at the direction of or on behalf of the physician or practice, and the physician and practice is responsible for the actions of employees.

If an employee of the medical practice performs an act that harms a patient, the physician and the medical practice can be held liable because the employee represents the physician and the medical practice. A patient may elect to sue the physician, medical practice, and even the employee. Generally, claimants will sue the party or parties that have the most to lose: typically, the physician and the medical practice, although it is also possible that an employee may be sued if he or she has some responsibility for the situation in question. An assistant should be very careful to perform only those job duties that have been assigned and should be careful to never say anything that might be construed as giving medical advice.

Consider the following inappropriate comments by someone without the proper training:

Patient phoning the office: "I'd like to make an appointment to see Dr. Anderson. My big toe is red and swollen and oozing pus around the toenail."

Untrained assistant: "You probably have an ingrown toenail. I can make an appointment for you this afternoon."

Such a comment could possibly be interpreted as practicing medicine without a license. If a patient calls with a question about how to treat a condition or asks what to do about a certain medical situation, the assistant must let the staff members who are specifically trained to respond to such situations do so.

Res Ipsa Loquitur

A Latin phrase meaning "the thing speaks for itself," *res ipsa loquitur* refers to the idea that evidence speaks for itself. If a patient has an infection because of a surgical sponge left in a surgical site, it is likely that the sponge was the cause of the patient's infection and that the patient would not have experienced such an infection if all sponges had been removed. An obvious mistake on the part of a health care provider is usually negligence, and it is enough evidence for a legal action.

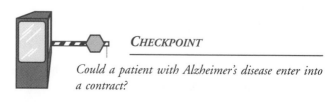

CHECKPOINT

Identify whether or not the following situations could be malpractice on the part of a health care professional:

1. A nurse gives the wrong dosage of a drug, and that dosage causes harm to the patient.
2. A patient phones the clinic with chest pain, and the nurse fails to inform the physician of the phone call. Later in the day, the patient suffers a massive heart attack while at home and dies.
3. A physician fails to notify a patient of normal laboratory results.
4. A physician fails to inform the patient of suspicious Pap smear results. The patient is not informed of the need for follow-up care, and 1 year later she is diagnosed with cervical cancer.

Contract Law

The basis for many civil suits, or civil **litigation,** involving medical practice is founded in contract law. A **contract** is a legal agreement between two parties that creates an obligation. Establishment of a contract creates a duty for one party to do something because another party has agreed to do something in return.

Essentials of a Contract

Many times, when someone hears the word *contract,* what usually comes to mind is something that is written and then signed by both parties. A contract may be written or verbal, however. The physician-patient relationship is based on a contractual agreement. Most physician-patient relationships are established through an oral contract.

A contractual agreement is said to exist if each of the following four criteria have been met:

Offer and Acceptance. This is the initial step in establishing a contract. **Offer** means that the first party has offered to provide something, such as a good or service. **Acceptance** means that the second party has accepted the first party's offer. Therefore, when a physician offers service to a patient and the patient accepts the service, the beginning steps of a contract have commenced.

Legal Subject Matter. The topic or subject matter of a contract must be a legal act or object. A contract would not exist if the subject matter was an illegal item nor would a contract exist if the action to be performed was illegal (e.g., prescribing illegal drugs to treat a condition).

Legal Capacity. **Legal capacity** refers to a party's ability to enter into a contract. Generally, an individual must be 18 years of age or older to enter into a contract. Minors (individuals younger than age 18) usually cannot enter into a contract. There are certain exceptions to this requirement. One exception is an individual declared by the court to be an **emancipated minor,** meaning that the individual is younger than age 18 but is capable of making adult decisions despite not having reached adulthood. Generally, an emancipated minor meets one of the following conditions:

- the minor is married, separated, divorced, or widowed;
- the minor is a parent;
- the minor is in the armed forces; or
- the minor resides away from home and supports himself or herself.

Some states recognize that minors are **statutory adults** and may consent to medical treatment at 14 years of age. Statutory adults also have the right to confidentiality in relation to their medical records, even though parents may be obligated to pay for a minor's medical care.

Other states recognize some minors as **mature minors** who are capable of making medical decisions without parental consent. Mature minors are generally unable to give consent for medical treatment except in cases involving pregnancy, requests for contraception, treatment for sexually transmitted diseases, substance abuse, and psychiatric care. Usually, if a minor is 14 years of age and seeks treatment for the aforementioned conditions, information regarding treatment must be kept confidential and cannot be released to the minor's parents without the minor's consent. Not all states recognize mature minors, statutory adults, or emancipated minors.

Another component of legal capacity is that an individual entering into a contract must be of sound mind and must be capable of making decisions that are in his or her best interest. If a patient is younger than the age of 18, a parent or guardian is usually needed to give consent for the examination. If the patient is not of sound mind (mentally incompetent) or is incapable of making his or her own decisions, a guardian or someone with legal authority will make the decision for the patient. A patient with a known psychiatric disorder or low IQ may not have the legal capacity to consent to treatment.

Consideration. To complete a contractual agreement, something of value is exchanged between the two parties. This is known as **consideration.** If a physician examines a patient and determines a diagnosis, the professional opinion or advice of the physician is something of value. The patient, after receiving the physician's treatment and diagnosis, will then pay the physician for the services provided. The physician's professional advice and patient's money are the items of value that are exchanged.

CHECKPOINT

Could a patient with Alzheimer's disease enter into a contract?

The Physician-Patient Relationship

A physician-patient relationship is present if the four criteria of a contract are met. If a patient alleges wrongdoing on the part of a physician, it will be important to establish the existence of a relationship or contract between the physician and the patient. If a relationship does not exist, the physician could, possibly, not be held liable.

Physicians are free to choose whom they will accept as patients. Obstetrics and gynecology physicians may have to restrict the number of obstetrics patients they accept in order to not overload their practice. If confronted with an emergency situation, however, a physician must provide care for the patient until care can be transferred to another physician or facility.

Once a physician-patient relationship has been established, it is important for the physician to provide services to the patient as needed. The establishment of the physician-patient relationship creates an obligation on the part of the physician to provide ongoing treatment to the patient if needed.

Terminating a Contract

If a physician can no longer provide services for a patient, the physician must notify the patient that he or she is no longer able to provide care for the patient.

A physician who finds it necessary to discharge a patient from care should consult an attorney as to the appropriate steps to take to terminate care. Usually, the physician is advised to send a letter notifying the patient of the termination via certified mail with a return receipt verifying delivery of the letter. The physician should specify in the letter the reason for dismissing the patient and should tell the patient that he or she can provide names of other physicians who may be available to provide care. The physician is obligated to provide care for a reasonable period (typically 30 days) until the patient can make other arrangements for medical care.

Sometimes, a patient decides to terminate the relationship with a physician. If a patient is currently being treated for a medical condition, it is important that the physician confirm the patient's wishes. The termination should be confirmed in writing to the patient to verify his or her intent to sever the relationship.

In all cases of termination of the physician-patient relationship before patient care is finished, the termination should be well documented by the physician in the patient's chart. No matter who initiated the termination, medical record documentation is vital to protect the physician and the practice should litigation arise from any treatment situation.

Abandonment. If a physician does not properly meet his or her obligation to treat the patient, the physician could be held responsible for abandoning the patient.

Abandonment might be alleged if a patient is admitted to the hospital and the physician does not see the patient in the hospital and makes no arrangements for another physician to take his or her place. A physician who suddenly closes the practice doors one day without notifying patients and making arrangements for subsequent treatment might also be found guilty of abandonment, as might a physician who is constantly unavailable for follow-up treatment of chronically ill patients. Even a physician who performs a surgical procedure and does not provide the necessary follow-up care could be found guilty of abandonment. A physician who does not provide follow-up care because a patient has a large outstanding balance on an account could also be found guilty of abandonment.

Legal Action against a Medical Practice

Occasionally in medical practice, a patient alleges that something has gone wrong in the physician-patient relationship. Because of an adverse outcome, a patient may assert that he or she has been injured because of the negligent actions of the physician or one of the physician's employees. If a patient decides to pursue **litigation,** or legal action, the patient (who initiated the suit) is known as the **plaintiff** and the physician, allied health employee, or practice (party or parties accused of wrongdoing), or both, is known as the **defendant.**

Statute of Limitations

Cases regarding medical malpractice must be brought forward within a reasonable period of time. This period is known as the **statute of limitations** and varies from state to state. If the state statute of limitations is 2 years for a medical malpractice suit, a patient may bring suit within 2 years of the alleged injury or when the patient becomes aware of the injury.

In the case of injury to a minor, the statute of limitations may be figured from the time the patient reaches the age of majority. For example, if a child is injured at 5 years of age and the statute of limitations is 2 years in the state where the child resides, the child may have a right to sue even at age 19 because the statute of limitations may not begin to run until the child reaches 18 years.

In some states, a plaintiff alleging medical malpractice is required to obtain expert opinions from another physician to support allegations made against a physician. If this is not done in a timely manner, the suit may be dismissed. Some states allow only 3 months for expert opinions to be obtained.

Effects of Medical Malpractice Suits

A medical malpractice case can be devastating to a physician, staff, and health care facility. Litigation places a physician's and facility's reputation at stake. Even if a physician wins, his or her reputation may be damaged by the publicity of the suit. Also, involvement in a suit can be a financial strain and can be emotionally draining.

Physicians may sometimes elect to settle the suit before it even reaches the trial stage. If the plaintiff will settle for a nominal amount, a physician may choose to settle instead of going to trial. Frequently, settlements do not admit wrong-doing but are made because they may be cheaper than defending a lawsuit. A physician's malpractice insurer may decide to settle with a plaintiff and may do so without the approval of the physician. Insurers will weigh the chances of successful outcome of the trial along with the potential cost of going to trial and determine whether it is prudent to settle the suit before trial.

Legal Proceedings

Once a patient has decided to pursue litigation against a physician or health care facility, an assistant should be prepared to receive legal requests for information. The pretrial phase of a lawsuit involves much information gathering on the part of both parties. Information regarding any malpractice case should not be given without consulting the attorney representing the physician or clinic. If the opposing party's attorney asks questions of any medical office employees, all employees must refrain from giving any information whatsoever to the attorney. The slightest comment could be potentially damaging.

A flow chart illustrating the process of a typical medical malpractice case is shown in Figure 3–1. At any time during the process illustrated in this Figure, the parties may agree to a settlement. An alternative to settlement or trial is the arbitration process. The parties who agree to have a case decided by arbitration do so knowing that the decision of the arbitrator will be final.

Interrogatories

Before a trial begins, a set of written questions may be asked of the opposing party by either the plaintiff or the defendant. These questions are known as **interrogatories.** The purpose of interrogatories is to obtain basic factual information such as dates of employment, education, and other pertinent professional qualifications. These questions are answered in writing under oath and should be answered in consultation with an attorney.

Depositions

Sometimes, a physician must be an expert witness (having treated the patient) and must give testimony regarding a patient's claim of injury against a third party. It is not always necessary for witnesses to testify in court. Expert testimony can be given outside the courtroom in a procedure known as a **deposition.** A deposition may be held in a medical facility or at an attorney's office, with the latter

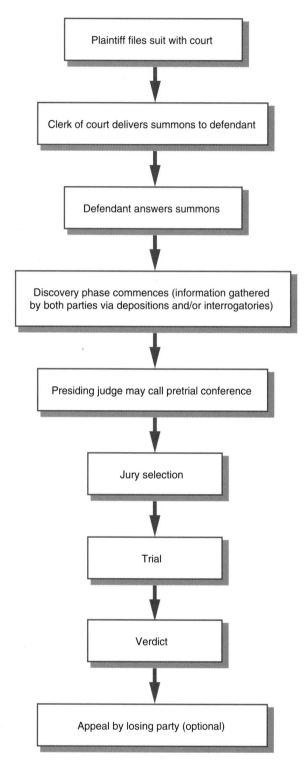

Figure 3–1. Flow chart of the possible sequence of a medical malpractice case.

being more common. Generally, it is preferred that depositions be held away from a medical office, to avoid drawing attention to a group of attorneys visiting the physician at the office.

Usually taken before trial, a deposition is a written record of the sworn testimony of a witness. This testimony, given in question/answer format similar to courtroom proceedings, is taken by a court reporter who has been retained by one of the parties to record the proceedings of the deposition. Before the deposition begins, the witness is sworn in just as if he or she were in a courtroom. Attorneys representing each party to the suit take part in the deposition and ask questions of the witness, the same as in a courtroom.

In a deposition of a physician, the opening questions usually relate to the physician's professional qualifications (e.g., where he or she attended medical school, whether he or she has board certification, where he or she practices). Once this foundation is laid, questions center around the patient's visits with the physician and the physician's professional opinion of the patient's injuries (Box 3–1).

After the deposition has concluded, the court reporter prepares an original and copies of the deposition in written form. The court reporter sends a rough draft of the deposition for review to the person who gave the testimony. Any necessary corrections (changes in testimony are not allowed) are made by the witness and returned to the court reporter.

Corrections are then made to the deposition, and the original of the deposition is filed with the court. Copies of the deposition may be ordered by the attorneys if they wish. The court reporter charges the attorney who arranged for the deposition for the original. If the physician is an expert witness in the case, the physician charges the attorney who arranged for the deposition for the testimony. Any additional copies ordered are charged to the ordering party. A physician who is a defendant in a case is not allowed to charge for testimony.

Subpoena

If a case goes to trial, it may be necessary to order an individual to appear in court. This order is known as a **subpoena.** A subpoena instructs an individual to appear in court at a certain time and place. If an individual fails to do so, that individual is subject to a penalty imposed by the court.

Physicians may appear in court for a variety of reasons. They may be called in a civil or criminal trial. Most commonly, they are called as expert witnesses to give their professional opinion about a party's injury. Remember, as an expert witness, a physician normally charges a fee for giving testimony.

Subpoena Duces Tecum

In cases involving a patient from a physician's practice, it will become necessary for the patient's medical records to be submitted into evidence at a trial. An order to produce medical records for use at a trial is known as a **subpoena duces tecum.** If records are subpoenaed, the assistant or another employee of the clinic who is responsible for the medical record may be called on to identify the record. A photocopy of the record is usually acceptable to submit into evidence, and the patient's original record remains in the clinic. In a legal case, it is acceptable to charge the patient's attorney for photocopying the patient's record.

The medical administrative assistant who has received a subpoena duces tecum will be expected to bring the patient's record to the court at the time and place specified. It is the physician's responsibility to give meaning to the record; it is the medical administrative assistant's responsibility to verify that the record belongs to a certain individual and that the content is original and has not been altered or falsified.

The Assistant as a Witness

When served with a subpoena, a medical administrative assistant should consult the legal counsel retained by the clinic or physician. An attorney will instruct the assistant about the proper procedures to follow to obey the subpoena.

When appearing in court as a witness, a medical administrative assistant should do the following:
- Answer only the question asked by the questioning attorney. Do not offer additional information.
- Answer each question truthfully.
- Be sure the question asked is understood. If not, state "I don't understand the question."
- If an answer to a question is unknown, do not be afraid to say "I don't know."
- Explain the facts in easy to understand terms.
- Never cover up any discrepancies in the record.
- Wear professional dress. Appearance adds to witness credibility.

Damages

When a case is filed with the court, damage amounts requested by the plaintiff are specified. **Damages** are monetary

---

Box 3–1 Portion of a Sample Deposition*

Q: When did you first see Jennifer Singer as a patient?
A: June 16, 1998.
Q: And what was her chief complaint at that visit?
A: Pain and swelling of the right knee.
Q: What was the condition of her right knee at that time?
A: She had significant infrapatellar swelling and erythema. Her range of motion was restricted.
Q: What did she say caused her injury?
A: She reported she was in a motor vehicle accident and her knee struck the dashboard.
Q: Were her injuries consistent with a motor vehicle collision?

*Q, questions by an attorney; A, answers by a physician.

amounts requested by a plaintiff in consideration for injuries the plaintiff alleges to have received.

If the defense of a malpractice case is unsuccessful and a physician or practice loses the case, damages to be awarded to the plaintiff will be specified by the jury. Common damages sought in actions against a medical practice or physician (or both) are compensatory and punitive damages.

Compensatory damages are awarded to compensate the plaintiff for injuries or losses suffered as a result of the wrongdoing of the defendant. These awards are meant to compensate for damages such as physical injury, loss of wages due to inability to work, emotional suffering, or loss of companionship, or both.

Punitive, or **exemplary,** damages are usually the most severe. Multimillion dollar awards one hears about in the media usually consist of substantial punitive damage amounts. Punitive damages are awarded to do exactly what the word punitive means: to punish. This damage award is given to punish a defendant for something that was very wrong. Large punitive damage amounts are intended to deter others from similar conduct and are intended to make an "example" of the case. Because punitive damages can be so high, some states have set limits as to the punitive damage amounts that can be awarded. Punitive damages may be awarded along with compensatory damages.

LEGAL TOPICS RELATING TO THE MEDICAL OFFICE

The Practice of Medicine

To legally practice medicine, a physician must be licensed to practice in each state in which he or she practices medicine. The State Board of Medical Examiners in each state is responsible for the physician licensure process.

What constitutes the practice of medicine in each state is established by the state's Medical Practice Act. It is important for an assistant to note that anything that could be construed as medical advice should never be given to a patient. An assistant should be careful to never say such things as "You probably have strep throat" or "Take two aspirin and call back tomorrow morning." By such actions, an assistant is giving medical advice or a diagnosis and could very likely be accused of practicing medicine without a license.

Consent

To treat patients, a physician must obtain consent for medical treatment from the patient. Consent is either expressed or implied by the patient. To give **consent** for medical treatment is to give approval for medical treatment.

Expressed consent is a statement from the patient that the physician should provide medical treatment for the patient. Expressed consent may be given by the patient either verbally or in writing. The nature of the proposed medical treatment will determine whether or not the consent should be written. Consent for routine care, such as examinations and basic diagnostic tests, is usually given verbally. If medical treatment is invasive or if it requires administration of a medication, a written consent is usually given. Written consent is used for such procedures as surgery, administration of immunizations, and removal of lesions and for certain laboratory or radiologic examinations, such as testing for the human immunodeficiency virus and computed tomographic scans requiring use of contrast medium.

Implied consent is given very often in a medical office. Patients may not even realize when they are giving implied consent. Implied consent is evidenced by a patient's actions. If a physician asks a patient to open his mouth and say "Ah," and the patient does it, the patient is giving consent to the physician to examine his throat. Even the very act of arriving for an appointment with a physician is implied consent: implying that the patient wants to be treated.

In a life-or-death situation, consent is not required to treat a patient. It is implied, or assumed, that a patient would want his or her life saved. Even if a patient cannot communicate, the medical staff will commence and continue treatment until the patient is out of danger. The consent of a patient or relative is not necessary to begin life-saving treatment.

To give consent, patients must have full knowledge of their medical condition and the proposed treatment for the condition. Whenever consent is given by patients, it must be an **informed consent.** Informed consent means patients have been given information about their medical condition, the treatment alternatives for their condition, and why treatment is recommended. They must be told of the potential benefits and risks of each treatment and likely outcomes related to each treatment. They must also be informed of what may happen if they choose not to treat the condition, and they must receive this information in language that they understand.

Let's apply informed consent to the following examples:

- A patient suffers from elevated blood pressure. The physician gives in detail the treatment options (e.g., various medications, dietary changes) and the risks associated with each option. The physician must also inform the patient of what may happen if the patient does not treat the condition (the patient may be at risk for serious health complications, such as a stroke).
- A patient has a suspicious mole. The physician may recommend an excision of the mole but must inform the patient of possible scarring, infection, and other consequences. The physician may also inform the patient that if he or she chooses to wait to remove the lesion and it is malignant, serious complications could occur.

Licensure

As mentioned previously, a physician must be licensed to practice medicine by the state in which he or she works.

Each state sets the requirements for licensure, which usually include successful completion of the United States Medical Licensing Examination (USMLE), graduation from an approved medical school, and completion of a residency.

If a physician moves out of state, he or she may be able to meet the requirements for licensure in the new state by demonstrating a current license from another state. This is referred to as *reciprocity*. In the reciprocity process, as long as a physician has met requirements to practice in one state, he or she may apply for a license in another state that has reciprocity with the first state.

Licensure is also required of individuals wishing to practice as a registered nurse (RN) or licensed practical nurse (LPN). As mentioned in Chapter 2, nursing professionals must pass national examinations to work as an RN or LPN and may then apply for licensure to work in their state.

Licensure in a medical field must usually be renewed every few years. To be eligible for renewal, most states require that a health professional have a minimum amount of continuing education units (CEUs) in order to renew a license in his or her field.

Certification and Registration

Not all professions require licensure. Some health professions have a certification or registration process. Certification or registration is not always required of an employee to work in certain fields.

Certification is administered by the national organization of each profession. An individual desiring certification must meet the organization's requirements for certification, which typically include taking a credentialing examination. On successful completion of the examination, the individual may use the "certified" designation. CEUs are usually required to retain certification. Some professions may have more than one certification examination.

The registration process for a profession involves meeting specific requirements. Those requirements may involve special educational requirements or may simply be payment of a registration fee.

Confidentiality

The concept of health care **confidentiality** means that communication between a patient and a health care professional must be kept confidential. Federal legislation known as the Health Insurance Portability and Accountability Act of 1996 provided the groundwork for the first federal protection of health care information. Individual states may have greater protection of a patient's medical privacy.

Without confidentiality, a patient may be reluctant to divulge important information that may have an impact on his or her health. For instance, if a physician asks about a patient's social habits and the patient answers no to questions of illegal drug use, this could have a serious impact on the patient's treatment for his or her condition.

There are some instances when a physician is required to release confidential information about the patient, whether or not the patient has authorized its release. Note that the exceptions listed here apply to physicians only, not to an assistant. An assistant is expected to keep all health information confidential unless a written authorization to release information is obtained from the patient. A physician may release confidential information about a patient in the following instances:

- If it is legally required to be released. Injuries as result of a crime are required to be reported.
- If the patient has certain communicable or infectious diseases.
- If the patient is a serious threat to someone (including themselves) or to society, (e.g., the patient threatens to harm someone [Box 3–2]).
- If the physician is subpoenaed.

Under no circumstances should any health care professional **ever** discuss a patient's medical treatment or diagnosis with anyone (the patient's family or anyone else) unless it is vital for providing continuing care to the patient. This includes all health care professionals in the medical office. Adult family members are not entitled to information about other adult family members unless the patient gives permission.

As mentioned previously, minors may receive treatment in certain instances without parental consent. Those instances include treatments for pregnancy, contraceptive prescription, sexually transmitted diseases, drug and other substance abuse, and psychiatric problems. Information regarding those treatments cannot be released to the parent without the approval of the minor. Because these conditions are so serious and fundamental to the well being of the minor, this information is kept confidential.

Imagine how many minors with concerns related to these conditions would seek treatment if they knew their parents would know everything. Treatment of minors is often a "sticky" situation, and a physician in conjunction with legal counsel should establish guidelines consistent with state law for the entire medical office staff.

Details regarding any patient's visit should be discussed with other health care personnel only if the details are necessary to provide continued care or a service to the patient. Possible situations in which this would apply might be (1) giving information to the billing personnel within the office for completing the billing process or (2) asking the nurse to verify a patient's medications because the physician's dictation is inaudible. More information on legal issues as they pertain specifically to a patient's health information can be found in Chapter 9.

Mandated Reportable Injury, Disease, and Occurrences

To protect the public from outbreaks of disease, the government requires certain medical occurrences to be reported to the state health department.

Box 3-2 Tarasoff v. Regents of University of California; Morgan v. Fairfield

Following are examples of why confidentiality may need to be breached by a physician or other health care providers. These are real cases.

Tarasoff v. Regents of University of California

Poddar, an adult male, became obsessed with a student named Tatiana Tarasoff. A friend encouraged Poddar to get professional help. Poddar saw a psychiatrist, was given medication and scheduled for weekly appointments with a psychologist. During the appointments, Poddar confessed to having fantasies about harming, maybe killing, Tarasoff. A friend told the psychologist Poddar planned to buy a gun. Poddar stopped therapy and the psychologist asked campus police to question Poddar. When questioned, Poddar denied a plan to harm Tarasoff.

Two months later, Poddar stabbed Tarasoff to death. Poddar was convicted of murder but due to a technicality the conviction was overturned. Poddar then left the country.

Tarasoff's family filed a civil suit against the university, psychiatrist, psychologist, and campus police for negligence. The court found for the plaintiff and concluded that the therapists had a duty to warn Tarasoff of possible impending danger.

Morgan v. Fairfield

In a more recent case, Morgan v. Fairfield (1997), the Ohio Supreme Court ruled against Dr. Brown, a psychia-trist/consultant, and the Fairfield Family Counseling Center. A psychiatric patient, Matt Morgan, had made threats against his father and was subsequently hospitalized and diagnosed with a schizophreniform disorder. After being released from the hospital, he received follow-up care from Dr. Brown, who later discontinued Matt's medication. Matt's mother repeatedly reported to the doctor that her son's condition was deteriorating. The parents made repeated attempts to have Matt involuntarily committed but were unsuccessful. On July 25, 1991, Matt Morgan shot and killed his parents and seriously injured his sister. The plaintiffs alleged that the doctor did not obtain an adequate medical history, improperly discontinued the patient's medication, and failed to monitor the patient's condition. The case reached the Ohio Supreme Court, where the Court ruled in favor of the plaintiffs.

These cases illustrate the point that confidentiality should not be protected if society or an individual is in danger. In instances such as these, the need for society or an individual to know of the threat is greater than the need to protect the patient's confidentiality.

Tarasoff v. Regents of University of California, 17 Cal. 3d 425, 551 P. 2d 334, 131 Cal. Rptr. 14 (1976)
American Association of Community Psychiatrists. AACP Newsletter, Vol. 11, No. 3, Summer 1997

Public health laws in every state require physicians to report certain occurrences of disease, injury, and other medical events. The requirements for reporting vary from state to state. These occurrences include such items as the following:

- Births and deaths
- Suspected abuse (child, adult, or elderly)
- Treatment of patients with injuries from a violent act, such as stabbing, shooting, or poisoning
- Communicable or infectious diseases (Box 3–3)

Information received by the state health departments is then compiled on a national scale by the Centers for Disease Control and Prevention (CDC) in Atlanta. Each week, the CDC publishes the *Morbidity and Mortality Weekly Report*, which reports instances of certain diseases and death statistics from every state.

Advance Directives

No individual can ever be certain that he or she will always be capable of making all of his or her health care decisions. At one time or another, everyone will probably know someone who is no longer able to communicate wishes for medical treatment. This may happen as a result of an accident or serious illness at any time in someone's life.

What happens when patients are so ill or incapacitated that they cannot make health care decisions for themselves? **Advance directives** are legal documents that establish a patient's wishes for medical care when he or she is no longer able to make those decisions. Almost all states recognize advance directives.

In the absence of any written instructions for health care decisions, physicians consult with the patient's relatives to obtain consent for medical treatment. A patient's relatives may not be aware of the patient's wishes for medical treatment. An advance directive will inform family members of a patient's wishes if the patient has failed to do so.

The Joint Commission on Accreditation of Healthcare Organizations (JCAHO), an organization that reviews practices and procedures of hospitals and other health care facilities, requires hospitals to ask every patient when admitted if he or she has an advance directive. If the patient has an advance directive, a copy must be placed in the patient's chart.

There are two forms of advance directives: living wills and Durable Power of Attorney for Health Care.

Box 3–3 Conditions Reportable to State Department of Health (From the State of North Dakota)

Anthrax*
Botulism*
Brucellosis*
Campylobacter enteritis*
Cancer, all invasive and in situ carcinoma
Chickenpox (varicella)
Chlamydial infections
Cholera*
Cryptosporidiosis
Diphtheria*
Encephalitis
Enteric Escherichia coli infection*
Enterococcus, vancomycin resistant (VRE)*
Foodborne or waterborne outbreaks
Giardiasis
Gonorrhea
Hantavirus*
Haemophilus influenzae infection*
Hemolytic uremic syndrome
Hepatitis (specify type)
Human immunodeficiency virus (HIV) infection, include acquired immunodeficiency syndrome (AIDS)*
Influenza
Lead blood level greater than or equal to 10 μg/dL
Legionellosis
Listeriosis*
Lyme disease
Malaria*
Measles (rubeola)*

Meningitis, bacterial*
Meningococcal disease
Mumps
Nosocomial outbreaks in institutions
Pertussis*
Plague*
Poliomyelitis*
Q fever*
Rabies (animal or human*)
Rocky Mountain spotted fever
Rubella*
Salmonellosis*
Scabies outbreaks in institutions
Shigellosis*
Staphylococcus aureus, methicillin resistant (MRSA)*
Staphylococcus aureus, vancomycin resistant (VRSA)*
Streptococcal infections*
Syphilis
Tetanus
Toxic-shock syndrome*
Trichinosis
Tuberculosis*
Tularemia*
Tumors of the central nervous system
Typhoid fever*
Unusual disease cluster or outbreak
Weapons of mass destruction suspected event

* Requires sample submitted to public health laboratory.
(From North Dakota State Department of Health, 2000.)

A **living will** specifies the type of treatment the patient would or would not like if in a terminal, irreversible condition. A living will communicates the patient's wishes with regard to having life-sustaining treatment.

A **Durable Power of Attorney for Health Care** is a document that is broader in nature and covers more possible types of medical situations. A Durable Power of Attorney for Health Care is a legal document that gives authority to an individual who will make health care decisions for a person if that person is no longer able to make those decisions. If the patient is comatose or is mentally incapacitated and cannot make decisions for himself or herself, the individual designated as the durable power or attorney for health care will make the patient's decisions.

A living will is different from a durable power of attorney in that the living will communicates the patient's wishes if the patient should have an irreversible or terminal illness. Many medical situations can arise that may impede an individual's ability to decide, but all of those situations are not necessarily irreversible or terminal.

A living will identifies whether or not the patient desires tube feeding, cardiopulmonary resuscitation, or other extraordinary measures to save his or her life. Once the patient is attached to a life-sustaining or prolonging device, it is often very difficult to have that device removed. If a living will has been prepared by the patient, it may spare the patient and the family from an undesirable, unpleasant medical situation.

Advance directives are legal documents and must be witnessed by individuals who do not stand to benefit from the patient's medical condition. Hospital or health facility employees, blood relatives, and anyone named in a patient's will could not be a witness to that patient's advance directive. Health facility employees may benefit if a patient is kept on life support and large bills result. Relatives or people named in wills may benefit from a patient's demise. It is easy to see why a witness to an advance directive must be free from those connections to a patient. Although a relative may not be a witness, a relative can be named to make decisions as a power of attorney.

Patients who have or desire advance directives should be sure to communicate their wishes to the health care provider. Copies of the directives should be placed in the patient's medical record, and the record should be clearly marked that the patient has an advanced directive. Patients should also inform family members about the existence of their advance directive.

Uniform Anatomical Gift Act

The Uniform Anatomical Gift Act was passed in 1968 and governs the donation of body parts. Common parts of the body that are donated include heart, lungs, kidneys, liver, and corneas. An individual wishing to donate body parts on his or her death may specify exactly which parts may be donated.

Because of the advancement of medical technology and the ability to transplant body parts from one individual to another, it became necessary to control the transplantation and donation process. This is often the case with law pertaining to medicine: Technological advances in medicine make it necessary to enact laws to protect society.

The basic principles of the Uniform Anatomical Gift Act are the following:

1. An individual 18 years of age and of sound mind may donate any or all parts of his or her body upon his or her death.
2. If an individual has not specified donation, a relative of a deceased individual may donate any or all body parts. The relative making the decision is usually based on the following order: spouse, adult children, parents, adult brothers and sisters.
3. Gift recipients (recipient of the donation) are restricted to certain medical-related facilities (e.g., hospitals, medical schools) or to a specific individual in need.
4. An individual may revoke his or her donation at any time.
5. The facility or person designated to receive the donation has a right to reject the donation.

Controlled Substances Act of 1970

The Controlled Substances Act (CSA) is part of the Comprehensive Drug Abuse Prevention and Control Act of 1970. The purpose of this legislation is to control the manufacture and distribution of narcotics, stimulants, depressants, hallucinogens, anabolic steroids, and chemicals used to produce a controlled substance. Drugs that are regulated by the CSA are placed on one of five schedules according to their potential for abuse. Schedule I includes dangerous drugs with no recognized medical use and great potential for abuse; schedule V drugs have the least potential for abuse.

Physicians and other health professionals who are authorized to dispense, prescribe, or administer drugs identified under the CSA must identify their DEA number on a patient's prescription when one of these drugs is prescribed. All individuals and companies that are authorized to handle these drugs are required to maintain a complete, accurate inventory and records of the substances and their related transactions as well as proper security measures for storing the substances.

Good Samaritan Statutes

Good Samaritan statutes are designed to protect health professionals who stop to render aid at the scene of an accident. Good Samaritan statutes are present in all 50 states. The intention of the statute is to protect trained medical personnel from liability if they stop at the scene of an accident to render aid (Fig. 3–2). As is the case with many accidents, if a trained passerby arrives on the scene before an emergency response team, treatment without delay can mean the difference between life or death.

Good Samaritan statutes do not protect health care professionals from negligent, reckless behavior. A good Samaritan is usually not held liable for injury to the patient unless the health care professional's behavior was not within standards of care and contributed to further injure the patient. The Good Samaritan Act also does not apply to emergency cases within a medical facility.

Health Insurance Portability and Accountability Act of 1996

The Health Insurance Portability and Accountability Act, otherwise known as HIPAA (pronounced hip pah) became law in August 1996. Included in this act was the requirement that Congress develop national medical record privacy standards by August 21, 1999. Because Congress did not meet the deadline, HIPAA then required the Department of Health and Human Services to establish and enforce

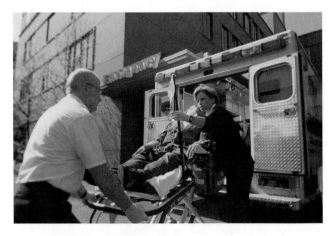

Figure 3–2. Good Samaritans who stop at the scene of an accident may be able to administer life-saving care to a patient. Seconds can count before emergency personnel arrive.

national standards for medical record privacy. The HIPAA regulations apply to all personal health care information, including oral, paper, and electronic information. Most health care organizations and insurance plans have until April 2003 to come into full compliance with HIPAA regulations. Of course, the regulations may be voluntarily complied to before that date.

The HIPAA regulations are composed of the following five basic standards:

- **Consumer Control.** Health care consumers have new rights in regard to control of their health information. These rights include an individual's right to obtain a copy of his or her medical record and the right to receive information on how a patient's private health care information is used.
- **Boundaries.** For the most part, disclosure of heath information is limited to a patient's treatment or payment for health care treatment. Employers are not allowed access to health care information that could be used for hiring and firing or to determine promotions unless the individual authorizes such access. Health care facilities may use personal health care information for patient treatment, educational purposes (teaching and conducting research), and for quality assurance. To provide the best possible medical care, physicians and other health care providers still have access to a patient's entire health record when providing treatment for a patient.
- **Accountability.** For violations of a patient's right to privacy, civil and criminal penalties may be imposed. Criminal penalties are imposed when violators knowingly disclose health care information improperly or if health care information is obtained using deceptive practices.
- **Public Responsibility.** Standards are established that allow access of information for public health purposes such as public health protection, medical research, health care improvement, and health care fraud and abuse. Examples include access to health care information for emergency circumstances, health care facility patient directories, and national security and defense activities.
- **Security.** Health care organizations have a responsibility to protect the privacy of health care information. Organizations must establish clear written procedure to protect privacy, and within the organization, a privacy officer must be designated to monitor privacy issues.

If state and federal laws conflict in regard to privacy issues, the privacy standard that is greater would pertain. Some states have more stringent laws relating to health care records such as HIV/AIDS information and mental health records.

Risk Management

To serve patients in an appropriate manner, a medical administrative assistant must be aware of the legal and ethical responsibilities that affect the medical office and its staff. This knowledge will help minimize the risk of any possible legal cases being pursued against the practice. The concept of **risk management** means minimizing the potential for legal action being taken against the practice.

Keep the following in mind to minimize the chance of litigation involving the office:

- Always remember that the patient is the reason everyone is employed in the medical office.
- Always keep the patient's best interest at the forefront of your actions.
- When assisting a patient, keep in mind how a simple action or statement may be viewed by the patient. Every action of the assistant is assumed to be done at the direction of the physician.
- Health care employees who have a good rapport with patients reduce the risk of lawsuits against the practice.
- Take immediate steps to resolve any patient conflict; notify the physician if necessary.
- Keep all medical information confidential.
- Be aware of the physical environment of the facility. Things such as wet floors, loose carpeting, malfunctioning doors, and dangling electrical cords have the potential to cause physical injury to the public.
- Report any incidents or injuries to the physician, and complete any necessary paperwork to report those events. An incident report should always be completed to document any incidents or injuries that occur in the office.

A main concept of risk management is that all employees of the medical office should be aware that the treatment or service provided for a patient should never give the patient a reason to sue. In the day-to-day operations of a medical office, tasks may become familiar, and it is sometimes easy to forget that patients of the office could potentially sue the office in the future. So the moral of the story is *never, ever give a patient cause to even consider legal action against the office.*

SUMMARY

The law has many applications in the practice of medicine. Laws governing medicine are created by legislators, case law precedent, and federal agencies designated to supervise the medical practice. If a situation would ever arise in the medical office that could have legal implications, it is extremely important for an assistant to notify the physician if there is ever a question of potential liability on the part of the medical office or staff.

Knowledge of the laws that govern medicine and awareness of potential legal troublesome areas within the clinic will help a medical administrative assistant to serve patients better and will help avoid the possibility of litigation against the medical office. All employees of the medical office can be sued and can play a role in preventing legal action. Positive patient relations and good customer service go a long way toward reducing the possibility of litigation.

Bibliography

Brent NJ: Nurses and the Law, A Guide to Principles and Applications. Philadelphia, WB Saunders, 1997.

Flight M: Law, Liability, and Ethics for Medical Office Professionals, 3rd ed. Albany, NY, Delmar, 1998.

Huffman EK: Health Information Management. Berwyn, Ill Physician's Record Company, 1994.

Judson K, Blesie S: Law and Ethics for Health Occupations, 2nd ed. New York, Glencoe McGraw-Hill, 1999.

Lewis MA, Tamparo CD: Medical Law, Ethics and Bioethics for Ambulatory Care. Philadelphia, FA Davis, 1998.

Medical Records Briefing, vol. 11, No. 8. Opus Communications, Marblehead, Mass. August 1996.

U.S. Department of Labor, Bureau of Labor Statistics: 1998–99 Occupational Outlook Handbook.

Internet Resources

Consumer Guide to Advance Directives: Group Health Cooperative of Puget Sound, September 1997.

U.S. Drug Enforcement Agency.

U.S. Food and Drug Administration.

U.S. Office of Personnel Management, Federal Employees Health Benefits FAQ.

U.S. Department of Health and Human Services.

3

REVIEW EXERCISES

Exercise 3–1 LEGAL CONCEPTS AND TERMS

Read each statement and choose the answer that best completes the statement. Record your answer in the blank provided.

_____ 1. Type of law governing the relationship of individuals.
    (a) Criminal law   (c) Statutory law
    (b) Administrative law   (d) Civil law

_____ 2. Laws established by the legislative branch of government.
    (a) Common law   (c) Statutory law
    (b) Case law   (d) Administrative law

_____ 3. Laws established by the court.
    (a) Common law   (c) Statutory law
    (b) Administrative law   (d) Criminal law

_____ 4. Legal concept establishing that evidence speaks for itself.
    (a) Advance directive   (d) Respondeat superior
    (b) Res ipsa loquitur   (e) Expressed consent
    (c) Standards of care

_____ 5. A physician who fails to properly terminate a physician-patient relationship may be liable for
    (a) Consideration   (c) Res ipsa loquitur
    (b) Abandonment   (d) Respondeat superior

_____ 6. Name of party initiating a legal action against another.
    (a) Plaintiff   (c) Statute
    (b) Defendant   (d) Mature minor

_____ 7. Federal agencies are responsible for establishing and enforcing
    (a) Administrative law   (c) Case law
    (b) Common law   (d) Criminal law

_____ 8. Health care professionals are required to perform consistent with the expectations of their profession. This is a legal concept known as
    (a) Abandonment   (c) Malpractice
    (b) Standards of care   (d) Litigation

_____ 9. The Latin phrase *respondeat superior* means
    (a) An assistant may be held liable for the actions of another staff member of the medical office.
    (b) An assistant is required to keep medical information confidential.
    (c) A physician may be liable for the actions of his or her employees in the medical office.
    (d) The evidence speaks for itself.

_____ 10. If a physician terminates care of a patient, which of the following is incorrect?
    (a) A certified letter with return receipt should be sent to the patient informing the patient of the termination of care.
    (b) The physician must provide care for a reasonable period of time.
    (c) The patient is not required to pay his or her outstanding bill.
    (d) Termination should be documented in the patient's medical chart.

_____ 11. Which of the following is not required to prove a physician's negligence?
    (a) Physician failed to provide proper care for the patient's medical condition.
    (b) Patient suffered damage or injury.
    (c) Physician's failure caused patient's injury.
    (d) Patient paid physician for medical treatment.
    (e) Physician had an obligation to provide service to the patient.

_____ 12. A legal agreement between two people that creates an obligation.
    (a) Contract   (c) Subpoena
    (b) Deposition   (d) Statute

_____ 13. Establishes a time period during which legal action must commence.
    (a) Litigation   (c) Deposition
    (b) Statute of limitations   (d) Interrogatories

_____ 14. Which of the following health information could not be released by a physician?
    (a) Information legally required to be released.
    (b) Reporting an infectious disease to a state health department.
    (c) Information about a minor's treatment for a sexually transmitted disease.
    (d) Reporting a patient who threatens to physically harm someone.

_____ 15. If an assistant is called to court as a witness, the assistant should
    (a) Offer additional information without being asked.
    (b) Cover up discrepancies in the record to protect the physician.
    (c) State "I don't know" if an answer to a question is not known.
    (d) Pretend to know everything.
    (e) Dress in jeans or other comfortable clothing because a day in court can be long.

_____ 16. Which of the following is **not** part of informed consent?
    (a) Patient is given information about his medical condition.
    (b) Patient is informed of alternative treatments for his medical condition.
    (c) Patient is told of potential benefits and risks of different treatment options.
    (d) Physician communicates in language that patient understands.
    (e) Patient is informed of costs of treatment.

_____ 17. Which of the following is **not** good risk management practice?
    (a) Develop a good rapport with patients.
    (b) Ignore upset patients and give them a chance to cool down.
    (c) Keep information confidential.
    (d) Be alert to the physical environment of the office.
    (e) Document incidents or injuries immediately

_____ 18. Which of the following is **not** true about a license to practice medicine?
    (a) Each state sets its own requirements for licensure.
    (b) A currently licensed physician may be eligible for a license in another state through a process called reciprocity.
    (c) CEUs are usually required to renew a license.
    (d) A physician involved in a malpractice suit is not allowed to practice.
    (e) The USMLE is the United States Medical Licensing Examination.

Exercise 3–2 LEGAL TERMS

In each group, match each term above with the definition below that best matches the term. Record your answer in the blank provided. Each answer is used only once.

    (a) Subpoena   (d) Living will
    (b) Subpoena duces tecum (e) Durable Power of Attorney for Health Care
    (c) Deposition

_____ 1. Testimony given outside a courtroom.

_____ 2. An advance directive specifying a patient's desired treatment if in a terminal irreversible condition.

_____ 3. An order for an individual to appear in court.

_____ 4. An advance directive giving authority to an individual to make medical decisions for an incapacitated patient.

_____ 5. An order to produce medical records for trial use.

    (a) Offer and acceptance   (c) Legal capacity
    (b) Legal subject matter   (d) Consideration

_____ 6. The act or service to be performed is lawful.

_____ 7. Individual is an adult of sound mind.

_____ 8. One party agrees to do something, and another party accepts.

_____ 9. Something of value is exchanged.

(a) Implied consent   (c) Consent

(b) Expressed consent   (d) Informed consent

_____ 10. To give approval for medical treatment.

_____ 11. Patient is given full information about medical condition, alternative treatments, and associated risks, as well as potential benefits of each treatment.

_____ 12. This consent is evidenced by the patient's actions; that is, a patient opens her mouth when the physician asks her to do so.

_____ 13. The patient either verbally or in writing communicates the desire to have medical treatment.

Exercise 3–3 TRUE OR FALSE

Read the following statements and determine whether the statements are true or false. Record the answer in the blank provided. T = true; F = false.

_____ 1. Risk management means reducing the possibility that a patient will sue the practice.

_____ 2. Establishing a good relationship with patients helps to reduce the chance of litigation in the future.

_____ 3. Everything an assistant says or does is believed to have been done at the direction of the physician.

_____ 4. If a patient is upset about services received in the office, it is best to point out to the patient why the patient is wrong.

_____ 5. If a patient is injured in the office, it should be reported to the physician immediately.

_____ 6. If a patient is injured in the office, a report should be completed to document the incident.

_____ 7. An assistant has little effect as to whether or not a patient could potentially sue a medical practice.

_____ 8. Any employee of a medical office can be sued.

_____ 9. Keeping all medical information confidential is an important risk management practice of the medical office.

_____ 10. A patient suing a physician for malpractice may be required to obtain the testimony of an expert physician who will support the plaintiff's allegations.

_____ 11. A malpractice suit against a physician may be brought at any time during the patient's life.

_____ 12. The Uniform Anatomical Gift Act regulates gifts a physician is allowed to receive from health industry corporations.

_____ 13. A physician may be sued for malpractice if he or she fails to act.

_____ 14. Punitive damages are awarded to compensate for lost wages.

_____ 15. Some states may set limits on the amount of punitive damages that may be awarded.

_____ 16. Compensatory damages and exemplary damages may both be awarded in a legal case.

_____ 17. Certification examinations are offered by a profession's national organization.

_____ 18. A wife can be a witness to her husband's advance directive.

Exercise 3–4 LEGISLATION AND ADVANCE DIRECTIVES

Read the following statements regarding the following legal topics and determine whether the statements below each topic are true or false. Record the answer in the blank provided. T = true; F = false.

Uniform Anatomical Gift Act of 1968

_____ 1. This act governs the donation of body parts.

_____ 2. An individual must donate all body parts in order to be an organ donor.

_____ 3. Relatives of a deceased individual may donate any or all of the deceased's body parts.

_____ 4. Once an individual has made the decision to be an organ donor, the decision is permanent and may not be revoked.

_____ 5. A medical school, hospital, or a specific individual in need may be a recipient of an organ donation.

Controlled Substances Act of 1970

_____ 6. This act governs the manufacture and distribution of potentially addictive substances.

_____ 7. Narcotics are regulated by the Controlled Substances Act.

_____ 8. Controlled substances under this act are classified on a scale of 1 to 10 with 10 being the most addictive.

_____ 9. Physicians must include their DEA number on a prescription when prescribing a controlled substance.

Good Samaritan Statutes

_____ 10. Less than half of the 50 states have Good Samaritan statutes.

_____ 11. Good Samaritans are free from all liability if they stop at the scene of an accident.

_____ 12. Good Samaritan statutes protect all health care professionals working in an emergency room.

_____ 13. The purpose of Good Samaritan statutes is to protect health care professionals from liability when they stop at an accident scene to render aid.

Advance Directives

_____ 14. A living will covers more possible health care situations than does a Durable Power of Attorney for Health Care.

_____ 15. More or less, advance directives communicate a patient's wishes for health care treatment before a serious medical situation may arise.

_____ 16. Advance directives help inform a patient's family members of the patient's desire for medical treatment.

_____ 17. Every patient of a medical office must have an advance directive.

_____ 18. A living will communicates a patient's wishes for life-sustaining treatment such as tube feeding or ventilator use.

_____ 19. Once a patient is comatose, a living will is null and void.

_____ 20. Copies of a patient's living will or Durable Power of Attorney for Health Care should be placed in the patient's chart.

_____ 21. A patient's relative can be a witness to the patient's advance directive.

Health Insurance Portability and Accountability Act of 1996

_____ 22. HIPAA allows physicians to have complete control over the release of a patient's medical information.

_____ 23. Knowingly releasing private medical information in an improper manner is a criminal offense.

_____ 24. A patient may obtain a copy of his or her medical record.

_____ 25. When hiring an individual, an employer may access the individual's entire medical record.

ACTIVITIES

ACTIVITY 3–1   Research cases involving medical practice in your state. Many state sites have links to the state's judicial system. Find at least four cases involving medical practice, and briefly summarize each case and identify the decision of the court.

ACTIVITY 3–2   Find examples of a living will and a Durable Power of Attorney for Health Care. To find an actual form for an advance directive, search for *advance directive form* using a common Internet search tool. For information on advance directives, the American Association of Retired Persons and the American Bar Association Commission on Legal Problems of the Elderly have general information on advance directives.

ACTIVITY 3–3   Investigate the state health department of your state. What diseases or medical occurrences are reportable in your state?

ACTIVITY 3–4   Research medical malpractice on the Internet. Can you find the answers to the following questions?

1. Which professions have the greatest incidence of malpractice involvement?
2. What places a particular specialty at more risk for malpractice litigation?
3. How many physicians are sued for malpractice each year?
4. What are a physician's chances of being accused of malpractice at some point during his or her career?

ACTIVITY 3–5   Visit a courtroom and observe a trial in progress.

ACTIVITY 3–6   Research the medical practice act and the State Board of Medical Examiners in your state.

3

DISCUSSION

The following topics can be used for class discussion or for individual student essay.

DISCUSSION 3–1   Explain why a health care provider cannot guarantee medical treatment.

DISCUSSION 3–2   Explain how a medical administrative assistant can help reduce the chances of litigation involving the medical office.

DISCUSSION 3–3   Read the quotation at the beginning of this chapter. How does this quotation apply to a medical administrative assistant?

DISCUSSION 3–4   Discuss the following statement in the chapter: "Technological advances in medicine make it necessary to enact laws to protect society."

DISCUSSION 3–5   Discuss the importance to a patient of each section of the Health Insurance Portability and Accountability Act of 1996. For additional information, consult the U.S. Department of Health & Human Services Web site.

CHAPTER OUTLINE

LEARNING OUTCOMES

*On successful completion of this chapter the student
will be able to*

1. Define ethics and differentiate law and ethics.
2. Describe the Hippocratic Oath.
3. Identify ethical behavior of physicians.
4. Identify ethical behavior of medical assistants.
5. Describe confidentiality and protection of confidentiality.
6. Describe common ethical issues in health care.
7. Identify an assistant's appropriate responses to
ethical dilemmas in health care.

CMA COMPETENCIES

1. Identify and respond to issues of confidentiality.
2. Perform within legal and ethical boundaries.

RMA COMPETENCIES

1. Know the principles of medical ethics established by the American Medical Association.
2. Define terminology associated with medical
ethics.
3. Identify the ethical response for the various
situations in a medical facility.
4. Recognize unethical practices.

VOCABULARY

abortion
confidentiality
ethics
euthanasia
medical ethics

MEDICAL ETHICS

The moral test of government is how it treats those who are in the dawn of life—the children; those who are in the twilight of life—the aged; and those who are in the shadows of life—the sick, the needy and the handicapped.

—Hubert H. Humphrey

Patients receiving medical care and providers giving medical care are often faced with ethical dilemmas. An understanding of the ethical matters that patients and their providers face helps medical administrative assistants have empathy for patients as well as an understanding of the complicated medical decisions that face patients and their providers. An understanding of these issues allows an assistant to provide patients with the best possible service.

DEFINITION OF ETHICS

What exactly are ethics? According to the *Miller-Keane Encyclopedia & Dictionary of Medicine, Nursing, & Allied Health,* **ethics** are "rules or principles which govern right conduct," and **medical ethics** are "the values and guidelines governing decisions in medical practice."

But because this definition includes the word *right,* it is difficult to definitively define behavior as right or wrong, ethical or unethical. What is deemed to be right or wrong can vary among different groups in society. Even within the medical field, each patient and treatment situation is unique, and, therefore, what may be right in one situation may not be right in another.

LAW VERSUS ETHICS

In Chapter 3, we learned that laws are societal rules or principles established by various branches of government. Ethics are also rules or principles, but they are rules or principles that define right conduct. Again, because people have different perceptions of what is right and wrong, it is sometimes very difficult to determine what is ethical behavior. Although laws and ethics are both rules, laws establish a minimum expectation of behavior. Typically, if someone violates the law, fine or incarceration, or both, may result. Ethics, on the other hand, are often inspired by law but establish a much higher standard of behavior. Professional organizations desiring to promote high-quality behavioral standards among their members typically have a code of ethics for their members. Members deviating from the ethical standards established by an organization will usually find themselves stripped of membership rights.

HISTORY OF ETHICS

The topic of medical ethics is not a new one. Some early discussions of medical ethics occurred as long ago as 400 BC, when Hippocrates, the father of medicine, wrote the Hippocratic Oath (Fig. 4–1), to which today's physicians still pledge.

HIPPOCRATIC OATH

I swear by Apollo the physician, by Aesculapius, Hygeia, and Panacea, and I take to witness all the gods, all the goddesses, to keep according to my ability and my judgment the following oath:

To consider dear to me as my parents him who taught me this art; to live in common with him and if necessary to share my goods with him; to look upon his children as my own brothers, to teach them this art if they so desire without fee or written promise; to impart to my sons and the sons of the master who taught me and the disciples who have enrolled themselves and have agreed to the rules of the profession, by to these alone, the precepts and the instruction.

I will prescribe regimen for the good of my patients according to my ability and my judgment and never do harm to anyone. To please no one will I prescribe a deadly drug, nor give advice which may cause his death. Nor will I give a woman a pessary to procure abortion.

But I will preserve the purity of my life and my art. I will not cut for stone, even for patients in whom the disease is manifest; I will leave this operation to be performed by practitioners (specialists in this art). In every house where I come I will enter only for the good of my patients, keeping myself far from all intentional ill-doing and all seduction, and especially from the pleasures of love with women or with men, be they free or slaves.

All that may come to my knowledge in the exercise of my profession or outside of my profession or in daily commerce with men, which ought not to be spread abroad, I will keep secret and will never reveal.

If I keep this oath faithfully, may I enjoy my life and practice my art, respected by all men and in all times; but if I swerve from it or violate it, may the reverse be my lot.

Figure 4–1. Hippocratic Oath.

Hippocrates was a Greek philosopher who had tremendous insight (even at that early time) into the practice of medicine. He did much to influence the practice of medicine. In examining the Hippocratic Oath, the following influences on modern-day medicine are seen:

- Physicians will share their knowledge of the medical profession with others.
- Physicians will not provide advice or drugs to any patient that may cause that patient's death.
- Physicians will not provide a device that accomplishes an abortion.
- When appropriate, physicians will refer patients to a specialist.
- Physicians will practice for the good of their patients.
- Patients' medical information that comes to physicians in the practice of medicine will be held confidential.

The Hippocratic Oath is an ethical code of conduct giving physicians a guide for what is "correct" professional behavior. Although the Oath is not law, it is often used to judge the behavior of physicians.

CHECKPOINT

Physicians often provide treatment at no cost to their fellow physicians and their families. Is this in keeping with the Hippocratic Oath?

ETHICAL BEHAVIOR FOR PHYSICIANS

The American Medical Association (AMA), founded in 1847, is a professional organization for physicians dedicated to excellence in the practice of medicine. The AMA membership establishes policies that influence and further the practice of medicine in the United States. The AMA and its membership continually work to promote high quality standards in health care delivery and to significantly influence the development of health law in the United States.

The AMA has developed a list of general principles regarding medical ethics. The AMA Principles of Medical Ethics (Fig. 4–2) were developed with the patient as the primary focus in the patient-physician relationship. These statements are not laws but are standards of ethical conduct expected of AMA members. If a physician deviates from these ethical standards, he or she may likely become involved in civil litigation initiated by a dissatisfied patient and the physician may risk losing membership rights with the AMA, as well.

American Medical Association Council on Ethical and Judicial Affairs

The AMA's Council on Ethical and Judicial Affairs (CEJA) establishes the organization's position on ethical behavior of

Figure 4–2. American Medical Association Principles of Medical Ethics. (From Code of Medical Ethics. Current Opinions with Annotations of the Council on Ethical and Judicial Affairs of the American Medical Association. Copyright 1997, American Medical Association.)

AMERICAN MEDICAL ASSOCIATION

Principles of Medical Ethics

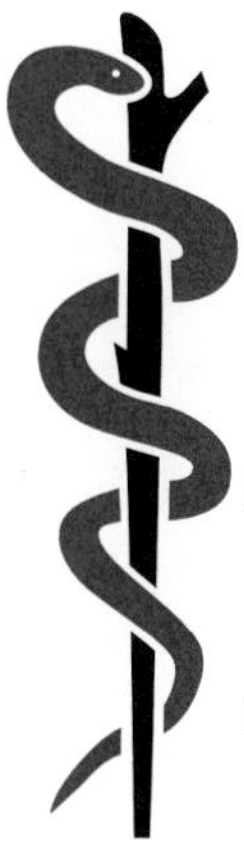

I. A physician shall be dedicated to providing competent medical service with compassion and respect for human dignity.

II. A physician shall deal honestly with patients and colleagues, and strive to expose those physicians deficient in character or competence, or who engage in fraud or deception.

III. A physician shall respect the law and also recognize a responsibility to seek changes in those requirements which are contrary to the best interest of the patient.

IV. A physician shall respect the rights of patients, of colleagues, and of other health professionals and shall safeguard patient confidences within the constraints of the law.

V. A physician shall continue to study, apply and advance scientific knowledge; make relevant information available to patients, colleagues and the public; obtain consultation; and use the talents of other health professionals when indicated.

VI. A physician shall, in the provision of appropriate patient care, except in emergencies, be free to choose whom to serve, with whom to associate, and the environment in which to provide medical services.

VII. A physician shall recognize a responsibility to participate in activities contributing to an improved community.

physicians. The Council develops positions on ethical matters involving physicians and comments on judicial matters that involve or influence the practice of medicine. These positions are known as opinions and are periodically reviewed and updated to reflect changes in the patient-physician relationship and the delivery of health care. They are meant to serve as a guide for appropriate physician conduct.

Current Opinions of the Council on Ethical and Judicial Affairs

The Current Opinions of the AMA's Council on Ethical and Judicial Affairs describe in more detail what is appropriate behavior for a physician. Topics such as social issues and medical practice issues are addressed in the Current Opinions. Even though the Current Opinions are quite detailed, they still cannot individually address every potential situation that may arise in the practice of medicine. Remember, each treatment experience with a patient is unique, and no two situations are exactly the same. Therefore, the Current Opinions are meant to serve as a guide for all physicians in the practice of medicine. A general explanation of some of the Council's Current Opinions is listed in Box 4–1, and a complete listing of the Opinions can be found in the ethics section of the AMA Web site.

Failure to Abide by Ethical Standards

Because the AMA is an organization of discretionary membership, it may choose who may be a member of the organization and who may not. Members who may have violated ethical standards will probably be reviewed by the AMA. After due notice and a hearing, members in violation of the AMA's standards may be censured, suspended, or expelled from the organization's membership.

In addition, physicians involved in legal proceedings may find themselves in a disciplinary hearing with the AMA on conclusion of the proceedings. A physician may even be acquitted in a civil or criminal proceeding, yet he or she may still face discipline by the AMA. Even though a physician has been acquitted in a legal proceeding, the physician may lose membership rights in the AMA.

Checkpoint

Examine the following examples of conduct, decide whether the conduct is in keeping with the information given about the AMA Principles of Medical Ethics, and state the reason for your answer.

1. Dr. Gonzalez is an obstetrician practicing in a large metropolitan city. Dr. Gonzalez has decided that she will not accept any new obstetrics patients in her practice.
2. Dr. Smith is an internist practicing in a state that has a law against physician-assisted suicide. Dr. Smith believes patients should have the right to choose physician-

assisted suicide if they are terminally ill, so he helps a patient commit suicide.
3. Dr. Anderson is aware of a physician in her health care facility that often bills Medicare for services that have not been performed. She does not report the physician's activity to the board of directors or to Medicare officials.
4. Dr. Kowalski has developed a new technique for suturing operative wounds. He demonstrates this new technique to colleagues at the AMA's national convention.

ETHICAL BEHAVIOR FOR MEDICAL ADMINISTRATIVE ASSISTANTS

The code of ethics developed by the American Association of Medical Assistants (AAMA) (see Fig. 1–4) serves as a guide for moral and ethical conduct for individuals employed in the medical assisting profession. These ethical standards have been developed to help medical assistants determine appropriate professional behavior in the health care workplace. Although a widely accepted ethics code is not available for medical administrative assistants, the AAMA's code of ethics can serve as a guide for ethical behavior.

Whether or not a code of ethics exists for a particular group of employees, any employee of a health care facility is expected to perform his or her duties in a professional manner and, above all, should keep all patient information confidential.

Checkpoint

A medical administrative assistant is confronted daily with situations to which she or he must decide how to respond. The AAMA's code of medical ethics provides a framework for the assistant to determine appropriate behavior. Consider the following instances and determine whether or not the assistant's behavior is in keeping with the code of ethics.

1. An assistant volunteers for a local nonprofit health care organization.
2. An assistant attends additional training to upgrade job skills.
3. An assistant unnecessarily discusses a patient's medical condition with a fellow employee.

CONFIDENTIALITY

All information regarding a patient's medical treatment is considered confidential information. **Confidentiality** in the medical office setting means that the information is to be kept secret or private and that patient information is to be kept among those providing care for the patient and may not be divulged to anyone else without the permission of the patient. Assistants must keep everything confidential that they see, hear, and do in the office.

Box 4–1 Summary of Several Current Opinions of the Council on Ethical and Judicial Affairs

- A physician's first concern should be the quality of care for the patient.
- A physician is allowed to participate in legal abortions.
- A physician should report instances of child, spousal, or elder abuse.
- A physician may not participate in a legally authorized execution.
- A physician may participate in research, provided the study has met acceptable standards of scientific research.
- A physician should not disclose genetic testing results to insurance companies. Such information may preclude a patient from obtaining insurance (if the patient is identified as being predisposed to a certain disease) and should be kept apart from the patient's medical record so it could not be accidentally included in a release of medical information.
- In the organ donation process, members of the deceased's or donor's health care team cannot participate as a member of the transplant team. These team members must be free from conflict of interest.
- In treating patients who are terminally ill or seriously debilitated, the best interest of the patient is of utmost importance, not the burden of the patient's condition on family members or society.
- A physician is dedicated to preserving life and easing patients' suffering. When these two are not compatible, the wishes of the patient are of primary importance. Participation in euthanasia conflicts with the position of the physician to "never to do harm to anyone" (as identified in the Hippocratic Oath, see Fig. 4–1).
- A physician may advertise his or her medical practice, but such advertisement should not be deceptive or misleading.
- A physician may not talk to the media about a patient without the consent of the patient. The physician may only release authorized information. Questions about violent acts should be referred to law enforcement authorities.
- A physician shall keep patient information confidential. It may be necessary for the physician to disclose confidential information if in the best interest of society. If a patient threatens to harm himself or herself or another individual or is a threat to society, the physician has a duty to warn the individual who is threatened and the appropriate authorities.

- A physician may treat a minor patient without parental consent unless the law forbids it. The physician should encourage the minor to discuss the nature of medical care with parents.
- A physician may not collect a fee for referring patients to another physician. A physician also may not collect any type of fee or compensation from health care suppliers for prescribing their products.
- A physician should never place his or her own financial interest above a patient's best interest. Financial interest in a company should not influence a physician's decision making.
- A physician should send a patient for consultation when medically necessary or when the patient requests it.
- A physician has a right to choose whether or not to accept an individual as a patient except in cases of emergency. A physician may not refuse to accept patients because of their race, national origin, or religion.
- A physician should not engage in a romantic or sexual relationship with a patient.
- A physician should not practice medicine while under the influence of a substance that could impair the physician's medical judgment.
- A physician should not treat himself or herself or family members except in an emergency situation.
- A physician has a duty to report colleagues who are incompetent or impaired in the practice of medicine or who engage in unethical behavior.
- A physician should report incidents in which he or she believes the use of a drug or device may be harmful.
- A physician has a duty to provide necessary health care for the poor and unfortunate.
- A physician should share his or her knowledge to advance the practice of medicine. Physicians are allowed to patent medical devices that they develop, but they are not allowed to patent medical procedures.
- A physician with an infectious disease should not put his or her patient at risk of transmission of the disease.

From American Medical Association: Current Opinions of the Council on Ethical and Judicial Affairs.

Even though federal regulations pertaining to confidentiality of health information do not take effect until April 2003, it is still expected that an assistant keep all health care information confidential. Whether or not confidentiality is legally mandated, it is ethically mandated.

Confidentiality Agreements

Every health care professional should be required to sign a confidentiality agreement (Fig. 4–3). These agreements are signed by employees at the beginning of employment and should be signed at every employment anniversary. Even those volunteering at a health care facility should be required to sign a confidentiality agreement. When signed, such an agreement acknowledges the assistant's understanding of the facility's policy regarding confidentiality of health information. After signing, the agreement should be placed in the employee's file in the human resources office.

The importance of protecting patient confidentiality cannot be stressed enough. In the course of business in a medical office, an assistant and all other employees are frequently required to deal with sensitive, personal information

**Horizons Healthcare Center
Confidentiality Agreement**

All information regarding patients and their health care that is acquired during the course of employment at Horizons Healthcare Center shall be considered confidential.

Confidential information must never be disclosed for non-employment related purposes. Disclosure of confidential information outside of an employee's assigned duties will constitute unauthorized release of confidential information and can be grounds for dismissal.

By signing this document, I acknowledge that I understand this statement.

SAMPLE

_____   _____
Employee name   Date

_____   _____
Witness name   Date

Figure 4–3. Sample of a confidentiality agreement.

about a patient's health care treatment. A patient's right to complete confidentiality must be protected. An assistant who does not respect confidentiality of medical information will be out of a job.

Release of Confidential Information

From time to time, it becomes necessary to release information regarding a patient's medical care to a third party. In most cases, a patient's medical information should be released only with the patient's written consent. It is inappropriate and unethical to release any information regarding a patient's health care treatment or services without that consent. There are a few exceptions to this as referenced in Chapters 3 and 9, but it is generally held that each patient owns the right to decide who may have access to his or her medical record. Release of information from a patient's medical record is discussed in greater detail in Chapter 9, Health Information Management.

Protecting Patient Confidentiality

In a medical office, an assistant must be aware of several possible locations in which health care confidentiality may be breached. Several precautions can be taken to guard against the possibility of a confidentiality breach in a typical medical office setting.

Photocopiers. Various types of documents are copied in the medical office: a patient's medical record for release, an insurance claim form, or an appointment schedule. Sometimes, after making a copy, originals are inadvertently left in the copier (Fig. 4–4). When making copies, an assistant should double-check the area around the copier to be sure no items are left. If copies are made in error, they should be disposed of properly.

Information Disposal. Anything that has a patient's name, chart number, or any other identifying piece of information could bring about a breach in confidentiality. Carbon copies of laboratory slips, copies of the appointment schedule, photocopies made in error, and anything else with identifying information on it could identify a patient, the procedure he or she had undergone, or the patient's diagnosis. A patient's name on a slip of paper may seem harmless, but imagine the personal implications for the patient if the slip of paper had a health care facility name, such as *Valley Mental Health Clinic.*

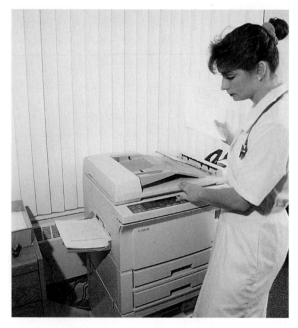

Figure 4–4. An assistant must be careful to remove all medical documents from a copier after photocopies have been made. (From Chester GA: Modern Medical Assisting, Philadelphia, WB Saunders, 1999.)

Anything with information that identifies a patient (e.g., name, chart number, phone number, address) must be destroyed. It is not enough to throw the information away—the information must be destroyed so that it cannot be read. A shredder is an easy way to be sure that information is destroyed before it leaves the clinic. Some offices may choose to incinerate their disposable paper, but the paper usually must be transported by an outside company to an outside facility for incineration. If an office decides to use such an outside company, a confidentiality agreement should be signed with the company as an added safeguard.

If a shredder is used, it should be placed in an area of the office where it is not seen by patients. A patient who sees an assistant shredding documents may get the wrong idea about the use of the shredder and may believe that vital information is being shredded. The shredder is used solely for the purpose of destroying sensitive medical documents that are no longer needed.

Computer Equipment. The arrival of the information age has brought some new concerns about safeguarding information stored in a computer system. There are several problem areas when a computer is used in a medical office.

If a computer system includes all of the basic office tasks, such as billing, appointment scheduling, registration, and medical records, access to different areas of the system is usually restricted. Employees should be given access only to those parts of the system they will need to accomplish their job duties.

For example, in a large clinic with several different departments, an assistant working in the billing and insurance area would probably not need access to the appointment scheduling portion of the system. An assistant working in patient registration would have access to the registration and appointments section of the system but not to the billing portion. Physicians should have access to everything within the system.

Every computer system should be password protected. Every employee should be required to log on with a unique employee identification and should use a password that only he or she knows. Using the employee identification, a computerized system then tracks all of the areas the employee visits and what is accessed. If a confidentiality breach occurs, a system log helps identify where the breach might have occurred. In a password-protected system, each user should change his or her password frequently to help avoid any security breaches. At no time should an assistant allow his or her identification and password to be used by anyone else.

Computer systems that are networked and contain sensitive areas should be protected from outside computer hackers. Hackers intentionally try to "break in" to computer systems to gain sensitive information or to destroy information contained in the system.

Computer screens should be pointed away from areas where the public could view the screen, and screen savers should be used to cover up the screen if information is left on it. Screen savers should be activated shortly after the computer becomes idle.

Printers are used to produce appointment schedules, patient statements, insurance forms, and other office documents. They should be located in a secure area that is consistently monitored by the office staff. Print jobs should be stopped while the assistant is away from the printer area.

Telephones. Everyone in the medical office should be aware of telephone conversations near public areas. Staff members at the nurses' station or front desk might be within earshot of the public. Confidential information should never be given when it may be overheard by the public. Additional information regarding telephone and fax machine confidentiality is addressed in Chapter 6, Interpersonal Communications.

Elevators and Hallways. Sometimes, staff members become "too comfortable" with patient information and may discuss a patient's treatment while in a public area of the clinic. A patient's medical information should never be discussed in such settings. Staff members should be very careful not to use patients' names when in public areas. Another person in the elevator or hallway may know the patient. A breach of confidentiality such as this would probably result in dismissal of the staff member who divulged the information.

ETHICAL ISSUES IN HEALTH CARE

Ethical dilemmas regarding health care treatment, procedures, and related scientific research are often in the news. One can hardly pick up a newspaper or turn on the television without seeing an item involving medical ethics. Because health care is a multibillion dollar business and touches so many lives, hardly a day goes by without the media informing us of a new medical breakthrough (Fig. 4–5). Technologic advances in medicine often provoke society's discussion of proposed limits or boundaries for medical science. Technology has enabled such advances as the ability to further sustain life (e.g., organ transplants, synthetic body components) and create life (e.g., in vitro fertilization, artificial insemination). Such rapid advances are the basis of many ethical dilemmas in the health care field because as technology advances, the legal and ethical boundaries that define the practice of medicine must address those technologic changes.

The Study of Ethical Issues in Health Care

When studying medical ethics and when encountering ethical issues in medicine it is important to remember that no two persons have exactly the same views on what is ethical or "right" behavior. Although many people would agree that basic principles such as cheating, lying, and stealing are wrong, individuals differ in their definitions of the terms.

Consider the following example:

A patient phones the office and asks to speak to the doctor. The doctor has instructed the assistant to take messages for all calls unless the call is a potential emergency. If the assistant replies that the doctor is with a patient, and the doctor is not with a patient, is that a lie? Some people may believe so and

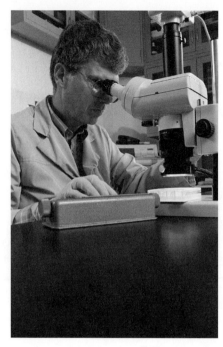

Figure 4–5. Technologic advances frequently push the ethical boundaries of medicine.

reply instead, "I'll need to take your name and number and pull your chart. The doctor or nurse will call you back after they have your chart." Some people may have no problem saying "The doctor is with a patient" regardless of whether or not the physician is with a patient. What is considered ethical behavior for one person may not be ethical behavior for another.

A medical administrative assistant is confronted daily with patients who are coping with ethical issues. It is important for an assistant to recognize and understand the ethical issues that patients face and to respect each patient's decision without bias. An assistant must have this understanding in order to provide optimal service for patients and to treat all patients with dignity and respect.

What follows is a glimpse into some of the ethical issues in health care today.

Abortion

Abortion is defined in the *Miller-Keane Encyclopedia & Dictionary of Medicine, Nursing, & Allied Health* as the "termination of pregnancy before the fetus is viable." *Viable* means *able to sustain life.* Oftentimes, when a person hears the term *abortion,* an image is produced of a willful procedure to remove a fetus from the womb. In the health care setting, the term *abortion* may be used to identify the aforementioned procedure (induced abortion), but abortion is also used to describe the miscarriage of a fetus (spontaneous abortion).

The ethical dilemma lies with induced abortion. The United States Supreme Court has provided for the intentional termination of pregnancy with the 1973 landmark decision in the case of *Roe v. Wade.* In this case, the Supreme Court's ruling essentially declared that many state

laws regarding abortion were unconstitutional. The Supreme Court defined the parameters for abortion as follows:

- During the first trimester, the abortion decision is between the mother and her physician.
- During the second trimester, the state may regulate abortion if the regulation is in the interest of the mother's health.
- Once the fetus is viable, the state may regulate or prohibit abortion except when abortion is necessary to protect the mother's health or life.

Although the judicial system provided women with the right to seek an abortion, an executive order issued by the Reagan administration and upheld by the George H.W. Bush administration said that federal funds could not be used for abortion counseling or to provide abortions. When President Clinton entered office in 1993, he removed the Reagan administration's executive order banning abortion counseling at federally funded clinics.

Abortion is not merely a legal problem. Technologic advances are enabling a fetus to survive outside the womb at 26 weeks' gestation or with a weight of just 1 pound. Whereas a fetus delivered 20 years ago weighing 1 pound had no chance of survival, medical miracles are now providing chances for life in such situations.

The major crux of the ethical dilemma with regard to abortion is the status of the fetus developing in the womb. Pro-life groups argue that a developing fetus has the rights of a person and should be regarded as such from the moment of conception. Pro-choice groups say that a woman has the right to choose what to do with her body. Another part of public opinion lies in the area between pro-life and pro-choice: the belief that the right to abortion should be determined according to the circumstances of the pregnancy; that is, abortion should be allowed in cases of pregnancy due to rape or incest but otherwise should not be allowed.

Although there are legal provisions for abortions, physicians and their employees cannot be forced to participate in abortions if they do not wish to participate.

Many people may think that the abortion issue has come to the forefront because advances in medical technology have made abortion possible. In actuality, the history of abortion reveals that abortion was a means of birth control in ancient times. In the early 1800s, there were no laws against abortion in the United States. In 1821, Connecticut passed the first law against abortion. By 1900, almost every state had laws against abortion. From the first part of the 1900s until the *Roe v. Wade* decision in 1973, women obtained illegal abortions. Thus, whether or not abortion was legal, women continued to have abortions.

The issue of abortion is therefore not new but is certainly controversial. It is important for medical administrative assistants to remember that it is not the assistant's place to judge. Instead, it is the assistant's place (1) to understand the law as it applies to abortion, (2) to understand the ethical viewpoints that may influence a patient's decision to seek or not to seek abortion, and (3) to understand that the choice of abortion is the patient's decision to make.

CHECKPOINT

Consider the following case and determine the appropriate action that you as a medical administrative assistant should take:

Sue Adams, an unmarried pregnant patient of the office, cannot decide whether or not she should have an abortion. Sue asks Dr. Johnson what she thinks should be done. How would Dr. Johnson reply?

Reproductive Rights

Reproductive capabilities have been greatly influenced by advances in medical technology. Such topics as artificial insemination, in vitro fertilization, amniocentesis, and surrogacy often spark debate as to what lengths women and men should be allowed to go to have a child.

Artificial Insemination. Artificial insemination involves injecting either the husband's sperm or donated sperm into a woman's vagina, cervical canal, or uterus with the hope of that process resulting in a pregnancy that otherwise would not be possible.

Many questions arise with this reproductive issue. Should any woman be allowed to have a child using artificial insemination? Some people may argue that the possibility of pregnancy should be left to a higher being and disagree with any interference from medicine. Others may want to put "conditions" on the procedure. They may want only women who are married to be eligible to receive insemination.

How well are donors screened and their identity protected? Should a sperm clinic set a maximum number of successful pregnancies with each donor? Many clinics do set a maximum number of times a donor is used for successful pregnancies. Imagine the problems that could occur if unlimited donation were allowed. One male donor might technically father hundreds of children.

Amniocentesis. Amniocentesis is a surgical procedure in which a needle is inserted into the amniotic sac and a sample of amniotic fluid is withdrawn. Tests can be conducted on that fluid to determine whether the developing fetus has certain abnormalities, such as Down's syndrome. This type of testing is routinely performed in pregnant women 35 years and older. Amniocentesis can also reveal the sex of the fetus. Should amniocentesis be required of all pregnant women 35 years and older? Do the benefits of this procedure outweigh the risks associated with it? If a woman undergoes amniocentesis or any other type of testing during pregnancy and the testing reveals what doctors believe to be a serious abnormality, should the woman be forced to abort or deliver the fetus prematurely? So far, courts have generally held that a woman of sound mind cannot be forced to undergo medical treatment against her will.

In vitro Fertilization. In vitro fertilization involves fertilizing an ovum in a test tube or Petri dish. The fertilized embryo is then implanted in the woman's uterus with the hope that the process will result in a full-term pregnancy.

It has been many years since the first test tube pregnancy occurred, and in vitro fertilization is becoming quite commonplace in treating infertility. Yet ethical issues relating to this method still arise. Should a woman be implanted with more than one embryo at a time to ensure a successful pregnancy? What if five embryos are implanted and all are successful? Should abortion procedures be used to eliminate some of the successful embryos to give the others a better chance at survival? What happens to frozen embryos that are no longer wanted?

Surrogate Motherhood. Many couples around the world today are infertile. Some of these couples for one reason or another choose not to adopt a child. With the advent of in vitro fertilization came the possibility of one woman carrying another woman's child. Such a possibility is called *surrogacy*. A woman can serve as a surrogate mother in one of two ways.

1. A husband and wife unable to have children because of the wife's infertility may ask another woman (a surrogate) to be artificially inseminated with the husband's sperm. The child is then half biologically related to the couple. On delivery of the infant, the surrogate gives the infant to the couple.

2. A woman unable to conceive or carry a child to term because of a uterine abnormality may first have her egg fertilized with her husband's sperm by means of the process of in vitro fertilization and then have the fertilized embryo implanted in a surrogate. The fetus is in no way biologically related to the surrogate in this case. On delivery of the infant, the infant is given to the biologic parents.

Although no one can buy or sell another human being in the United States, a fee is usually given to the surrogate in exchange for expenses and for providing a service. Should a woman be allowed to literally "rent" her uterus for a pregnancy? How are surrogate mothers screened? What happens if the surrogate decides she cannot give up the baby once it is delivered? The courts have seen many cases relating to the question of custody of a surrogate child.

It is plain to see that many questions arise when dealing with reproductive issues in medicine. Many patients will go to great lengths to conceive a child or to become parents. When serving patients in the medical office, medical assistants should be mindful of the emotional struggles that patients endure with regard to reproductive issues. Many questions frequently weigh heavily on the minds of both patients and their providers as they face these ethical dilemmas. In most instances, there is no "right" answer to many of these questions.

Issues Near the End of Life

Just as the question "When does life begin?" can create an ethical dilemma, so can the question "When does life end?" Does life end when the brain function ceases, or does it end when the heart stops beating?

The Patient Self Determination Act of 1992 made it necessary for every patient to be asked on admission to a hospital or nursing facility whether he or she has an advance directive or wants to have one. As mentioned in Chapter 3, an advance directive is a legal document that allows a patient's wishes for medical treatment to be known in the event the patient cannot speak for himself or herself.

In a way, an advance directive allows a patient to communicate what he or she feels is a "quality of life." For example, when a patient states he does not wish to have tube feeding, he is communicating that if he should be ill and would require tube feeding in order to survive, then—for him—it would not be worth surviving.

Sometimes, when faced with the end of life, a patient's choice may be to end his or her life. This choice, known as **euthanasia** may be either passive or active. Active euthanasia involves actually taking an action that will cause someone's death. With passive euthanasia, the "right to die" is present. Sometimes, a patient may refuse life-preserving medical treatment for an incurable, terminal disease. Such action is described as passive euthanasia. With passive euthanasia, a patient might be described as "losing the will to live."

Assisted suicide is different from active euthanasia in that assisted suicide involves one individual helping another individual to commit suicide. The first individual does not actually inject a lethal dose or place a mask over the other's face but gives instructions to the individual on how to accomplish the intended task. In the late 20th century, many cases of assisted suicide made headlines in the United States. Generally, courts have held that it is unlawful to assist an individual in committing suicide, although two states, Washington and Oregon, have given legislative support for assisted suicide.

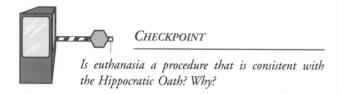

CHECKPOINT

Is euthanasia a procedure that is consistent with the Hippocratic Oath? Why?

AIDS, HIV

One of the leading health care headlines in the last part of the 20th century was the proliferation of the human immunodeficiency virus (HIV), which can lead to acquired immunodeficiency syndrome (AIDS).

Because an HIV infection has such serious implications for those infected, health care facilities must take special precautions to safeguard the privacy of patients with HIV. When an HIV blood test is done, a patient should be asked to sign a consent form indicating that he or she is giving informed consent to have the test. Patients should be counseled as to the implications of negative and positive results of the test and need to be aware of the mandatory requirement to report a positive result.

The social stigma faced by patients with HIV and AIDS is significant. Some individuals choose to label HIV-positive patients and may think that how the patient contracted the disease is important. There is not a "good" or "bad" way to contract the disease, just as there are no "good" or "bad" patients

with HIV. How a patient contracted the disease is irrelevant and does not change the fact that he or she has the disease. A positive diagnosis of HIV is usually devastating to a patient. Patients fear the loss of their jobs, their loved ones, and their life.

Ethical standards in health care demand that we treat all patients with compassion and that we do not discriminate because of a patient's circumstances. Serving a patient with HIV is no different from serving any other patient.

SUMMARY

During a typical workday, a medical administrative assistant deals with office situations that may involve a medical ethical issue. All members of the health care staff must exhibit ethical conduct at all times. When dealing with any issue in a health care setting, such conduct is expected in all situations that may arise.

When faced with a medical decision, patients bring with them their own, unique set of experiences and circumstances that have an impact on the decisions they make. Whatever a patient may decide with regard to his or her health care treatment, it is of the utmost importance for every health care professional to remember that, ultimately, the patient must decide for himself or herself what the treatment will be. After all, it is the patient who must live (or possibly die) with the decision.

YOU ARE THE MEDICAL ADMINISTRATIVE ASSISTANT

1. Julie Smith, a 16-year-old pregnant patient, has been a regular patient for years at your clinic. Her family members are regular patients of your clinic, as well. Julie is very tearful today and approaches you at the reception desk. She confides in you that she is pregnant and does not know what to do. She asks you for the name and number of the local abortion clinic in your city. (You know the name and number of the abortion clinic.) What do you do?
2. You just finished filing laboratory reports in patients' records. Among the reports was a pregnancy test for your best friend who has long hoped for a child. The results are positive. The nurse has notified your best friend of the results. You are having dinner with your friend this evening. What do you say?

Bibliography

Brent NJ: Nurses and the Law: A Guide to Principles and Applications. Philadelphia, WB Saunders, 1997.

Huffman EK: Health Information Management. Berwyn, Ill, Physician's Record, 1994.

Lewis MA, Tamparo CD: Medical Law, Ethics and Bioethics in the Medical Office, 3rd ed. Philadelphia, FA Davis, 1993, p 253.

O'Toole M: Miller-Keane Encyclopedia & Dictionary of Medicine, Nursing, & Allied Health, 6th ed. Philadelphia, WB Saunders, 1997.

Purtillo R: Ethical Dimensions in the Health Professions. Philadelphia, WB Saunders, 1993, p 162.

Exercise 4-1 TRUE OR FALSE

Read the following statements and determine whether the statements are true or false. Record the answer in the blank provided. T = true; F = false.

_____ 1. The Hippocratic Oath is a legal doctrine that must be adhered to by all physicians.

_____ 2. When a professional organization has a code of ethics, it is easy to determine whether a particular behavior is ethical or unethical.

_____ 3. The Hippocratic Oath still influences medicine today.

_____ 4. The Hippocratic Oath supports physician-assisted suicide.

_____ 5. The Hippocratic Oath supports abortion.

_____ 6. In the United States, abortion had not been legal until 1973.

_____ 7. A miscarriage is also known as an induced abortion.

_____ 8. An organization's code of ethics serves as a guideline for professional behavior.

_____ 9. The AMA establishes law that governs the practice of medicine.

_____ 10. There are no state laws protecting the confidentiality of patient's medical information.

_____ 11. Health care employees are usually required to sign a confidentiality agreement with their employer.

_____ 12. Volunteers at a health care facility should be required to sign a confidentiality agreement with the facility.

_____ 13. Oral consent of the patient is usually sufficient for release of his or her medical information.

_____ 14. A paper shredder should be placed in a visible area so that patients can see that medical information is destroyed before being thrown away.

_____ 15. A computer system in a medical office can track what parts of the system have been accessed by each user.

_____ 16. To protect confidential information on a computer system, access can be restricted for users.

Exercise 4-2 ETHICAL CONDUCT OF MEDICAL ADMINISTRATIVE ASSISTANTS

Read each of the following examples involving medical administrative assistant conduct. Using the AAMA code of ethics (see Fig. 1-4) as a guide for ethical conduct, determine whether the conduct is ethical or unethical. Record the answer in the blank provided. E = ethical; U = unethical.

_____ 1. Shredding copies of a patient's insurance form that are not needed.

_____ 2. Postponing handling records requests for patients who do not speak English until all other requests have been handled.

_____ 3. Volunteering at a blood drive in the community.

_____ 4. After seeing test results, informing a friend of another friend's serious illness.

_____ 5. Sending medical records to a patient's employer without the patient's consent.

_____ 6. Conversing with a patient regarding his medical condition within earshot of a lobby full of patients.

_____ 7. Attending a regional conference for medical office personnel.

Exercise 4-3 ETHICAL CONDUCT OF PHYSICIANS

After completing Activity 4-1, read each of the following examples involving physician conduct. Using the AMA Principles of Medical Ethics and the Current Opinions of the Council of Ethical and Judicial Affairs (located at the AMA's Web site) as a guide for ethical conduct, determine whether the conduct is ethical or unethical. Record the answer in the blank provided. E = ethical; U = unethical.

_____ 1. Physician grows and smokes marijuana for medicinal purposes.

_____ 2. Physician bills for services not rendered.

_____ 3. Physician refers a patient to a specialist when needed.

_____ 4. Physician refuses to speak to the press about a famous patient because the patient has not authorized release of information.

_____ 5. Physician donates services to a local homeless shelter.

_____ 6. A physician specializing in obstetrics and gynecology decides to stop taking obstetrics patients so that she can concentrate her practice in gynecologic pathology.

_____ 7. Physician has a personal problem with alcohol abuse.

_____ 8. Physician fails to report suspected abuse to law enforcement authorities.

_____ 9. Physician works with legislators to encourage new laws governing patients' rights.

_____ 10. Physician suggests a pharmacy to a patient by name because the physician has part ownership of the pharmacy.

_____ 11. Physician accepts educational medical literature and a scale anatomic model (of nominal value) from a pharmaceutical company for use with patients in the clinic.

_____ 12. Physician advertises her family practice clinic in a local newspaper. Information about location and hours is provided in the advertisement.

_____ 13. Physician performs a legal abortion.

_____ 14. Physician refuses care for an emergency patient.

ACTIVITY 4–1 Complete information on the AMA's Current Opinions of the Council on Ethical and Judicial Affairs can be found at the AMA's Web site. Review and discuss information found in sections 2 through 9 in the Current Opinions.

ACTIVITY 4–2 Research a medical ethical issue and identify why the issue is an ethical one by identifying the various viewpoints pertaining to the topic. Present the findings in a paper or presentation.

ACTIVITY 4–3 Several other ethical codes for medicine have been written throughout history. Research a medical ethical code not presented in this chapter and write a one- to two-page paper comparing the code to the Hippocratic Oath.

ACTIVITY 4–4 Several films have been made regarding ethical issues in medicine. View one or more of the following films and write your reaction regarding the movie's portrayal of the ethical issue. The paper should be one to two pages long and should contain a short summary of the medical ethical issue and your reaction to the portrayal.
- *Philadelphia* (Tom Hanks)
- *One Flew over the Cuckoo's Nest* (Jack Nicholson)
- *One True Thing* (Meryl Streep, William Hurt, Renee Zellweger)

ACTIVITY 4–5 Role play the following situations. What is the appropriate response to the situation given?
1. You are working in the medical records room at a medical office. A patient who was in today had a pregnancy test result that was positive. A nurse returns the patient's chart and comments, "The last thing she needs is another baby." How do you respond?
2. An acquaintance of one of your coworkers is pregnant and is a patient at the clinic. Your coworker knows that the acquaintance was in for an ultrasound scan because of the possibility of a twin pregnancy. Your coworker talks about going to get the scan results because she is so excited for the patient and can "hardly wait to find out the results." How do you respond?

4
DISCUSSION

The following topics can be used for class discussion or for individual student essay.

DISCUSSION 4–1 Why is it important for a medical administrative assistant to have an understanding of medical ethical issues? What might be different if an assistant did not study these issues?

DISCUSSION 4–2 Why should an employee be required to sign a confidentiality agreement?

Interacting with Patients

CHAPTER OUTLINE

LEARNING OUTCOMES

On successful completion of this chapter, the student will be able to

1. Identify cultural considerations when interacting with patients.
2. Reduce language barriers.
3. Identify appropriate interactions with various types of patients.

CMA COMPETENCIES

1. Instruct individuals according to their needs.

RMA COMPETENCIES

1. Employ appropriate interpersonal skills in the workplace

VOCABULARY

culture

THE DIVERSE COMMUNITY OF PATIENTS

Never look down on anybody unless you're helping them up.

—Rev. Jesse Jackson

People believe and value various things. With an increasingly mobile society, many cultural differences are present in the United States today. A medical administrative assistant should have great respect for all types of patients treated in the medical office and should be prepared to handle all sorts of situations. An assistant must respect each patient who comes to the practice, regardless of religion, sex, ethnic background, and other differences related to a person's lifestyle or beliefs.

It is expected that we not discriminate against people who are different from us. Not only is nondiscrimination politically correct—in many instances, such as in granting credit, it is unlawful to discriminate against another individual. Human rights issues have been debated throughout history and will probably continue to be debated, but the staff of a medical office—regardless of what laws might be in place—should provide patients with care and service free of bias or prejudice.

INFLUENCE OF CULTURE

What is culture? It is those beliefs, behaviors, and attitudes that are shared by a particular group of people and passed from one generation to the next. Culture is learned from various events and the social environment that a patient experiences.

A patient's nationality will have a great impact on his or her culture. For example, there is varying opinion around the world today about the status of women in society. Some nationalities believe women should be treated as equal to men. Other nationalities believe that women should not have as many rights as men do or believe that they should have very few rights at all.

The extent of a patient's religious upbringing will also have a great impact on the patient's beliefs and attitudes regarding health care. Some religions have strong convictions about procedures such as abortion or blood transfusions. A patient's religious convictions have a significant effect on his or her utilization of health care services.

Interactions with Patients of Different Cultures

Madeline M. Leininger conceived a nursing theory known as culture care diversity and universality. Its basic philosophy is that a patient's culture should be considered when one provides nursing services to a patient. The reasoning behind the theory is that the care a nurse provides should be consistent with a patient's cultural beliefs.

This theory is important for other staff members in the office, as well. To provide the best patient services possible, assistants working in the medical office should be well aware that patients hold a number of different beliefs regarding what they believe is appropriate medical care. This knowledge will help an assistant be "in tune" with many of the

needs and desires of patients and will help prevent the assistant from making mistakes when communicating with patients. Awareness of differing cultural beliefs is necessary to avoid insulting or offending patients. Saying or doing the wrong thing could adversely affect a patient's relationship with the clinic staff.

An assistant must understand that no culture is the "correct" culture and must recognize and respect cultures different from his or her own. To avoid the tendency to stereotype people belonging to a particular culture, this chapter does not attempt to categorize people by identifying a particular behavior with a culture but merely points out different beliefs regarding health care treatment.

When a medical administrative assistant serves a patient, the assistant should begin the encounter without a predetermined set of cultural expectations of patient behavior; he or she should merely serve a patient with the same respect and dignity given to all other patients.

For example, if a patient has a last name that appears to be of a particular cultural group (whether a nationality or a religion) the assistant should not assume that because of this culture the patient will behave in a particular manner. All people of one culture do not behave uniformly, although there are some beliefs that are held by many individuals within a cultural group. Although some behaviors are widespread throughout a culture, people of that culture do not hold a uniform set of values or beliefs. For the most part, the assistant should be aware that the behavior of a patient is likely a result of his or her own cultural influences.

A person's culture influences beliefs about the use of health care services and medicine in general. The following are common patient beliefs and behaviors about health care treatment:

- Reluctance to have surgery or other medical procedures.
- Refusal to have blood drawn or transfused.
- Strong belief in use of home remedies.
- Aversion to taking medication.
- Elders as decision makers of the family.
- Support for use of alternative treatments such as herbs or acupuncture.
- Refusal to allow any touching by a stranger.
- Frequent use of touch in interactions.
- Eye contact may be considered disrespectful.
- Men may be given preferential treatment.
- Condition of a terminal illness may not be shared with the patient.
- Certain types of food may not be eaten.
- Sexual inequality may be the norm.
- Use of alcohol or tobacco is strongly discouraged.

EXPECTATIONS WHEN SERVING PATIENTS

In dealing with patients in general, it is important to remember that many of the patients coming through the clinic doors are doing so because they are sick. Most of the time, illness can cause patients to behave differently. Regardless of whether they have special cultural considerations or other concerns, they may not respond to questions or instructions as an otherwise healthy individual would.

Often, patients experience physical discomfort or emotional distress because of illness. Parents of ill children or care givers of patients may behave differently because of stress precipitated by illness. Illness is often accompanied by pain, varied patterns of sleeping/eating, and by general anxiety about the prospect of recovery. Patients or care givers may be quick to react or respond in a negative way. They may be short in their responses, and an assistant should remember to not take it personally.

Because of illness, a patient may not be able to remember directions to an appointment in a particular department or may forget care instructions. It may be necessary for an assistant to repeat something several times, write it down, or escort the patient to a different location in the clinic.

An assistant may never know what problems a patient may be dealing with, but it is important to be caring and compassionate even in the most difficult situations.

Perhaps one of the most helpful things you, as an assistant, should remember in dealing with people is to consider how you would like to be treated if you were in the patient's situation. If the patient is a loved one, how would you expect that patient to be treated? When the focus is on what is patient friendly and respectful, the services provided will be appropriate.

LANGUAGE BARRIERS

Language barriers can create an interesting challenge. A language barrier exists if two people (e.g., a patient and an assistant) cannot communicate effectively using a common language. If a language barrier exists, it will take extra effort on the part of the medical administrative assistant to make sure the patient's needs are met.

English as a Second Language

If a patient's English is hard to understand, there are some communication options for the office staff. If the patient has learned English as a second language (ESL), a foreign language dictionary may help reduce the chance of miscommunication. Some medical dictionaries have translation tables included in the appendices.

An interpreter may also help bridge a language barrier. Frequently, a family member may serve as an interpreter for a patient who has limited English skills. Professional medical interpreters are often employed by large medical facilities that draw patients from all over the world. If a professional medical interpreter is not available at a facility, a general interpreter may be able to translate. A drawback to using a general interpreter is that the interpreter may have limited knowledge of medical procedures.

In geographic areas in which there are many ESL patients, medical offices may employ bilingual health care workers to reduce the language barriers between patients and medical office staff.

Speech Difficulty

On some occasions, a patient may know English but may have difficulty speaking. In this case, the patient may be able to write his or her request.

If the patient is unable to write, he or she may be able to respond to yes or no questions. If the medical administrative assistant asks a question that could be answered yes or no, the patient may be able to nod or shake the head appropriately. For instance, instead of "When would you like your next appointment?" try saying "Would Monday work for your recheck appointment?" and "Would you be able to come in the afternoon?"

Medical Terminology

Everyone does not speak the language of the medical office fluently. A medical administrative assistant should avoid creating a language barrier with a patient by inappropriate use of medical terminology. An assistant should use technical medical terms in a conversation only if the patient has used them first. For example, a patient may understand *bladder infection* but not *urinary tract infection,* or *sore throat* but not *pharyngitis.* An assistant should take conversational cues from patients and instruct patients to their level of understanding. If a patient uses particular technical terms, it is likely that the patient has a good understanding of those terms. Otherwise, keep the conversation uncomplicated until the patient demonstrates comfort with more complex medical terms.

SPECIFIC PATIENT GROUPS

Elderly Patients

Elderly patients are frequent users of health care services and have special concerns that must be considered. These patients are served in almost every specialty (a notable exception, of course, is pediatrics), and an assistant must be alert to the needs of some patients in this group.

The definition of an elderly patient, as given by the *Miller-Keane Encyclopedia & Dictionary of Medicine, Nursing, & Allied Health,* is an individual 65 years and older who has a functional impairment or any individual 75 years and older.

Several things to consider when communicating with an elderly patient are the following:
● Talk directly to the patient whenever possible (Fig. 5–1). Sometimes, a family member may have the habit of speaking for the patient when the patient is perfectly able to communicate. Sometimes, members of the patient's

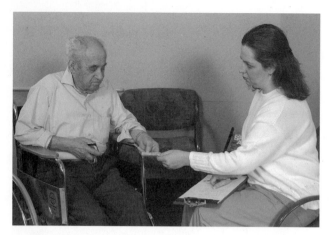

Figure 5–1. Whenever possible, the assistant should talk directly to an elderly patient.

family may even take over the conversation when the patient is talking. An assistant should not talk to family members as though the patient was not there. The patient should remain the main focus of the conversation.

- Be sure the patient understands all information given. Some patients may have disabilities that have impaired their ability to understand and make medical decisions.
- Sometimes, elderly patients develop problems with brain function. Dementias cause a patient's thinking to be confused. The patient may have trouble remembering certain things, events, and instructions given by the office staff. Written instructions may need to be given to the patient, and, in some cases, it may be necessary to communicate the instructions to a family member.
- Remember that the patient is an adult and should be treated as one.
- An elderly patient may also be hard of hearing. Do not assume that a patient is hard of hearing unless you are told so. Be careful to not shout at a patient. Remember, conversations within the public areas of the clinic should be kept confidential.

Children

Children are frequent visitors to clinics, either as patients or accompanying adults. Children may sometimes need special attention from the office staff. They may or may not be comfortable with the clinic surroundings. If possible, an assistant should try to include children in conversations. Welcome them to the clinic, and leave them with a friendly impression of the office staff. If a child speaks first, continue the conversation.

Occasionally, children must be left in the lobby while a parent is seeing the physician. Although it is certainly not a medical administrative assistant's job to provide daycare services, it may be necessary to supervise children and ensure their safety while a parent is having medical treatment. Although most offices would prefer that children are not left alone in the lobby, an assistant may need to be aware of children that have been left in the lobby while the parent is seeing the physician.

To keep children occupied while in the clinic, activities such as storybooks, toys, videos, and coloring books can be kept in the lobby and in examination rooms. Toys should be safe for children of all ages and should be sanitized routinely by the office staff to reduce the spread of infection.

Patients with Disabilities

Patients with physical or mental disabilities may require special attention. It is important to remember to talk directly to the patient. Do not ignore the patient and talk to family members unless it is apparent that the patient is unable to communicate.

Patients who have been injured in an accident may struggle with the operation of a wheelchair and may require the assistant's aid. If appropriate, assistance should be offered to the patient (Fig. 5–2). Many patients are capable of moving around on their own, but, if they seem to be having difficulty, an assistant may offer assistance by saying something such as "Could I offer any assistance, sir?" Then, wait for a response before proceeding. The patient may not need or desire any assistance.

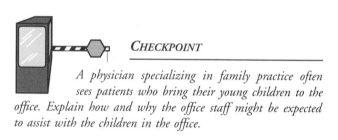

CHECKPOINT

A physician specializing in family practice often sees patients who bring their young children to the office. Explain how and why the office staff might be expected to assist with the children in the office.

Angry Patients

Angry patients may appear in the clinic occasionally. It is important to realize that their anger may or may not be directed toward the staff. Their anger may have been triggered earlier, and an assistant could then become the recipient of

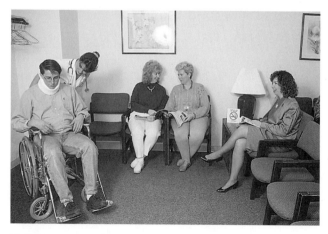

Figure 5–2. Assistance should be offered to patients who may have difficulty moving around the office. (From Chester GA: Modern Medical Assisting. Philadelphia, WB Saunders, 1998.)

the anger. Some medical conditions, such as psychiatric disorders and illnesses or injuries involving brain function, can contribute to a patient's angry or aggressive behavior. Even healthy people who are under a great deal of stress may become angry. Patients may be angry for a myriad of reasons, most of which an assistant may never be aware.

Defusing an Angry Patient

No matter what the reason for the patient's anger, do not avoid the anger. The anger will probably not go away by itself. Listen intently to the patient's concerns. Take notes if necessary. If the patient's concerns are not forthcoming, ask the patient what his concerns are. Ask the patient what he would like to have done about the situation. People are usually surprisingly reasonable and will probably not "ask for the moon." If a patient does, he should be referred to the assistant's supervisor. The assistant should offer to help the patient as much as possible without exceeding his or her authority in the office.

When speaking with an angry patient, remember to remain calm. Speak softly and directly to the patient. An assistant should never, ever raise his or her voice. Doing so would likely make the patient angrier and put the patient on the defensive. Once on the defensive, the patient will probably not listen to much more that the assistant has to say.

In dealing with an angry patient, think of the old adage "The customer is always right." Remember, the patient is a customer.

It does no good to point out that the patient is wrong. The patient will remember a response, and that may make the difference as to how the situation is ultimately resolved. The assistant should try to resolve the situation and make sure the patient understands what can be done. Above all, the assistant should be professional. The assistant should assure the patient that everything that can be done will be done to resolve the situation. The assistant must then follow through with his or her promise. Failing to follow through could damage relations with the office and could increase a chance of future litigation. Nothing should be promised that cannot be done.

When talking with an angry patient, an assistant should avoid having conversations at the front desk in the presence of other patients in the office. It is a good idea to ask a patient to go into a less crowded office area so that the assistant can give the patient full attention.

Violent Patients

Depending on their skills in dealing with difficult situations, angry patients do have the potential to become violent. Although this is a rather rare occurrence in most medical offices, the office should plan for a possible occurrence, and the assistant should be prepared to handle the situation if it arises. The assistant should never try to handle a violent person alone and should always remain within earshot of other staff members. The assistant should be careful to not back into a corner or position the patient between herself and the door. Any sudden moves could provoke the patient. Ask for help from another staff member if needed. If the patient begins to get physical (throwing or hitting things) or if the assistant feels in danger, a call to 911 may be warranted. This, however, should be done after all else fails and should be the last resort and used only when imminent danger is apparent.

Anxious Patients

Anxiety can manifest in a variety of ways. Patients may appear nervous or restless or may overreact to a situation. They may speak quickly and in a very random fashion. They may also be fixated on an idea. The patient may even come right out and tell an assistant that he or she is anxious or nervous. Anxiety usually develops because of a patient's fear of the unknown.

In talking with an anxious patient, convey a calm and caring attitude. This may help ease the patient's anxiety. If a patient is anxious about a medical condition or treatment, an assistant must be careful to avoid any conversation in which he or she may be interpreted as giving medical advice. Listening intently to the patient and giving as much time as possible will help the assistant relieve whatever anxiety he or she can and may help the patient's anxiety subside.

Depressed Patients

Depression is an illness often treated with medication. It is important to remember that depressed people are not weak—they are ill. Most people would not choose to be depressed. A depressed patient may experience a major depressive episode or may be chronically depressed during a long period of time. Whatever the case, the patient needs medical treatment and cannot just "snap out of it."

Depressed patients are usually not very talkative. If a patient talks of being depressed, do not dismiss the patient's complaints with a statement such as "Oh, everything will be fine. Don't worry." If a patient makes any comments about injuring himself or herself, these comments should be taken seriously and should be communicated directly to the physician. Because self-injury and suicide are a very real possibility with depressed patients, a medical administrative assistant needs to be sure to notify the medical staff of any pertinent incidents involving the patient.

Dying or Grieving Patients

Assisting patients who are dying or grieving the loss of a loved one presents a special challenge to everyone in the medical office. This is a very difficult time for patients and their families, and the medical office staff must be sensitive to their needs. The office staff should be prepared for a myriad of emotions from these patients and their families.

In the 1960s, Dr. Elizabeth Kübler-Ross, a physician who treated hundreds of terminally ill patients, researched the

Box 5–1 Kübler-Ross Stages of Loss

Denial

The patient cannot believe something has happened to him and may feel as though "it just can't be true." The situation may seem like a bad dream.

Anger

The patient becomes very upset with the situation and may feel as though "it just isn't fair." The patient may lash out and be angry with others who are not in the same situation.

Bargaining

This stage typically has a religious connection. Faced with a situation, the patient attempts to make a deal with a higher being, saying, for example, "If I get better, I promise to . . ."

Depression

In this stage, the patient may have tried many things—yelling, pleading, ignoring—and nothing is changing the situation for the better. Depression is a normal stage in the loss process. Hope of any improvement may be totally lost, and professional treatment for depression may be warranted.

Acceptance

Once the patient reaches acceptance of a situation, there is acknowledgement of the situation. The patient will likely want to say goodbye to those he loves and will get personal business affairs in order.

medical staff to be genuinely affected by a patient's loss, but this is also a time when patients need understanding and compassion. The assistant should strive to be kind, empathetic, and considerate of the patient's situation.

SUMMARY

A medical administrative assistant's workday consists of interactions with a wide variety of patients. Patients' beliefs are quite diverse, and an assistant must be respectful of people's differences and must take great care when communicating with patients to be sure their needs are met. Also, patients may have special physical needs of which the assistant must be aware. Elderly patients or patients with disabilities may require additional special attention of the assistant. While in the office, patients may also be experiencing various emotions, and the assistant should strive to provide services that provide comfort to patients.

YOU ARE THE MEDICAL ADMINISTRATIVE ASSISTANT

An 18-year-old's mother is upset about her son's treatment in the medical office. Her son came in with a reaction to an antibiotic and is having difficulty breathing. The mother is upset because she knew her son was allergic to an antibiotic but, because her son is an adult, was not asked about any allergies. The mother is talking very loudly, is becoming nearly hysterical, and is insisting on being taken back immediately to the treatment room to speak with the doctor. The treatment room is quite full, with medical staff working with the patient. What should you do?

thought processes associated with the loss or grieving process and defined five stages of loss (Box 5–1) that often serve as the basis for caring for people suffering from terminal illness, the loss of a loved one, the loss of bodily function due to disease or injury, or even the loss of someone or something significant in their lives.

An assistant should be aware that a patient will experience the various stages of loss in a very personal way. Not all individuals experience all stages. Some may never reach acceptance; others may go back and forth between stages. Some patients spend more time in one stage compared with another or may never experience one or more stages. An assistant who understands the stages of loss will be more understanding when assisting people dealing with loss.

Each person deals with loss in his or her own way. A sympathetic ear, kindness, and compassion can help ease the patient's experiences in the medical office. An assistant should never avoid a patient because the assistant is uncomfortable with the situation. It is perfectly normal for the

Bibliography

Adams CH, Jones PD: Interpersonal Communication Skills for Health Professionals, 2nd ed. Columbus, Ohio, Glencoe McGraw-Hill, 2000.
O'Toole M: Miller-Keane Encyclopedia & Dictionary of Medicine, Nursing, & Allied Health, 5th ed. Philadelphia, WB Saunders, 1992.
Sieh A, Brentin LK: The Nurse Communicates, Philadelphia, WB Saunders, 1997.

Suggested Reading

A winner of the National Book Critics Circle Award for Nonfiction, *The Spirit Catches You and You Fall Down* (Noonday Press, Farrar, Straus & Giroux, 1997), by Anne Fadiman, tells the story of a Hmong child who is diagnosed with epilepsy and the doctors who treat her. The book includes a reader's guide that offers questions for discussion or essay topics.

Exercise 5–1 TRUE OR FALSE

Read the following statements and determine whether the statements are true or false. Record the answer in the blank provided. T = true; F = false.

_____ 1. A patient's culture has an influence on his or her beliefs regarding health care treatment.

_____ 2. Knowledge of varying cultural beliefs can help an assistant avoid offending a patient.

_____ 3. An illness can cause a patient to be anxious.

_____ 4. The culture of the United States is easy to identify.

_____ 5. Care givers of ill patients may act differently than usual because of stress associated with the patient's illness.

_____ 6. An assistant may need to repeat instructions for an ill patient.

_____ 7. An assistant should strive to be respectful of the patient, no matter what the circumstances.

_____ 8. Patients who are unable to speak usually communicate through an interpreter.

_____ 9. While serving an elderly patient, the assistant should be sure to phone all instructions to a son or daughter of the patient.

_____ 10. Children should not be left in a clinic's lobby, and an assistant should insist that all children accompany their parents to an examination room.

_____ 11. The best way to handle an angry patient is for the assistant to become equally angry.

_____ 12. Culture can be defined as beliefs or attitudes that are shared by a group of people and are passed from generation to generation.

_____ 13. Some cultures may object to blood transfusions being used to treat patients.

_____ 14. Leininger's theory of culture care diversity and universality basically states that care givers should take a patient's culture into consideration when providing health care.

_____ 15. A patient's illness can affect his or her interactions with members of the medical office staff.

_____ 16. It would be unusual for an extremely ill patient to be upset.

_____ 17. Family members may serve as interpreters for patients who do not speak English.

_____ 18. An assistant should use medical terminology with all patients of the medical office.

_____ 19. It may be necessary to shout at an elderly patient who is hard of hearing.

_____ 20. Instructions for disabled patients should always be given directly to a care giver, not to the patient.

_____ 21. A patient who has been paralyzed may experience some or all of the five stages of loss.

Exercise 5–2 CHAPTER CONCEPTS

Read the following questions or statements and choose the answer that best completes the statement or question. Record the answer in the blank provided.

_____ 1. Which of the following is inappropriate when dealing with an angry patient?
    (a) Offer to help if possible.
    (b) Keep a calm voice.
    (c) Ask the patient what he would like done about the situation.
    (d) Record the conversation on tape.
    (e) Don't avoid the patient's anger.

_____ 2. If a patient becomes violent while in the office, which of the following should *NOT* be done?
  (a) Phone police if danger is imminent.
  (b) Take the patient to a rear office, shut the door, and try to calm the patient.
  (c) Ask for help from another staff member.
  (d) Remain within hearing distance of other office employees.

_____ 3. Which of the following is *NOT* true of anxious patients?
  (a) They are dangerous.
  (b) They may appear restless.
  (c) They may talk fast.
  (d) Anxiety may be caused by the patient's fear of the unknown.

_____ 4. Which of the following is *NOT* true of depressed patients?
  (a) They are ill.
  (b) They are usually very talkative.
  (c) An increased potential for suicide exists.
  (d) Depression can be treated with medication.

_____ 5. Which of the following is *NOT* true when serving patients in the medical office?
  (a) After age 75, most elderly patients will need assistance when making health care decisions.
  (b) Illness can be a stress factor for patients or care givers.
  (c) A foreign language dictionary may help an ESL patient explain a medical condition.
  (d) All patients of the office should be treated with dignity and respect, no matter what their culture.

Exercise 5–3 STAGES OF LOSS

Match the five stages of loss with the description of those stages. Record the answer in the blank provided.
  (a) Denial
  (b) Anger
  (c) Bargaining
  (d) Depression
  (e) Acceptance

_____ 1. Patient is extremely sad about the situation and may lose hope.

_____ 2. Patient does not believe what is happening to him.

_____ 3. Patient is extremely upset and furious about his situation.

_____ 4. Patient acknowledges his situation.

_____ 5. Patient tries to make a deal to get out of the situation.

ACTIVITIES

ACTIVITY 5–1   To understand how health care beliefs can vary from patient to patient, complete the following questions regarding health care. *Do not* write your name on this assignment. Give the completed sheet to your instructor and your instructor will tabulate the class results. Your instructor will then share the total results with the class.

1. I smoke cigarettes.   Yes   No

2. I drink alcohol at least once a week.   Yes   No

3. There are certain foods I will not eat at certain times because of my religious beliefs.   Yes   No

4. I use home remedies whenever possible.   Yes   No

5. I would accept a blood transfusion if I needed it.   Yes   No

6. I have seen a chiropractor for treatment.   Yes   No

7. I have taken herbal remedies to treat a health condition.   Yes   No

8. I have tried acupuncture to treat a health condition.   Yes   No

5
DISCUSSION

The following topics can be used for class discussion or for individual student essay.

DISCUSSION 5–1   Have you ever been in one of the following situations:
- Seriously ill
- Care giver of a seriously ill person
- Relative or close friend of a seriously ill person

Write an essay or participate in group discussion involving the following points:
- Was your life altered as a result of this experience? If so, how?
- Were the five stages of loss evident in this situation?
- Were any of the common patient beliefs identified in the chapter present in this situation?

For those who have never experienced any of the situations, listen to the discussion or read a published account of such a situation and give your reaction to it (verbally or in writing).

DISCUSSION 5–2   Research an issue relating to health care for geriatric patients. Present a synopsis of the issue in a one- to two-page report or in a presentation to the class.

CHAPTER OUTLINE

LEARNING OUTCOMES

1. Describe the basics of communication.
2. Identify effective and ineffective communication styles.
3. Identify proper communication with patients and coworkers.
4. Identify and use proper telephone communication skills.
5. Describe telephone equipment and services.
6. Apply proper written communication skills when preparing business correspondence.
7. Describe mail processing in the office.
8. Describe postal and delivery services.
9. Identify confidentiality issues related to patient communication.
10. Prepare business letters and memos.

CMA COMPETENCIES

1. Respond to and initiate written communications.
2. Recognize and respond to verbal communications.
3. Recognize and respond to nonverbal communications.
4. Demonstrate telephone techniques.
5. Identify and respond to issues of confidentiality.

RMA COMPETENCIES

1. Know terminology associated with medical secretarial and receptionist duties.
2. Answer and place telephone calls using proper etiquette.
3. Manage telephone calls requiring special attention (including laboratory and x-ray reports, angry callers, and personal calls).
4. Employ effective intra-office oral communication skills (including employee supervision and patient handling).
5. Compose correspondence according to acceptable business format.
6. Manage mail.
7. Use effective written communication skills.
8. Use computer for word processing.

VOCABULARY

communication
electronic mail (e-mail)
feedback
protocol
voice mail

6

INTERPERSONAL COMMUNICATIONS

I never learn anything talking. I only learn things when I ask questions.

—*Lou Holtz*

COMMUNICATION CONCEPTS

Excellent communication skills are essential for everyone in the medical office. Communicating with patients in a professional, business-like, yet caring manner fosters trust between the medical office staff and the patient and lays the foundation for a strong, trusting, and long-lasting relationship between the patient and the practice. Even the most glamorous physical surroundings cannot make up for a staff member lacking proper communication skills. A medical administrative assistant who has frequent interaction with patients has a great impact on the success of the practice. Whether an assistant is communicating with a patient face to face, on the telephone, or in writing, the assistant's communication must be professional and should reflect the image that the practice wishes to project.

Communication Basics

When applying professional communication techniques to interactions with patients, it is important to understand basic communication concepts. The *Miller-Keane Encyclopedia & Dictionary of Medicine, Nursing, & Allied Health* defines **communication** as the "sending of information from one place to another." One of the cornerstones in understanding communication is the idea that communication involves getting that information, idea, or thought from one individual to another.

Communicating Effectively

The vast majority of people in this world can talk, but can they communicate? Are they understood?

Consider this example. If you and a friend are outside one day, and your friend remarks, "The sky is blue today," you know that your friend thinks the sky is blue and not green. If your friend says, however, "Look at the sky," you may be able to guess that your friend wants you to notice that the sky is blue, but it is possible that you may be looking for something in the sky, such as an airplane or a bird. Or perhaps you may notice a cloud with an interesting shape. This example illustrates how important word selection can be.

Consider this next example. A patient enters the office and begins speaking to you in German. The patient is talking, but if you do not know German, very little communication will occur.

From the examples mentioned, the basic components of communication may be identified: a sender, a receiver, a message, and **feedback.** The sender and receiver are the two parties to the proposed communication, the message is the information from the sender, and the feedback is information the receiver gives the sender about the message.

Let's look at another example in a medical office setting. Suppose a patient phones the office and reports to the assistant that he is not "feeling well." This statement does not give the assistant a clear indication of what the problem might be. Consequently, if the assistant relayed this information to a nurse or to a physician, it would not be very helpful to them either because it is not very descriptive. If the patient reports, however, that he has a sharp, stabbing-like pain in his lower right side and that he has had it for two days, this gives a much more accurate picture of the patient's condition.

Unfortunately, not every patient may describe symptoms this well, which is why medical administrative assistants benefit from cultivating good communication skills.

When communicating with a patient, it is imperative to obtain a clear picture of what the patient is trying to say. One of the most important things a medical administrative assistant can do, and one of the most essential components of effective communication, is to listen to the other person while he or she is speaking. Be attentive by looking directly at the patient (if the patient is in the office) or by giving complete attention to the patient on the phone. Don't plan what might be said next while the patient is speaking. Give the patient plenty of time to say what he or she needs to say. After the patient is finished speaking, ask any questions that may be necessary to clarify the situation. Using the previous example, let's see how a medical administrative assistant might handle a patient's comment of not feeling well.

Patient: I'm not feeling well.
Assistant: What kind of symptoms are you having?
Patient: I threw up this morning.
Assistant: Is that the only symptom you've had?
Patient: I've also had a sharp pain on my lower right side.
Assistant: How long have you had the pain?
Patient: A couple of days.
Assistant: And have you had any other symptoms?
Patient: Just a slight fever.

The medical administrative assistant in this case has obtained just enough information to convey a picture of the patient's condition to the nurse or physician. It is not necessary for the assistant to get every last detail from the patient—the assistant simply needs enough information to give the medical staff a clear picture of the patient's condition. In this case, the patient might have appendicitis, which is a serious condition that must be brought to the attention of the physician immediately. If the assistant had stopped asking questions after the patient reported vomiting, he or she would not have been given enough information to illustrate the seriousness of the situation.

The assistant must be extremely careful to identify any serious or potentially life-threatening conditions *without alarming the patient* but must obtain this information and transmit it to the physician without delay. Identifying and handling emergency calls are discussed later in this chapter.

This example illustrates clearly the importance of communication in the medical office. Because of the nature of the calls that come into the office, good communication may in some cases mean the difference of life or death to a patient.

When speaking with patients, follow these basic guidelines for effective verbal communication:

- Speak clearly. Avoid chewing gum or eating lunch while at the desk.
- Speak loud enough so that patients can hear but not so loud that everyone else hears.
- Pronounce words correctly.
- The sound of your voice conveys a message. Others can tell whether you are genuine in your responses or whether you are hiding something. What kind of feeling does your voice convey? Is it one of caring, or is it one of indifference?
- Monitor the speed of your speech. Don't speak too fast or too slowly.
- Direct your words to the individual to whom you are speaking.
- When speaking with patients, be aware that you are a representative of the practice. Patients may interpret something you say as coming directly from the physician.
- Ask enough questions to identify the needs of the patient. Don't ask so many questions that it may appear you are prying into the patient's private health matters.
- *Never, ever* suggest to a patient what might be wrong. This is practicing medicine without a license and is punishable by law!
- Clarify the patient's needs by repeating the patient's request or statement. Clear up any misunderstandings. Say to the patient, "Let me make sure I have this right . . ."
- Don't interrupt. Give the patient ample opportunity to convey thoughts without interruption.
- As mentioned in Chapter 5, use of technical medical terms and jargon is best avoided unless the patient uses them in conversation.

Nonverbal Communication

Communication does not have to be a spoken or written message. Communication can occur without anyone speaking or writing anything. This type of communication is nonverbal communication and is more commonly known as body language. Nonverbal communication, or body language, is a sign or signal given by the body. These visual clues may have a greater impact on the conversation than may the words that are spoken.

Take a look at the interactions pictured in Figure 6–1. One of the interactions is much friendlier than the other. Note how each individual is interacting nonverbally with eyes, arms, and other parts of the body. An individual's appearance and body language communicate interest or disinterest to another individual.

Individuals receive many body signals subconsciously. We may not know what gives us a certain feeling about a person, but we often get that feeling from the body signals that are being sent. A frown, slumping posture, or eyes that wander create a negative image and demonstrate disinterest toward another individual.

Think about your own body language. Is it positive, or is it sending bad messages? Note the following recommendations for developing positive body language habits:

- Establish eye contact. Nothing conveys sincerity in a conversation more than a person who looks directly at someone else.
- Be conscious of your arm position. Are your arms crossed in front of your body, creating an almost protective barrier between you and another person, or are they casually at your sides or in use?

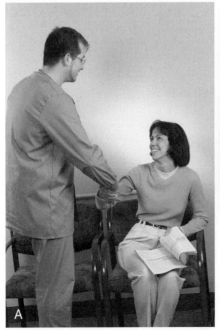
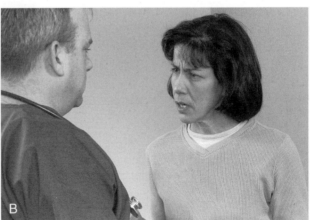

Figure 6–1. An individual's body language communicates a message.

- Smile, smile, smile at all times *when appropriate*. Cheerfulness goes a long way in making the patient feel welcomed in the office.
- Watch your posture. The front of your body should be directed toward the patient. Don't talk with your back to the patient.
- Watch facial expressions. Frowning sends an obvious negative message.
- Be aware of a patient's comfort zone. Leaning in too far to speak to a patient or positioning yourself closer than a few feet from a patient may invade his or her personal space and may make the patient feel uncomfortable.
- Be aware of the impact of personal attire and grooming. If necessary, refer to Chapter 1 for a refresher on professional appearance.

Personality Styles

Sometimes, we can be doing everything right in communicating with others, but we may have mixed responses from various people. These responses may be due to personality differences among individuals.

Maybe you are an outgoing person, or maybe you are more of an introvert. Maybe you enjoy the company of people, or maybe you prefer working alone. Perhaps a busy, hustle-bustle office is more to your liking than a quiet office. Not everyone has the same likes and dislikes and will respond differently to different situations. This does not mean there is anything wrong with you or them; it may just be that you have personality differences. As mentioned in Chapter 5, it is important to respect the opinions of others just as you would wish to have the same respect.

Personality differences may often lead to conflict in the office. When confronted with a conflict, it is important for each person to respect the rights of others who have differing opinions or different ways of looking at things and to accept those differences. Such action goes a long way in ensuring that the office environment will run smoothly.

Communication within the Health Care Team

Every medical administrative assistant will need to work with someone during the course of employment: an assistant may work alongside someone all the time or may have only periodic interactions with coworkers. In large offices, there may be several medical administrative assistants employed. These individuals need to develop a close working relationship with one another.

When communicating with coworkers, it is important for all coworkers to treat one another with respect and courtesy. Many conflicts in the office may start because of one person's feeling of superiority over another. All members of the health care team need to develop a good working relationship with one another, need to be tolerant of others' differ-

ences, and need to remember that all members of the health care team are important.

When communicating with physicians and other providers in the office, it is important for an assistant to realize that physicians and other providers (e.g., nurse practitioners, nurse midwives, physician assistants, therapists, and other individuals) are the ones chiefly responsible for generating the income of the practice. If the assistant can make providers' jobs easier and can help the office be as productive as possible, the practice will be well served.

Communicating with Your Supervisor

The best relationships between supervisors and staff are ones in which there is a healthy mutual respect. In some practices, the physician is the assistant's direct supervisor. In larger practices, an office supervisor is usually hired to oversee the business functions of the office. Regardless of who is the supervisor, the supervisor is in charge and is responsible for the operation of the office.

When communicating with the supervisor, an assistant must be respectful of the supervisor's position and should strive to meet the expectations of the supervisor. It is important for the assistant to bring to the supervisor's attention any problems or concerns that the assistant cannot handle. The assistant should not think that a problem will go away if it is ignored. The supervisor and the assistant who work together to help the office run smoothly will provide service for the good of the patient and will help to build a strong, successful practice.

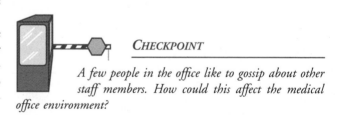

CHECKPOINT

A few people in the office like to gossip about other staff members. How could this affect the medical office environment?

TELEPHONE COMMUNICATION

The telephone is an indispensable piece of equipment in the office today. Most of a practice's business is conducted over the telephone. Appointments are made, patients call to inquire about health concerns, office staff members use the phone to conduct business, and a multitude of other office activities require the use of a telephone. However, just because someone knows how to pick up the phone and say hello, it cannot be assumed that the telephone will be used properly.

Proper Telephone Technique

The foundation for developing good telephone communication skills is to develop a good telephone personality. An individual's choice of words, volume, tone of voice, and general expression on the telephone has a tremendous impact on patients. A customer-friendly, service-oriented attitude is essential in telephone communication.

Many of us, at a very young age, learned to answer the telephone. What a thrill it was to hear the phone ring and run to answer it. Ah, if only it were that easy! Answering the phone in a medical office carries a great deal of responsibility with it. A patient may reveal sensitive, confidential medical information over the telephone. A patient may telephone the office with a potentially serious medical situation. Responsibility for answering the telephone in a medical office must be taken seriously, and an assistant must continually exhibit professionalism when communicating on the telephone.

Many of the same rules mentioned previously for good communication apply to communicating via the telephone. When speaking on the phone, keep in mind the following guidelines for professional communication:

● Tone and volume of voice. Speak in a tone that is thoughtful and caring. Speak loud enough for the patient to hear but soft enough so that others in the office will not hear. If appropriate, smile while talking on the telephone. Patients will notice the pleasantness of a smile reflected in your voice.

● Quality of your speech. Consider the words used in your conversation. Avoid slang, use proper grammar, and maintain professionalism while on the phone.

● Proper telephone posture. You should sit upright (no slouching!), hold the handset one to two inches away from the mouth, and be sure to enunciate clearly (Fig. 6–2). In most medical offices, there is considerable background noise, and to be heard well, you will need to be attentive to the patient on the other end of the line and speak directly into the handset. Proper posture at the telephone will help assure that you present your best self when speaking with a patient over the phone.

● Speed of your speech. Be careful to speak at a rate that will be understood by the caller. Depending on your interaction with the caller, you may need to adjust your speech rate to be sure that both of you are communicating. Routine information that is repeated many times to various patients may be well understood by an assistant, but it may be the first time the information is heard by a patient. Be sure to give information in a way that is understood by the patient.

Incoming Calls

Responsibility for managing the telephone traffic in a medical practice is an important matter. If more than one line is coming into the office, managing incoming calls can be very challenging. While an assistant is speaking on one line, one or more calls may come into the office on other lines. Depending on the size of the practice, one assistant may be assigned to handle the phone on a full-time basis. See Procedure 6–1 for a summary of how to demonstrate proper telephone techniques.

In addition to learning the proper telephone technique, there are special considerations that must be taken into account when answering the telephone in a medical office.

● Consider telephone location. The office telephone should be located on the assistant's desk within arms reach of the office computer. Many times, you may be speaking with a patient on the telephone and will need to access information from and input information into the computer

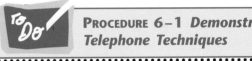

PROCEDURE 6–1 *Demonstrate Telephone Techniques*

Materials Needed

- Telephone set-up with two separate lines
- Pencil

1. Answer the telephone using the proper greeting.
   - Welcome
   - Identification of the facility
   - Identification of the operator
   - Offer to help
2. Determine the reason for the call.*
3. Identify the caller.
4. Determine the appropriate action based on the reason for the call.
5. Confirm the call.*
6. Close the call.

Optional

7. Demonstrate holding.
8. Demonstrate transferring a call.

Denotes a crucial step in the procedure. This step must be completed satisfactorily for the procedure to be completed satisfactorily.

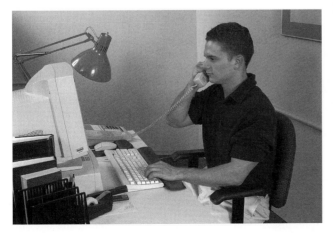

Figure 6–2. Proper posture while speaking on the telephone has an effect on speech.

during your conversation. If the lobby is close to the front desk, you will need to be careful that patients in the lobby do not hear your voice.

- Maintain confidentiality. Because the office is often a busy place with patients stopping at the front desk for assistance, you will need to be sure not to divulge a caller's complete name or disclose medical information in front of another patient. All phone conversations must be kept confidential.
- Keep conversations brief. Because many offices do get a tremendous volume of calls, be mindful of the time that is spent on the telephone. You must be sure to give the patient the time needed, but be sure that it is time well spent in getting information for a message or assisting the patient in another way.
- Don't ignore a ringing telephone. If the office is extremely busy and it is difficult to answer the phone, some practices may be arranged in such a way as to allow other staff members in the facility to give assistance in answering the phone when the phone traffic becomes too heavy.
- Answer incoming calls in three rings or fewer. If the call cannot be answered as soon as it rings, be sure to answer within a reasonable time of the call coming in. If the phone is allowed to ring four to five or even more times, many callers may begin to wonder whether the office is open or whether the practice cares about the patients who call.
- Don't give medical advice or ask questions that may lead a patient to believe you may be diagnosing the patient's condition. For example, if a patient calls reporting severe right lower quadrant abdominal pain, **never** say "It sounds like you have appendicitis" or "Have you ever had problems with your appendix?" Both of these statements could be interpreted as practicing medicine without a license (which is illegal) and could result in immediate dismissal from employment.
- Don't use the phone for personal business while on duty. This is unprofessional behavior. Always wait for a lunch or coffee break to make personal calls.

A Pleasant Telephone Greeting

If answering the telephone were as easy as it was when we were young, this chapter would have ended much earlier. However, because a practice's business is so dependent on the telephone, it is absolutely critical that patients hear a professional image every time they call. It simply is not enough to say "Hello" and then wait for the caller to answer.

Every call that comes into the office should be answered with a cheerful greeting consisting of three to four components: welcome, identification of facility, identification of operator (assistant's name), and an offer to help.

Appropriate greetings may sound like the following:

1. "Good morning, Horizons Health Care; this is Annie. How may I help you?"
2. "Thank you for calling Horizons Health Care; this is Mike. How may I direct your call?"

3. "Good afternoon, Horizons Health Care, this is Rosa. How may I help you today?"

When a call is answered in a medical office, an assistant should speak clearly and slowly. Many operators say the office greeting much too fast, and that can leave callers wondering what was really said.

Welcome

The welcome portion of a telephone greeting is a pleasant statement such as "Hello," "Good Morning," or "Thank you for calling." These introductions are a pleasant way to start a conversation with a caller and help to establish a pleasant foundation to the conversation with the patient.

Welcomes such as "Merry Christmas" and others with obvious ties to religious holidays should not be used in an office setting. Patients of one religion may be offended by a welcome that has ties to another religion.

Identification of the Facility

After the welcome, the operator should identify the facility by name.

1. "Good morning, Horizons Health Care . . ."
2. "Good afternoon, Country Care Associates . . ."
3. "Thank you for calling Horizons Health Care . . ."

Complete identification of the office name is necessary to help the patient be certain that the correct office has been reached.

Identification of the Operator and an Offer of Help

After identifying the facility, the operator states his or her name. The operator is the individual who answers the call.

In smaller facilities, very often the operator is the assistant who takes the call and performs tasks necessary to complete the handling of the call. If a patient leaves a message, schedules an appointment, or makes another request, it is likely that the assistant will directly assist the patient. The assistant's name is given so that the patient will be able to identify the individual who provided assistance if future questions should arise in regard to the patient's call.

Larger facilities that handle a tremendous volume of calls usually have a central switchboard setup in which one or more individuals answer incoming calls. In this type of medical facility, incoming calls are usually answered with a welcome, identification of the facility, and an offer of assistance. The switchboard operator does not give his or her name because the operator does not directly deal with the call other than to transfer the call to someone who will assist the patient. A greeting such as "Good afternoon, Horizons Health Care. How may I direct your call?" would be appropriate, although a facility may prefer that the operator be identified in order to give a personal touch to the conversation.

Telephone Protocol

Because there are many different types of situations that arise in the medical office, use of an established telephone **protocol** will give a medical administrative assistant a guide to follow when processing incoming calls. Protocol refers to instructions to use in response to an event. Protocol gives an individual a guide to use in response to a situation. Each office should establish specific protocol to handle the calls that come into the office. An example of telephone protocol is given in Table 6–1 and provides a sample of the numerous types of calls that come into a practice and a possible response to each call. Table 6–1 is not a definitive list of calls, and before a telephone protocol is put into use in any practice, it must be reviewed and approved by the practice physician or physicians.

Reason for the Patient's Call

As mentioned previously, every call is answered with a greeting. After the greeting, the most important piece of information needed by the medical administrative assistant is the reason the caller has phoned the office.

In almost every other type of business, typical phone practice is to identify the caller first. That is not the case in the medical office. Because you will be working in a medical office, the reason for the call may be a medical emergency. If a patient is calling with an emergency situation, the call must be handled quickly, because seconds may make a difference. Identification of common emergency calls is addressed later in this chapter.

Caller Identification

Once the reason for the call has been identified, the assistant will then ask for the caller's name. Once the reason and caller have been identified, the assistant will be able to decide how to handle the call based on protocol that has been established for the office (see Table 6–1).

Action

After the assistant has determined why the caller is calling and who the caller is, it is time to take action. At this point, the assistant decides what needs to be done (transfer the call or assist the patient directly), and that action is then taken. Occasionally, the assistant may need to handle a patient's request later in the day (as in the case of release of medical records to another facility) when the business of the office has slowed down.

Call Confirmation

Once the caller has been assisted, it is important to confirm any necessary information. If an appointment is scheduled, the provider, date, and time of the appointment should be confirmed with the caller. If a message was taken, the message written should be repeated verbatim to the caller to be sure it accurately reflects the wishes of the caller. Whatever the assistant is going to do for the caller, the assistant should inform the caller of the action that will be taken.

Closing the Call

After the call has been confirmed, the assistant should ask if there is anything else that the caller needs. If not, the assistant should say goodbye with an appropriate closing. Possible closings are the following:
1. "Thank you for calling."
2. "I'll take care of this right away."
3. "Have a nice day."
4. "Thank you."

Holding

Frequently, not all calls can be handled without asking a caller to hold. Of course, it would be best if no callers were ever asked to hold. Some calls, however, simply cannot be handled without having the caller hold.

The most important thing to remember when asking callers to hold is that the caller *must be asked* if he or she is able to hold. As mentioned previously, some calls may be an emergency and should not, of course, be placed on hold.

The appropriate way to ask a caller to hold would sound like the following:

Operator: Good morning, Horizon's Health Care. This is Amy. Are you able to hold?

At this point, the operator *must wait* for a response. If it is an emergency, this gives the caller a chance to say so. If it is not an emergency, the caller can say either "yes" or "no."

The caller may say "no" to holding for various reasons. Maybe the caller only needs to be transferred or, possibly, the caller is calling long-distance.

A caller should *never* be "told" to hold, as in "please hold." This statement gives absolutely no opportunity for the caller to respond if he or she is not able to hold. Always give the caller a choice.

If a caller is placed on hold, a reasonable period to expect a caller to hold is no longer than one minute. One minute can seem quite long. After one minute, if the call needs to be on hold for a little longer, the assistant should answer the line again and ask the caller if he or she can continue to hold or if the assistant may call the caller back. Some telephone systems even have a feature that re-rings a call that has been on hold for a specific length of time. When returning to answer a call that has been on hold, an appropriate introduction would be, "Thank you for holding. How may I help you?"

When the office is busy and incoming calls may need to hold, an assistant should wait until just after the third ring to answer the call and then should ask the caller to hold. If the assistant answers on the first ring and asks the caller to hold, that might give the impression that calls are not a big priority of the practice. By waiting just past the third ring, the caller is aware that the practice may be busy at the moment.

Table 6–1. Sample Telephone Protocol

Type of Call	Action Taken by Medical Administrative Assistant	Call Handled by Whom
Patient requests appointment	If not a potential emergency, schedule appointment	Medical administrative assistant
Patient requests prescription refill	Take a message with medication name and patient's pharmacy name. Send message with patient's chart to physician.	Physician will call pharmacy if approved; nurse will phone patient to inform the patient as to action taken by the physician (refilled or not refilled)
Patient asks to talk with physician or nurse because patient is ill or needs some medical information	Take a message, send message with patient's chart to physician or nurse. (Depending on the severity of the patient's illness, the call may need to be transfer immediately to the physician or nurse.)	Physician or nurse
Patient is returning a call to the physician or nurse	Transfer call directly to physician or nurse as requested	Physician or nurse
Another physician calls for the physician	Transfer call directly to physician as requested; no need to ask the reason for the call	Physician
Outside laboratory calls with test results	Transfer call directly to individual requested by the laboratory	Identified staff member
Patient is uncomfortable identifying the reason for calling	Ask the patient if the call is an emergency. If not, ask the patient if you can have the nurse return a call to the patient.	Nurse
Patient calls for test results	Take a message, send message with patient's chart to physician or nurse.	Physician or nurse
Patient calls with insurance or billing question	After confirming the identity of the patient and if the patient is entitled to the information, answer the patient's question. Some information may not be able to be released over the phone and may need to be mailed directly to the patient's home.	Medical administrative assistant
Insurance company calls requesting information on a patient	Identify requested information and identity of caller. Usually, only limited information may be given over the phone, and the caller may need to send in a written request for information that has been authorized by the patient.	Medical administrative assistant
Personal calls for a member of the office staff	Transfer directly to the staff member. If the call is for the physician and the physician is with a patient, notify the caller of that fact, and ask if you should interrupt, i.e., "The doctor is with a patient right now; would you like me to interrupt?"	Identified staff member
Administration calls for a member of the office staff	Transfer directly to the staff member. If the call is for a physician and the physician is with a patient, notify the caller of that fact, and ask if you should interrupt, i.e., "The doctor is in with a patient right now; would you like me to interrupt?"	Identified staff member
Patient has a complaint	Attempt to handle the situation if at all possible; otherwise, take a message or transfer the call to the appropriate individual. If necessary, notify physician of complaint.	Medical administrative assistant or identified staff member
Patient has been poisoned	Immediately give patient telephone number of poison control center and obtain identification of patient. Poison control centers are properly equipped to handle poisonings in a rapid manner.	Notify physician, and document call in patient's medical chart
Pharmaceutical sales representative wants appointment to give sales talk to physician and nurse	Make appointment under the guidelines established for the office	Medical administrative assistant
Office supply sales representative	Take message and give to staff member chiefly responsible for buying office supplies.	Identified staff member

Two Calls at the Same Time

If a practice has a multiple telephone line system, sooner or later two lines will ring at virtually the same time. Instead of answering and holding in the order the calls are received (e.g., line 1, then line 2, then going back to answer line 1), holding can be cut 50% by picking up one line, asking the caller whether he or she is able to hold, and then picking up the other line and speaking with that caller directly. Either line 1 or line 2 can be picked up first. Callers will not know whether they are on line 1 or line 2.

Transferring Calls

Some incoming calls will require transfer to another staff member. When transferring, the assistant should ask the caller whether he or she can hold so the call can be transferred. The assistant should let the caller know to whom he or she will be transferred.

A proper call transfer might sound like this.

Assistant: Are you able to hold while I transfer you to Dr. Pearson's nurse, Donna?

Caller: Yes.

(Caller is then placed on hold.)

Assistant: (signals nurse's station) Donna, Jane Doe is on line 1.

Some important things to remember when transferring are

- Ask the caller if you may transfer the call.
- Explain to the caller what you are going to do; "Can you hold while I transfer you?"
- Announce the call: "Dr. O'Brian, Mrs. Johnson is on line 1."
- When signaling the nurses' station, remember not to speak loudly. People in the area may be able to hear.
- *Never, ever* give sensitive information over a speaker phone, for example, "Mary Johnson is on line 1 for the results of her pregnancy test." Obviously, this would embarrass some people, but, more important, it is a breach of confidentiality.

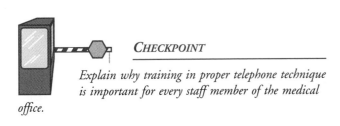

CHECKPOINT

Explain why training in proper telephone technique is important for every staff member of the medical office.

After Hours Calls

A practice may have patients who call after the clinic has closed. Most practices have an answering machine, voice mail, or an answering service to answer after-hours calls.

The use of one of these methods is essential to help the medical office communicate to patients what they should do if they need medical attention and the office is closed.

If the office has an answering machine, voice mail, or answering service, an assistant should not rely on these alternatives to answer the phone during business hours.

Answering Machine

An answering machine is probably the most affordable after-hours solution available. Single line phones and many phones with multiple lines can be connected to an answering machine. Answering machines generally cost between $30 and $50 and usually last for many years.

When using an answering machine to handle after-hours calls, the machine should be set to not allow messages to be recorded after hours. Individuals may call with a serious medical situation and may expect a return call if they leave a message. An outgoing message should be recorded that instructs the patient as to what should be done to get needed medical treatment until the office opens again. A message like the following might be used:

You have reached Horizons Healthcare Center. Our office is now closed. If you are calling about a medical emergency, please hang up and call 911. If you need immediate medical attention for a reason other than an emergency, 24-hour urgent care services are available at our facility located at 123 Main Avenue in Farmington. Our regular office hours are 9 AM to 6 PM weekdays and 9 AM to 12 PM on Saturday. Thank you for calling.

Voice Mail

A **voice mail** service may also be used to handle telephone traffic. Voice mail works like an answering machine in that a recorded message from the medical office plays when the phone line is not answered after a certain number of rings. Voice mail does allow incoming messages to be recorded when the line is not answered or when the line is busy. Messages may then be played back when the assistant accesses the voice mail system.

Answering Services

An answering service is an outside company that provides individuals who answer the office telephone (at an offsite location) when the practice is closed. This alternative is used by practices that prefer to not have a machine or recording answer the telephone. An answering service answers the telephone during off hours and may then give specific instructions to a patient regarding after-hours care or may relay a message from a patient to an on-call provider. Answering services charge a monthly fee for services rendered.

Telephone Screening

Because of the large volume of telephone traffic that most medical offices experience, screening incoming calls is an absolute necessity in the medical office.

The screening process involves obtaining enough information about the call to either handle it at the front desk or give the call to the proper department. Screening actually reduces the amount of calls that go back to the physician or nurse. If someone else in the office can handle a call, that makes the physician's time more productive. If at all possible, calls should be handled by the front desk.

Many patients will often call the medical office and ask to speak to the physician directly. It is not often that such a call is transferred directly to the physician. Nearly all physicians prefer to have a message taken and to then have the message attached to the patient's chart. Physicians must have the patient's chart to be familiar with the fine points of the patient's medical history and to document any call regarding medical treatment or advice given to the patient.

Identifying Emergencies over the Telephone

Occasionally, a patient (or relative of a patient) may telephone the clinic with a serious problem that may constitute an emergency regarding the patient's health. The person phoning in may not realize that the symptoms could cause a serious threat to the health of the patient. The medical administrative assistant must be aware of symptoms that could constitute a potentially serious health situation.

An emergency may be defined as a situation in which a patient's health might be adversely affected if immediate action is not taken. Box 6–1 outlines some critical symptoms of which an assistant should be aware. This list is not an all-inclusive list but is designed to introduce the assistant to some of the more common symptoms that may indicate an emergency situation. An assistant should review the list with the physicians in the practice to determine whether the list is inclusive enough for their office.

When you receive a questionable call in the clinic, you should be careful to not diagnose the patient, alarm the patient, or place the patient at undue risk. If a patient phones in with chest pain, before taking a message or making an appointment, an appropriate response by the assistant would be "I'd like to have you speak with the nurse before I take a message" or "I'd like to have you speak with the nurse before I make an appointment."

Box 6–1 Potential Emergency Situations

If you receive a call regarding a patient who is experiencing any of the symptoms listed here, a medical professional should assess the situation immediately.*

- Shortness of breath
- Chest pain or pressure
- Pain in upper left arm
- Extreme dizziness or complaints of vertigo
- Loss of consciousness
- Serious injury or trauma such as broken bones or head injury
- Sudden numbness or tingling
- Blurred vision
- Slurred speech
- Severe, unrelenting headache
- Profuse, uncontrolled bleeding
- Acute abdominal pain

*This list is not inclusive.

The patient should *never* be told she might be having a heart attack. That statement may be interpreted as diagnosing the patient. The assistant should also be careful to not ask too many questions, because the patient may feel the assistant is prying and because the amount of questions may frighten the patient. The patient should also not be told to go to the emergency room. Imagine what might happen if a patient gets in her car and drives to the emergency room. If she is having a heart attack, she could go into cardiac arrest while driving and die on the way to the hospital.

When the physician or nurse speaks directly to the patient and determines that the patient may be experiencing a life-threatening situation, the physician or nurse will instruct the patient to call 911 immediately.

If you are wondering whether or not a situation is a potential emergency, remember this rule: *When in doubt, check it out!* Don't be afraid to check with the physician or nurse regarding any situation you are unsure about.

Physician Out of the Office

If the physician is out of the office and unavailable, tell the patient that "Dr. Lopez is not in the office, but Dr. O'Brian is taking her calls" or "She's out of the office until (date). May I take a message or transfer you to . . .?" Don't mention that the physician is on vacation unless the physician approves. The physician may not want "the whole world" to know she is not at home.

Complaint Calls

No one enjoys answering complaint calls, but if you should happen to get a call from a patient who is unhappy, follow these general guidelines for handling complaints.

- Acknowledge there is a problem.
- Ask the patient what you can do to help. If you can help the patient, do so. If you cannot help, find someone who can.
- Don't "pass the buck." Help the patient if possible.
- Keep your cool even if the patient is angry.
- Don't make excuses such as, "We're short-staffed today" or, "The computer's down" or, "We're so busy." All these excuses convey is poor planning on the part of the practice.
- Do what you can to make sure the problem does not happen again. Take the problem and ideas for potential solutions to your supervisor if necessary.

Taking Messages

When reviewing the telephone protocol as presented in this chapter, you will note that many calls require that a message be taken. It is important that enough information be obtained in each message in order to handle the call. It is also important to remember that a message is taken to help the patient in some way and that complete, detailed information will be needed to assist the patient as much as possible.

Frequently, telephone messages become part of the patient's medical record. It is critical to realize that what you are writing on the message may some day be a part of a patient's permanent medical record. Because the message blanks themselves are sometimes included directly in the medical record, they are often a full half or quarter sheet of paper to allow the physician or nurse to document the action taken on the message (Fig. 6–3) and to allow the message to be easily affixed inside the chart.

When an assistant realizes that a message will need to be taken, a message blank should be obtained and the components of the message noted. Each telephone message will contain nine essential pieces of information necessary to process the message (Procedure 6–2).

1. **Date and time of call.** On every message, list the complete date (month, day, and year) that the call came in. If the practice is open extended hours, AM or PM should be identified with time.
2. **Caller's name.** The caller's complete name should be obtained.
3. **Patient's name.** If the patient's name is different from the caller's name, be sure to obtain the complete name of the patient. In the case of a parent calling on behalf of a child, the call will be returned to the parent, but the medical staff will need the patient's medical chart when speaking with the parent. If a caller is not the patient, the caller's relationship to the patient should always be noted.
4. **Chart number.** If the call involves anything in regard to the patient's health or medical history, the patient's chart will be needed. The physician may need to review

PROCEDURE 6–2 Demonstrate Taking Telephone Messages

Materials Needed

- Telephone set-up with two separate lines
- Message blanks
- Pencil

1. Determine that a message is needed for an incoming telephone call and obtain a message blank to record the message.
2. Record date and time on message blank.
3. Record caller's name on message blank.
4. Record patient's name on message blank.*
5. Obtain patient's chart number. If chart number is not available, obtain patient's date of birth to help locate the chart number.
6. Record name of individual to whom the call is directed—physician or another individual.
7. Record message narrative including action requested on message blank.
8. Record telephone number to return call.
9. Sign the message with your name or initials.

*Denotes a crucial step in the procedure. This step must be completed satisfactorily for the procedure to be completed satisfactorily.

MESSAGE FROM								
For Dr. Sanchez	Name of Caller Nancy Stevens	Rel. to pt. Mom	Patient Evan Stevens	Pt. Age 3	Pt. Temp. 100	Message Date 8/4/xx	Message Time 11:16 (AM) PM	Urgent ☐ Yes ☒ No

Message: Evan has had temp from 100–102 for 2 days –	Allergies
cough & thick green discharge from nose	

Respond to Phone # 555-3456	Best Time To Call any AM PM	Pharmacy Name/#	Patient's Chart Attached ☒ Yes ☐ No	Patient's Chart # 689723	Initials MAA

DOCTOR–STAFF RESPONSE

Doctor's/Staff Orders/Follow-up Action

Mom reports purulent nasal discharge, productive cough, ↑ temp and HA.

Instructed to make appt for today.

Call Back ☒ Yes ☐ No	Chart Mes. ☒ Yes ☐ No	Follow-up Date 8/4/xx	Follow-up Completed–Date/Time 8/4/xx 11:45 (AM) PM	Response By: MMS

Figure 6–3. A message blank may include a section for the physician or nurse to record how the call was handled. (Form courtesy of Bibbero Systems, Inc., Petaluma, California, 800-242-2376. Fax, 800-242-9330. Available at www.bibbero.com.)

patient's past medical history or medications and will need to make a notation in the chart regarding the disposition of the call. If the patient does not know his or her chart number, obtain the patient's date of birth to identify his or her record. If a patient calls with a medical question and is a new patient to the practice, obtain the patient's date of birth to check the practice's records for any possible information. It should then be noted on the message that the patient is new or does not have a chart with the practice.

5. ***Provider name or the person who is called.*** This identifies the individual to whom the call is directed.

6. ***Operator (person receiving the call—Assistant's name or initials)*** The assistant taking a message must sign each message. If the medical staff has a question about the message, they may need to talk directly to the assistant. In most offices, the operator may be identified with his or her initials.

7. ***Message narrative.*** Information given to the assistant in the conversation with the patient should be listed on the message. This includes the patient's concern or reason for calling the medical office. The assistant should also include action requested by the caller. Often, options for action are listed on the message blank. A box to check in front of items such as "please return call" or "urgent" may be included on the message blank. The assistant may also need to write a patient's request for action in the message narrative. An example would be a request that a prescription be filled at a particular pharmacy.

8. ***Telephone number.*** A telephone number where the caller can be reached should be obtained for each message. If the caller will be available only at a certain time, note the availability near the telephone number (e.g., "555-1122 after 3 PM"). Some callers may want to leave more than one number, such as a cell phone number or work number. If the office serves a large geographic area or is located near a state border, remember to include an area code with the telephone number.

Telephone Equipment

The telephone is not the only piece of telephone equipment in the medical office. Many other devices either work in conjunction with the office telephone or may operate independent of the office telephone.

Telephones

Many different kinds of telephones are readily available in the marketplace. The size of the practice will dictate just how much telephone equipment is needed. Most offices require a phone with speaker or intercom connections to allow calls to be transferred within the office easily.

A telephone with at least two lines is necessary (Fig. 6–4) for even the smallest of practices to ensure that patients call-

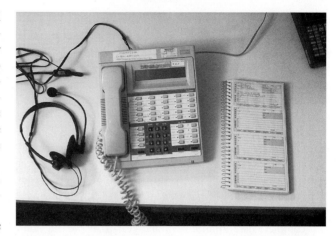

Figure 6–4. Multiline telephones are necessary for the medical office to accommodate patients calling in and staff calling out.

ing in will be able to reach the office and that office personnel (physicians and nurses) and communications equipment (fax machines and computers) have outside phone access.

Switchboard

Larger practices will likely have a switchboard system that allows calls to be answered by a central switchboard operator (Fig. 6–5). Computerized switchboard systems are now available to help track the flow of telephone traffic within the office.

Some switchboard systems allow calls to bypass the switchboard. This bypass can occur when the caller, instead of calling the main switchboard, dials an extension number directly. The call then goes directly to the intended recipient without having to be handled by the switchboard operator. Dialing an extension directly helps reduce the amount of calls handled by the switchboard. A direct-dial number might be used to allow a hospital laboratory department to reach a clinic laboratory directly or vice versa. This type of call would not need to be handled by the switchboard.

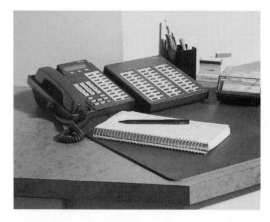

Figure 6–5. Large medical practices have a central switchboard that directs calls to the proper area in the practice. (From Kinn ME, Woods MA: The Medical Assistant: Clinical and Administrative, 8th ed., Philadelphia, WB Saunders, 1998.)

Pager

Very often, a physician may need to be contacted when not in the clinic. A pager can be used to reach physicians in such an instance.

To reach a physician using a pager, an assistant simply needs to call the pager's telephone number and leave a message. Depending on the type of pager service, the assistant may either leave a verbal message or may enter a telephone number for the physician to call. An important point to remember when leaving a verbal message is *patient confidentiality*. You will not know exactly where the physician may be when the message is played; do not leave any message that could cause embarrassment to a patient.

Cell Phone

Cell phones, too, can help the physician stay in touch with the office when the physician is away. Cell phones are very reasonably priced and allow physicians to stay in immediate contact with the practice.

Once a cell phone has been purchased, there are many different types of calling plans for cell phone use. For a monthly fee, the user purchases a certain amount of minutes and is then charged per minute if the monthly allotment of minutes is exceeded. Calling plans may include one or more cell phones that share minutes and may have special plans for callers using a large amount of long-distance minutes.

A major concern with cell phone use is that calls may be intercepted or overheard by others. Obviously, for this reason, confidential information should not be discussed over a cell phone.

Headsets

Headsets are small devices similar to headsets for a music player that fit over the operator's head (Fig. 6–6). Headsets, however, also contain a microphone that allows the operator to carry on a complete conversation with the caller. Headsets are particularly useful because they allow operators to use their hands while on the telephone. The devices plug directly into the telephone and can allow an operator to answer the telephone with either the handset or the headset.

Using a headset is a good idea if an assistant is spending a large amount of time on the telephone. It is very difficult to balance a handset on a shoulder and to try to write a message or type information into a computer at the same time. If a headset is not used, over a period of time, a "shoulder balancing" posture may cause an assistant to develop a neck injury as a result of repeated incorrect posture.

If a headset is used in a reception area where patients are assisted, many patients may not see the headset and may begin speaking to the assistant while the assistant is on the telephone. When a patient approaches the desk, the assistant will need to allow the patient to see that the assistant is speaking with a patient on the telephone.

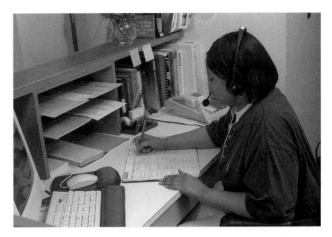

Figure 6–6. A headset allows a medical administrative assistant to write message and operate a computer while on the telephone with a patient.

Facsimile

A facsimile or fax machine (Fig. 6–7) is a valuable piece of equipment in the medical office. Fax machines allow printed data to be transmitted almost instantly to another location anywhere in the world. A document is read electronically by one fax machine at one location and transmitted to a fax machine at another location.

Confidentiality concerns also exist with the use of a fax machine. A patient's medical information should not be sent via fax without the patient's expressed consent. In the case of an emergency or life-threatening situation, faxed material may be sent without the patient's knowledge if the information is needed to treat the patient; however such a release of information occurs infrequently.

When transmitting medical information by fax, an assistant must exercise great care in entering the fax number. One incorrect number, and sensitive information could end up in the wrong hands.

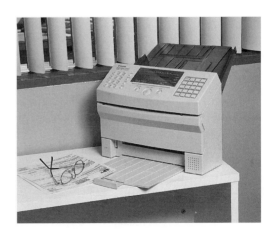

Figure 6–7. A medical administrative assistant should use a fax machine with caution in the medical office. (From Kinn ME, Woods MA: The Medical Assistant: Clinical and Administrative, 8th ed., Philadelphia, WB Saunders, 1998.)

Telephone Services

Several additional services may be available from local phone companies. These services may enhance the customer service that the office staff is able to provide. The practice will need to weigh the potential benefit of the services with the cost of the service. The following services may be of benefit to a medical office:

- **Caller ID.** A small device is attached to the phone or built into the phone. Caller ID displays the number and name of who is calling before the call is answered.
- **Three-way calling.** This feature allows three parties in three separate locations to speak simultaneously. This may be particularly helpful in phone conferences among one or more physicians, a patient, and one or more family members.
- **Call forwarding.** Calls are forwarded from one phone number to another. If a medical office is closed during a vacation, calls may be forwarded to another physician's office that may be taking calls for the physician.
- **Conference calls.** With this feature, several individuals at different locations may speak with each other simultaneously. Three or more parties at separate locations can all be connected on the same call.

Outgoing Calls

Although most of the practice's calls will be incoming calls, occasionally an assistant will need to call a patient.

If long-distance calls will need to be made, an assistant may wish to wait to make calls at a time that may be less costly to the practice. Depending on the long-distance calling plan of the practice, certain times of the day may be cheaper to make long distance calls. Plans are also sometimes available that have very low long-distance rates during daytime hours. Some practices have toll-free lines, but it may be cheaper to call long-distance and pay the per-minute charge and reserve the toll-free line for incoming long-distance calls.

Using a Telephone Directory

The traditional printed telephone directories contain a wealth of information about telephone service as well as information about the community. Information regarding calling features, area codes, and how to obtain services is available in most telephone directories. Community information, such as local area maps, local zip codes, and community services are also frequently found in many directories. An assistant should take the time to review the local phone directory to be familiar with the type of information that is available in the directory.

Web Directories

Many on-line directories are now appearing on the Internet. These electronic directories allow users to search for an address or telephone number for a business or a person in any state. The directories are available usually free to the user and are paid for by the advertisers who sponsor the site. Using an electronic directory can help save money, compared with having to use a long-distance directory service.

Developing a Personal Directory

A personal directory of frequently called numbers should be kept on hand at the front desk. It is the responsibility of the front desk staff to maintain a directory of telephone numbers for physicians and other staff members as well as for other businesses that are frequently contacted by the office. These numbers should be recorded in an easy-to-use reference, such as a computer list or a desktop rotary file. The directories should then be placed at the front desk and at other office telephones to allow easy accessibility.

Frequently called numbers can be stored in memory on many telephones. This storage can substantially reduce the amount of time it takes to dial a frequently called number. If the practice is continually calling a laboratory, another physician's office, or surgery center, storing these numbers in the telephone's memory can save a lot of time.

Leaving Messages for Patients

If a patient is not at home, the practice may wish that the assistant leave a message for the patient. Depending on the nature of the practice and the wishes of the practice's physicians, however, a message may be left asking a patient to return a call to the practice. Obviously, practices such as mental health clinics or human immunodeficiency virus treatment centers would not leave messages for patients because if the wrong person hears the message, the nature of the patient's treatment may be implied by the call.

When leaving a message, remember not to divulge any confidential information. Exercise extreme caution when leaving any message for a patient. There is no way of knowing who may listen to the message. Some practices prefer to never leave a message for a patient. A message as simple as "Call Amy at 555-3424 about your appointment" may seem harmless enough but may actually cause problems if the patient does not want a spouse to know about the appointment. It is best to consult with the practice's physicians to establish a policy on leaving messages.

WRITTEN COMMUNICATION

All business cannot be conducted over the telephone or in person, and, occasionally, an assistant will need to write a letter to a patient or a memo to office staff members. When communicating in the written form, it is imperative that proper grammar rules be followed. Your written word is a reflection of you and the practice.

When writing correspondence, a good set of reference materials are a must. A well-stocked office library would include medical and English dictionaries, medical word books, pharmaceutical references, and style references such as *The Gregg Reference Manual*. These references will be used frequently to look up spelling and appropriate usage of terms as well as style of written correspondence. Many electronic references are also available for computer systems. Many word processing packages have templates or sample formats available for easy letter and memo writing.

Business Letters

Letters in the medical office are written on 8 1/2" × 11" office letterhead. The letterhead contains the name and complete address along with the telephone number or numbers of the practice. Any practice logos are also present, and, if the practice is small, names of the providers are also included. Some very large practices with many physicians may choose to print the names of the physicians in a lighter ink on the back of the stationery. Copies of all letters to patients are filed in the appropriate patient chart, and copies of all other correspondence are filed in the appropriate office file. See Procedure 6–3 for a summary of how to prepare business correspondence.

Components of a Letter

All letters have the same basic components, beginning with the date the letter is written. After the date, the inside address (the address of the individual to whom the letter is sent) is listed, followed by the salutation or opening greeting of the letter. Next, the body of the letter begins with a subject line (if any) listed first. In a medical office, the subject line information is usually a patient's name and chart number for reference. The remainder of the body is information the sender wants to convey. Once the body is completed, the closing contains a complimentary closing, such as *Sincerely* or *Very truly yours*, the author's name, reference initials, computer file name notation (if applicable), enclosure notation, and copy notation. Examples of letters are shown in Figures 6–8, 6–9 and 6–10 with line spacing for each line noted on the left-hand margin.

Proper Format

There are various ways to format a business letter properly. Some of the more commonly used formats are the block style (see Fig. 6–8) and modified block style (see Figs. 6–9 and 6–10).

Most letters begin 2 inches from the top of the page. This spacing allows room for any letterhead that may be used. Occasionally, a letter may be lengthy and may begin closer to the top of the page to accommodate the letter on one page. Be sure to leave enough room at the top and bottom of the page to have a professional looking letter. Spacing for the various components of a letter appears on Figures 6–8 and 6–9.

Top and bottom margins should be set at 1 inch. Depending on the type of word-processing software you may use, default settings for side margins may vary from 1 inch to 1.25 inches. Margins can be adjusted for both short and long letters to make the letters look more appealing on the page.

Block Style

A block style letter is probably the easiest type of letter to produce. All letter components are flush with the left margin of the page. No indentations are used in this style, with the exception of any tables or other elements that may need to be set apart in the body of the letter. An example of a block style letter is shown in Figure 6–8.

Modified Block Style

The modified block style differs from the block style in that the date, complimentary closing, and author's signature begin in the center of the page. The remaining information is flush with the left margin (see Fig. 6–9). If the author prefers to indent the paragraphs in the body of the letter, this type of letter is known as a modified block style with indented paragraphs (see Fig. 6–10).

PROCEDURE 6–3 *Prepare a Patient Letter*

Materials Needed

- Computer with word processing software
- Printer
- Letterhead stationery
- #10 business envelope
- Reference materials as necessary (e.g., dictionary, grammar reference)

1. Prepare a letter to a patient using the proper format illustrated in Figures 6–8, 6–9, or 6–10.
2. Proofread the letter for proper grammar and punctuation.*
3. Print enough copies of the letter.
4. Address a business envelope using proper format for an OCR as shown in Figure 6–11.
5. Fold and insert letter in an envelope as shown in Figure 6–12.

Denotes a crucial step in the procedure. This step must be completed satisfactorily for the procedure to be completed satisfactorily.

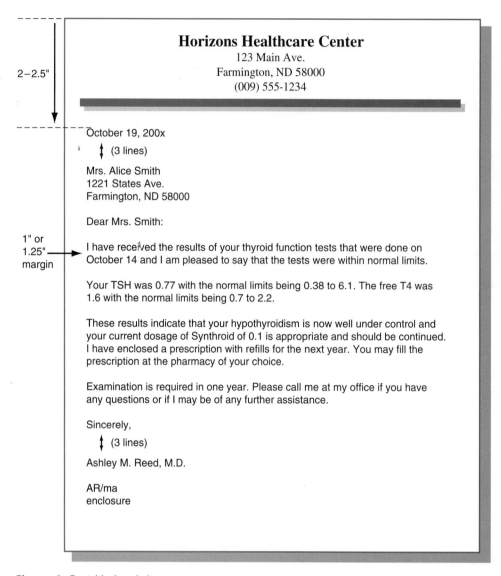

Figure 6–8. A block style letter.

Envelopes

Standard-size #10 business envelopes are used for business correspondence. Figure 6–11 demonstrates the proper format for addressing a business envelope. When addressing an envelope, capital letters and no punctuation are used to allow the address to be read by a machine called an Optical Character Reader (OCR) used by the U.S. Postal Service.

When placing the letter in an envelope, the letter should be folded in thirds and inserted as indicated in Figure 6–12. This method of folding allows the letter to be removed easily when received and to be read by the recipient.

Letter Portfolio

It is a good idea to develop a portfolio of the varieties of letters written in the medical office. Simply saving copies of letters in a printed file or computer file develops a letter portfolio. Later, when an assistant is asked to compose a letter, a portfolio provides excellent examples of letter "how-to's."

When compiling a letter portfolio, an assistant should delete any patient references in the letter—name, address, chart number, and any other identifying information–that may be confidential.

Memos

Memos are used internally in the office. A memo allows information to be communicated in an efficient format to other staff members in the office. Memos may be written on blank sheets of paper or letterhead. It is inappropriate to write to a patient using a memo format. An example of a memo is shown in Figure 6–13.

Components

The heading of a memo contains four basic pieces of information. The first item is *to* whom the memo is sent,

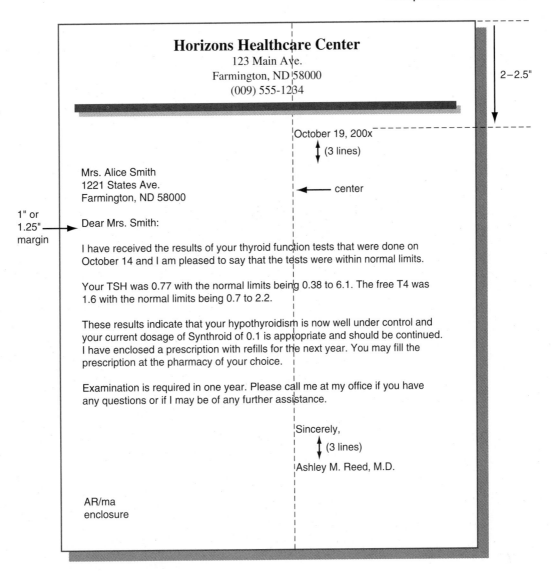

Figure 6–9. A modified block style letter.

usually followed by to whom the memo is *from*. Next, the *date* is listed, followed by the *subject* of the memo.

After the heading is completed, the body of the memo should begin on the third line below the last line of the heading. Occasionally, a signature line is added to the bottom of a memo, but it is also common practice for the memo's author to initial after his or her name on the *from* line.

Reference initials belonging to the person who keyed the memo and a computer file name can be added to two lines below the body of the memo.

Proper Format

Memos should begin 2 inches from the top of the page. Occasionally, letterhead may be too large, and the starting line may need to be moved a few lines down the page.

Side margins are similar to that of letters, either 1 inch or 1.25 inches, depending on the default settings of the office software. Margins may be adjusted to accommodate short or long memos (Procedure 6–4).

E-mail

An **electronic mail message,** or **e-mail,** is a quick, efficient way to communicate internally in the office. Almost instantly, a printed message can be sent virtually anywhere. E-mail can be sent to one individual or to a group of individuals. If the medical office sends e-mail to and receives e-mail from patients, the message system should be checked several times daily to keep up to date with messages from patients.

Because it is so easy to use, e-mail is sometimes overused. You should be careful not to e-mail anything unless it is necessary. Because of the volumes of e-mail some offices produce, it is not unusual for someone to be gone from the office for a couple of days and come back to find 50 or even 100 e-mail messages.

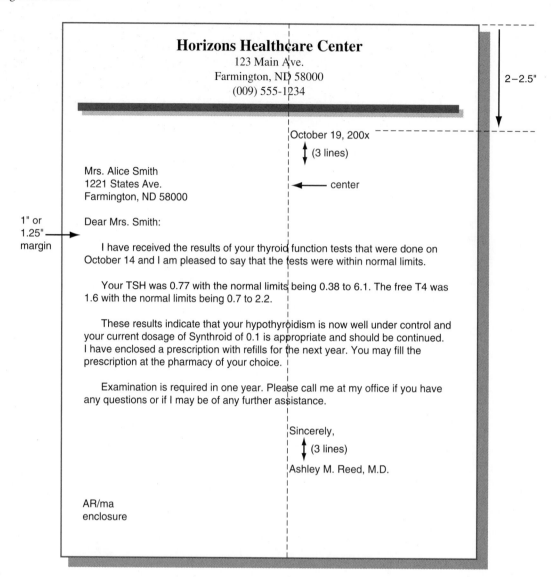

Figure 6–10. A modified block style letter with indented paragraphs.

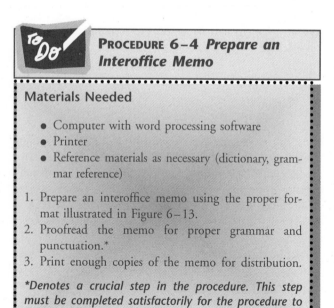

PROCEDURE 6–4 *Prepare an Interoffice Memo*

Materials Needed

- Computer with word processing software
- Printer
- Reference materials as necessary (dictionary, grammar reference)

1. Prepare an interoffice memo using the proper format illustrated in Figure 6–13.
2. Proofread the memo for proper grammar and punctuation.*
3. Print enough copies of the memo for distribution.

Denotes a crucial step in the procedure. This step must be completed satisfactorily for the procedure to be completed satisfactorily.

With the increased use of computers today, many patients may soon use e-mail to contact the medical office. Because the nature of the e-mail environment is not totally secure and messages can be easily passed back and forth, confidential information should not be included in e-mail communication with patients. A printed copy of all e-mail from a patient should be kept in the patient's chart.

As the use of e-mail continues to increase, e-mail users must be careful to use proper e-mail etiquette when writing messages. Proper etiquette for business use includes the following:

- *Never* type messages in solid capital letters (e.g., "THIS NEEDS TO BE DONE IMMEDIATELY"). The use of solid capital letters is equivalent to shouting at the other person.
- It is acceptable to use all lowercase letters for casual e-mail conversations. Everything, including the beginning of sentences, may be typed in lowercase letters. When communicating with patients, however, appropriate business grammar should be used.

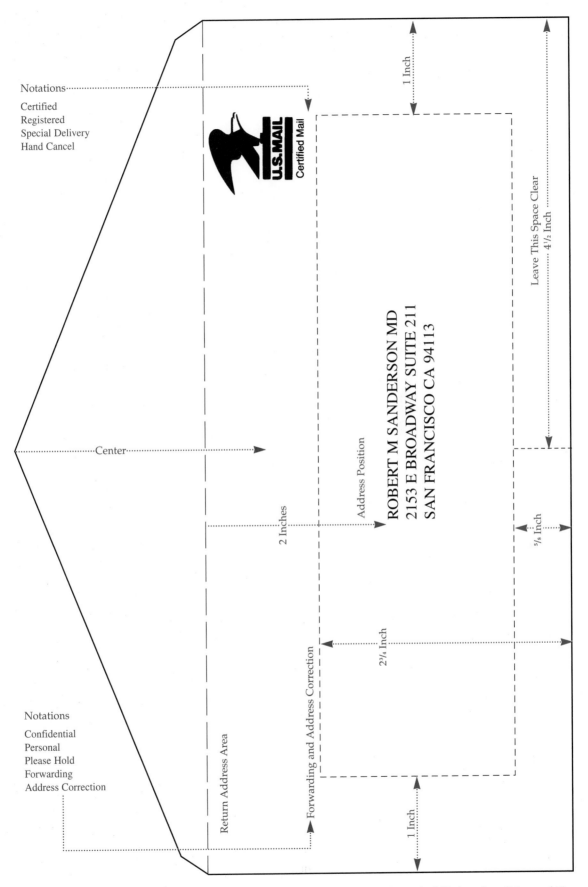

Figure 6–11. Proper format of a business envelope. (From Diehl MO, Fordney MT: Medical Keyboarding, Tying, and Transcribing, 4th ed., Philadelphia, WB Saunders, 1997.)

No. 10 Envelope (9-1/2 x 4-1/8 Inches)

_DO_ bring up the bottom third of the sheet, and crease. Fold down the upper third of the sheet so the top edge is a one-inch from the first fold, and crease. Insert the last creased edge into the envelope first.

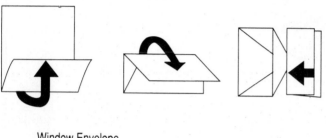

Window Envelope

Figure 6–12. Folding and inserting a letter into a business envelope. (From Fordney MT, Diehl MO: Medical Transcription Guide: Do's and Don'ts. Philadelphia, WB Saunders, 1990.)

_DO_ bring up the bottom third of the sheet and fold. Fold the top of the sheet _back_ to the first fold so that the inside address is on the outside, and crease. Insert the sheet so the address appears in the window.

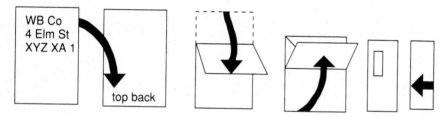

- Be brief and as precise as possible. Oftentimes miscommunication may occur because each individual may react differently to the same statement. Remember, as the message is read, the sender of the statement has no opportunity to see the reaction of the receiver.
- The use of symbols conveying feeling, sometimes known as _emoticons_, may help bridge a possible communication gap. A colon and right parenthesis—:)—signifies the sender's happiness during communication.
- Above all, avoid discussing sensitive issues or serious subjects via e-mail. The likelihood that the message will be misunderstood is great, and a more personal form of communication (in person or telephone call) should be used to avoid misunderstanding.

CHECKPOINT

Explain the importance of deleting patient references from sample letters even though the letters remain in the office.

United States Postal Service Delivery Services

The majority of the medical office's written correspondence will be handled through the U.S. Postal Service. The more common postal delivery methods used by medical offices include city delivery and post office box delivery.

With city delivery, mail is delivered directly to the front desk or central mailroom depending on the size of the practice. City delivery is convenient in that the postal carrier can leave the incoming mail, and outgoing mail may be picked up by the carrier to be taken to the post office.

Post office box delivery service is available for a nominal fee at most post offices. Up to five different sizes of boxes may be available from which to choose, and the size of the box determines the cost. Mail in a post office box may be retrieved any time that the post office lobby is open.

Processing Incoming Mail

In almost all offices, mail is received every day. As mentioned previously, it may be delivered directly to the office

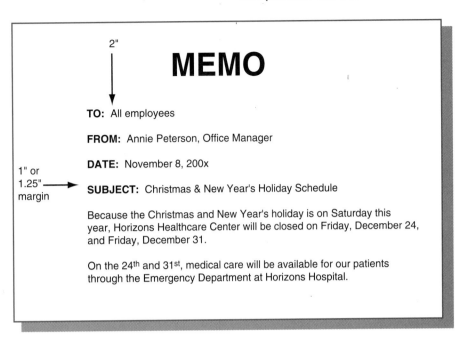

Figure 6–13. Proper format for an office memo.

2"

MEMO

TO: All employees

FROM: Annie Peterson, Office Manager

DATE: November 8, 200x

1" or 1.25" margin

SUBJECT: Christmas & New Year's Holiday Schedule

Because the Christmas and New Year's holiday is on Saturday this year, Horizons Healthcare Center will be closed on Friday, December 24, and Friday, December 31.

On the 24th and 31st, medical care will be available for our patients through the Emergency Department at Horizons Hospital.

or picked up at a post office box. Whatever the case, it is important that once the mail is received in the office, it must be handled in an expeditious manner.

Every piece of mail that comes into the office should be opened unless it is marked confidential. Confidential mailings should be opened only by the intended recipient.

On opening the mail, letters and other personal documents should be stamped with the date on which they were received. A machine or rubber stamp may be used to easily record the date on the document. In addition to the date stamp, sometimes a physician may prefer to have the envelope stapled directly behind the letter.

After the mail has been dated, any correspondence pertaining to a patient should have the patient's chart number noted on the correspondence. Letters and copies of medical records from other facilities that are received will need to be filed in the patient's chart. Therefore, the assistant will need to look up the patient's chart number and write the chart number on the correspondence.

After all chart numbers have been found, all correspondence that has been received will need to be attached to the patient's medical chart. Frequently, physicians ask their patients to obtain another facility's records for the patient's current medical record. The correspondence that is received should be paper clipped or attached in some way to the front of the chart and should be placed on the physician's desk for review.

After the mail has been dated, chart numbers have been found, and charts have been attached, the mail is now ready for distribution inside the clinic. Because the volume of mail in most offices is quite considerable, it is a good idea to sort the mail in designated bins or slots for each physician or recipient (Fig. 6–14). Often, you may need to stop and assist a patient in the middle of sorting the mail. For that reason, it is a good idea to use some type of organizing receptacle for sorting the mail and not to have it strewn all over the desk.

Medical information received about a patient should never be filed inside the patient's chart without the physician's review of the correspondence. If important information is filed in a patient's chart without the physician reviewing the information, a potential legal problem could result if the information is needed in the treatment of the patient. After reviewing the correspondence, the physician should initial and date the correspondence in a conspicuous place to indicate that the physician has reviewed the document. The correspondence may then be filed in the patient's chart.

Processing Outgoing Mail

Many types of services are available for sending mail. The postal rates vary considerably depending on the type of service you choose.

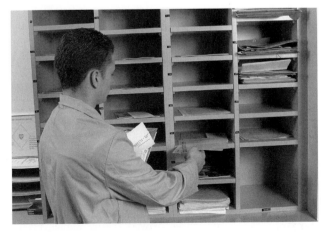

Figure 6–14. A central location for sorting mail and other office documents allows for easy distribution of all office correspondence.

```
UNITED STATES POSTAL SERVICE          ‖‖‖‖       First-Class Mail
                                                 Postage & Fees Paid
                                                 USPS
                                                 Permit No. G-10

        ● Print your name, address, and ZIP Code in this box ●

                    KENNETH B MERETTI MD
                    483 SO AUGUSTA STREET
                    MARINELAND CA 90000
```

SENDER:
- Complete items 1 and/or 2 for additional services.
- Complete items 3, 4a, and 4b.
- Print your name and address on the reverse of this form so that we can return this card to you.
- Attach this form to the front of the mailpiece, or on the back if space does not permit.
- Write *"Return Receipt Requested"* on the mailpiece below the article number.
- The Return Receipt will show to whom the article was delivered and the date delivered.

I also wish to receive the following services (for an extra fee):

1. ☐ Addressee's Address
2. ☐ Restricted Delivery

Consult postmaster for fee.

3. Article Addressed to:

W. B. SAUNDERS COMPANY
INDEPENDENCE SQUARE WEST
PHILADELPHIA PA 19106-3399

4a. Article Number

4b. Service Type
☐ Registered   ☐ Certified
☐ Express Mail   ☐ Insured
☐ Return Receipt for Merchandise   ☐ COD

7. Date of Delivery

5. Received By: *(Print Name)*

8. Addressee's Address *(Only if requested and fee is paid)*

6. Signature: *(Addressee or Agent)*
X

Is your RETURN ADDRESS completed on the reverse side?

Thank you for using Return Receipt Service.

PS Form **3811**, December 1994   **Domestic Return Receipt**

Figure 6–15. Sending a letter certified with return receipt gives the sender proof that a letter was received. (From Kinn ME: The Administrative Medical Assistant, 4th ed, Philadelphia, WB Saunders, 1999.)

First Class

First class mail rates apply to almost all of the mail that will be sent out by a medical office. First class mail covers letters, postcards, and the like. If mail is larger than letter-size, it should be marked "First Class" to ensure proper, more expedient handling.

Express Mail

Express Mail is the fastest delivery service offered by the U.S. Postal Service. Most Express Mail packages are guaran-teed delivery overnight. Usually, mail must be brought in by 5 PM to qualify for overnight express mail service. Delivery is then made by 3 PM the next day. Express Mail may be deposited in an Express Mail delivery box or may be picked up by the letter carrier. The U.S. Postal Service provides containers and mailing labels for Express Mail packages at no charge. Packages are allowed to weigh up to 2 pounds, and the rate stays the same no matter what the package weighs. Express mail is very costly compared with regular mail services and is used only if a package requires expedi-ent delivery.

Priority Mail

For larger packages that need quick delivery, priority mail provides delivery service for packages weighing up to 70 pounds. Local postal offices will provide Priority Mail boxes, stickers, and envelopes at no charge. Priority Mail should be well marked to ensure proper handling by the Postal Service.

Certified with Return Receipt

Sometimes, it is necessary to have proof that a letter has been mailed and received. In this case, the letter should be sent certified with a return receipt (Fig. 6–15). This service assigns a number to the delivery and requires that a signature be obtained at the time of delivery. This service is necessary to document important notifications to patients, such as withdrawal of medical services.

For complete information on all of the postal services that are available from the United States Postal Service, visit their Web site at www.usps.gov.

Postage Machines

Most offices today have some type of postage machine (Fig. 6–16) that stamps postage directly on envelopes or on postage meter adhesive strips. Postage meter strips are affixed to any larger packages that cannot fit through a machine. Postage machines have a descending meter that tracks how much postage is left in the machine. When the postage left in the machine reaches a certain amount (sometimes, less than $100), the machine automatically shuts off, and more postage must be purchased for the machine before it can be used again.

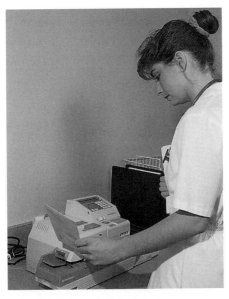

Figure 6–16. A postage machine allows postage to be affixed to letters and packages at the office. (From Chester GA: Modern Medical Assisting. Philadelphia, WB Saunders, 1998.)

A postage machine saves the office considerable time in that the mail may be weighed and stamped at the office and then deposited for delivery.

Presort Mail Services

For practices that process large amounts of mail to specific ZIP codes, discount rates may be available for first class delivery services if a presort mail service is used. Presort involves sorting the mail by ZIP code before it is delivered to the post office. Offices may save a few cents for each letter that is sent at the presort rate. It may not sound like much, but, in the long run, the savings really do add up!

Private Courier Services

Private courier services such as FedEx or United Parcel Service (UPS) provide alternatives to services offered by the U.S. Postal Service. Private couriers usually specialize in certain types of delivery, such as overnight delivery or package services. Different rates are available depending on what type of service is needed.

SUMMARY

As a medical administrative assistant, you will interact with patients and others every day in one way or another. It is absolutely critical that you use the proper communication skills and techniques to ensure a more effective and smooth running office environment.

The telephone is the central communication tool used between office staff members and patients, and professional telephone communication skills must be used by staff members to maintain the professional image of the medical office. A consistent telephone protocol will ensure that calls are handled in a professional and appropriate manner. Because the telephone is the key piece of equipment used by patients when contacting the medical office, attention must be paid to how callers are screened, asked to hold, assisted, and transferred. A variety of telephone communications equipment helps provide professional service to patients.

Sometimes, the office needs to communicate with a patient in writing. It is normally the medical administrative assistant's responsibility to type (and sometimes compose) a letter for a patient. Proper grammar and document formatting skills must be used when producing business correspondence. A medical office sends and receives correspondence each day that must be processed internally within the office before it is filed in a patient's chart or picked up for delivery.

Whether conversing with a patient in person, on the telephone, or via written correspondence, an assistant must be professional at all times and strive to meet the patient's needs whenever possible. Professional customer oriented communication is the foundation to a long-lasting relationship between the patient and the medical office.

Bibliography

Ballweg R, Stolberg S, Sullivan EM: Physician Assistant: A Guide to Clinical Practice, 2nd ed. Philadelphia, WB Saunders, 1999.

Diehl MO, Fordney MT: Medical Keyboarding, Typing, and Transcribing: Techniques and Procedures, 4th ed. Philadelphia, WB Saunders, 1997.

O'Toole M: Miller-Keane Encyclopedia & Dictionary of Medicine, Nursing, & Allied Health, 5th ed. Philadelphia, WB Saunders, 1992.

Calling 911. Postgrad Med: 154, 1994.

Sabin WA: Gregg Reference Manual, 8th ed. New York, Glencoe McGraw-Hill, 2001.

Sieh A, Brentin LK: The Nurse Communicates. Philadelphia, WB Saunders, 1997.

United States Postal Service: Available at www.usps.gov. Accessed December 1, 2000.

Exercise 6–1 TRUE OR FALSE

Read each statement and determine whether the statement is true or false. Record your answer in the blank provided. T = true; F = false.

_____ 1. An appropriate way to ask a caller to hold is to say "Please hold."

_____ 2. A proper way to answer a call is to say "Good morning, Skyway Medical Associates, this is Laura. How may I help you?"

_____ 3. Body language is a form of communication.

_____ 4. If the telephone traffic is very heavy, it is sufficient to answer the phone with just "Hello."

_____ 5. Confidential information may be sent over e-mail because it is a secure form of communication.

_____ 6. It is acceptable for an assistant to leave any message on an answering machine.

_____ 7. Announcing a transferred call means informing the recipient as to who the call is from.

_____ 8. A medical administrative assistant may need to recognize emergency symptoms over the phone.

_____ 9. When answering a call that is a possible emergency, an assistant should ask only those questions necessary to determine how to handle the call.

_____ 10. If a patient insists on speaking directly with the physician, you must transfer the call immediately.

_____ 11. A parent calling to request medical information regarding his 25-year-old son should be given the information.

_____ 12. The office telephone should always be answered immediately after the first ring.

_____ 13. E-mail is synonymous with express mail.

_____ 14. A caller should never hold more than 20 seconds.

_____ 15. First class mail is the standard delivery service used by the U.S. Postal Service for office letters.

_____ 16. Priority mail service guarantees letter delivery within 24 hours.

_____ 17. A certified letter with return receipt may be used if the medical office needs a record of the patient receiving correspondence from the office.

_____ 18. If a medical administrative assistant is responsible for entering computerized appointments for patients, a headset should be used while talking with patients over the telephone.

_____ 19. Because a medical administrative assistant is not licensed to practice medicine, an assistant answering the telephone does not need to be able to recognize symptoms common to a medical emergency.

_____ 20. If the office is very busy, an assistant does not need to ask whether a patient can hold; the assistant can place every call directly on hold if necessary.

_____ 21. A patient can communicate a message without speaking.

_____ 22. A response to a question is known as feedback.

_____ 23. If a patient is vague about symptoms, a medical administrative assistant may need to ask the patient a few questions about his or her symptoms.

_____ 24. Personality differences can affect communication.

_____ 25. If the office is extremely busy, it is acceptable to let the phone ring 10 times before answering.

_____ 26. If the office is extremely busy, an acceptable way to answer the phone is to say "Skyway Medical Associates."

_____ 27. If a caller is upset, the best thing to do is to ask him to call back another day when he is more calm.

_____ 28. A medical office needs a minimum of two telephone lines.

_____ 29. Voice mail will record a message if a phone line is in use.

_____ 30. Screening calls is necessary to decrease the number of calls handled by the physician or other clinical staff.

Exercise 6–2 COMMUNICATING WITH PATIENTS

When patients call the office, they often use lay person's terms to describe a medical condition. Identify the appropriate medical term for each lay person's term. Record the answer in the blank provided.

_____	1. Stitches	(a) Conjunctivitis
_____	2. Cold	(b) Gastritis
_____	3. Sore throat	(c) Otitis media
_____	4. Bladder infection	(d) Urinary tract infection
_____	5. Stomach ache	(e) Pharyngitis
_____	6. Pinkeye	(f) Rhinorrhea
_____	7. Nosebleed	(g) Upper respiratory infection
_____	8. Cut	(h) Hematuria
_____	9. Ear infection	(i) Sutures
_____	10. Runny nose	(j) Laceration
_____	11. Blood in urine	(k) Epistaxis

Exercise 6–3 TELEPHONE SCREENING

Identify whether or not a medical administrative assistant would be authorized or able to complete the following telephone requests. Record your answer in the blank provided. Y = yes; N = no.

_____ 1. Pharmacy calls for a prescription refill for a patient.

_____ 2. Patient wants to make an appointment.

_____ 3. Patient has a complaint about a bill.

_____ 4. Patient asks maximum dosage of ibuprofen that can be used per day.

_____ 5. Patient wants to know how much the practice charges for a mammogram.

_____ 6. Patient wants to know whether heat or ice should be used for an ankle sprain.

_____ 7. Patient needs to cancel an appointment.

_____ 8. Insurance company calls for additional information about a patient's claim.

_____ 9. Patient calls asking whether two particular medications can be taken simultaneously.

_____ 10. Patient calls asking for laboratory test results.

Exercise 6–4 CHAPTER CONCEPTS

Read each statement or question and choose the answer that best completes that statement or question. Record your answer in the blank provided.

_____ 1. After answering a call, the first thing the assistant should do is
    (a) Obtain the patient's name.   (d) Get the patient's chart number.
    (b) Offer an appointment.   (e) Any of the above could be done first.
    (c) Determine the reason for the call.

_____ 2. A correct way to transfer a call to a physician is
    (a) "Dr. Sanchez, line 2."
    (b) "Line 2."
    (c) "Kelly Garcia is on line 2. She wants to know whether she should keep taking her prescription of Xanax."
    (d) "Dr. Sanchez, Mrs. Garcia is on line 2."
    (e) None of the above.

_____ 3. Which of the following is not usually needed when taking a phone message?
    (a) Patient's name.   (d) Time of message.
    (b) Patient's insurance company.   (e) All of the above are necessary for every phone call.
    (c) Reason for calling.

_____ 4. Which of the following is inappropriate when speaking with a patient over the telephone?
   (a) Speak with a moderate rate of speed.
   (b) Confirm the conversation with the caller.
   (c) Hold handset 1 to 2 inches away from your mouth.
   (d) Use medical slang to convey your medical knowledge to the patient.
   (e) Exhibit proper posture.

_____ 5. Which of the following is not true regarding nonverbal communication?
   (a) Nonverbal communication has little impact on communication with a patient.
   (b) An assistant's posture can communicate a message.
   (c) A patient's comfort zone should be respected.
   (d) Lack of eye contact can communicate disinterest.

_____ 6. All of the following should be done when handling a complaint call except
   (a) Offer to help the patient if at all possible.
   (b) Let your supervisor know about the problem and identify ways the problem may be avoided in the future.
   (c) Deny that a problem exists.
   (d) Ask the patient what you can do, and do it if possible.

_____ 7. Which of the following may have the greatest potential for a possible breach of confidentiality?
   (a) Pager   (c) Answering service
   (b) Switchboard   (d) Cell phone

_____ 8. Which of the following is inappropriate in telephone communication?
   (a) Speak clearly.
   (b) Maintain patient confidentiality.
   (c) Confirm a call.
   (d) Obtain every possible piece of information about a patient's medical condition.

_____ 9. When transferring calls, the assistant should do all of the following except
   (a) Explain that the call needs to be transferred.
   (b) Give confidential information over a speaker phone.
   (c) Ask the patient whether he or she will hold while the call is transferred.
   (d) Announce the call.

_____ 10. When handling a possible emergency call, the assistant should
   (a) Tell the patient to drive to the nearest emergency room.
   (b) Transfer the call only if the assistant is sure it is an emergency.
   (c) Tell the patient to come to the clinic immediately.
   (d) Transfer the call immediately to a doctor or nurse.

Exercise 6–5 TELEPHONE PROTOCOL

You are working for Drs. Marks, O'Brian, and Sanchez as a medical administrative assistant at Horizons Health Care and receive the following calls. What is the best way to handle the call?

_____ 1. Mr. Stein (65 years of age) calls with indigestion and just a little shortness of breath after shoveling snow. You
   (a) Transfer the call directly to Mr. Stein's physician.
   (b) Take a message to give to the nurse.
   (c) Tell Mr. Stein to rest and that if he doesn't feel better within 30 minutes he should call back.
   (d) Give him an appointment later this afternoon.
   (e) Tell Mr. Stein to hire someone to shovel his snow.

_____ 2. A physician from the hospital emergency department calls to speak with Dr. O'Brian about her patient Alice Shepard who is currently in the emergency room. You
   (a) Determine the nature of the call by asking as many questions as necessary.
   (b) Never interrupt Dr. O'Brian when she is with a patient.
   (c) Take a message and tell the patient the doctor will call back when she is available.
   (d) Transfer the call immediately to Dr. O'Brian.

_____ 3. Maggie Pinkerton reports that her daughter, Laura, has a slight fever and has been extremely tired for 4 days. You
  (a) Give her an appointment this afternoon.
  (b) Give her an appointment next week. She might get better before then.
  (c) Tell her to give the child two children's nonaspirin tablets and let her rest for the remainder of the day.
  (d) Tell her to call her pharmacy for advice on over-the-counter medications to give for the child's fever.

_____ 4. Lisa Martin, a 20-year-old single female patient, had taken a home pregnancy test, and the result was positive. She is very upset and calls to request an appointment to see the physician about the pregnancy. She mentions she needs to come in soon because she may wish to terminate the pregnancy. You
  (a) Tell her no appointments are available for quite some time because you are morally opposed to abortion.
  (b) Give her the number of a local abortion clinic.
  (c) Accommodate her request for an appointment.
  (d) Tell her to come in to have another test to verify the home test.

_____ 5. Nancy Martin, Lisa's mother, telephones the office and asks to speak with the doctor. She is concerned that her daughter is possibly depressed. She asks if Lisa has been in the clinic lately for anything. You
  (a) Tell her Lisa phoned yesterday but you cannot tell her mother why Lisa phoned.
  (b) Tell her that information regarding a patient cannot be released without the patient's permission.
  (c) Tell her Lisa has not contacted the office for anything in the past 6 months.
  (d) Call Lisa and tell her that her mother phoned the office asking about her.

_____ 6. A pharmacy calls requesting an okay for a refill of a patient's medication. You
  (a) Check the chart, and, if any refills have been ordered, tell the pharmacy another refill should be okay.
  (b) Take a message for the patient's physician.
  (c) Tell the pharmacy all patients need to see their physician before any refills are made.
  (d) Tell the pharmacy the patient should bring the prescription bottle into the pharmacy so it can be checked.

_____ 7. Barb Baker, the practice's legal counsel, asks to speak with Dr. Marks. You
  (a) Transfer the call to Dr. Marks.
  (b) Tell Ms. Baker to phone Dr. Marks at home this evening.
  (c) Take a message and tell Ms. Baker that Dr. Marks cannot be interrupted.
  (d) Transfer the call to the office manager.

_____ 8. A patient calls asking for results from a recent laboratory test. You
  (a) Take a message for the physician or the nurse.
  (b) Find the results and give them over the telephone to the patient.
  (c) Transfer the call to the laboratory technician.
  (d) Tell the patient you will send the results by mail.

_____ 9. Mr. O'Brian, Dr. O'Brian's husband, calls to speak with Dr. O'Brian. She is currently with a patient. You
  (a) Tell Mr. O'Brian you must take a message.
  (b) Transfer the call directly to Dr. O'Brian.
  (c) Tell Mr. O'Brian the doctor is currently with a patient, and ask if he would like you to interrupt.
  (d) Ask Mr. O'Brian to call back right before lunch because all patients will be gone at that time.

_____ 10. Susan Walter, MD, the chief of the medical staff, calls for Dr. Sanchez. You
  (a) Transfer the call to Dr. Sanchez.
  (b) Take a message.
  (c) Ask what the call is about, and then determine whether a message should be taken.
  (d) Transfer the call to the practice manager because Dr. Sanchez is too busy.

_____ 11. Eileen Smith, an obstetrics patient, calls with medical questions relating to her pregnancy. You
    (a) Determine that the call is not an emergency and take a message for the physician or the nurse.
    (b) Tell her to call and ask the hospital where she plans to deliver.
    (c) Ask her whether she has consulted her prenatal guide provided by the doctor.
    (d) Check her chart to see whether you can answer her questions.

_____ 12. A patient calls and is too embarrassed to say why she is calling. You
    (a) Tell her to call back when she is not so embarrassed.
    (b) Tell her nothing will shock you.
    (c) Determine that the call is not an emergency and take a message for the physician or nurse.
    (d) Tell her to look for information on the Internet.

_____ 13. Dr. O'Brian's son calls and reports he is in trouble at school. You
    (a) Take a message and tell him the doctor will call the school after school is out.
    (b) Transfer the call to Dr. O'Brian.
    (c) Tell him to call his father.
    (d) Tell him to have the teacher call back during the lunch hour.

_____ 14. A patient calls with severe vertigo. You
    (a) Ask the patient whether she has been drinking any alcohol.
    (b) Check her chart to see whether she has had vertigo before.
    (c) Transfer the call to the doctor or the nurse.
    (d) Make an appointment next week for the patient.

_____ 15. An hysterical parent calls reporting that her toddler has drunk half a bottle of a children's pain reliever. You
    (a) Transfer the call to the pharmacy.
    (b) Tell her to take the child to an emergency room.
    (c) Tell her to make the child vomit the drug.
    (d) Give her the number of the poison control center, instruct her to call the number immediately, and obtain the patient's name before hanging up.

Exercise 6–6 APPLICATION OF KNOWLEDGE

To develop a greater understanding of office emergencies and how to recognize them over the telephone, look up the following medical conditions in a medical reference and identify the common symptoms associated with each condition. (All of the following conditions have the potential to become critical. This list is not inclusive of all critical conditions that may occur with patients.)

Medical Condition	Symptoms
Myocardial infarction (heart attack)	_____
Cerebrovascular accident (stroke)	_____
Asthma attack	_____
Appendicitis	_____
Pyelonephritis	_____
Migraine	_____
Volvulus	_____
Ileus	_____
Intussusception	_____
Perforated ulcer	_____
Aneurysm	_____
Osteomyelitis	_____
Meningitis	_____

6
ACTIVITIES

ACTIVITY 6-1   Using the message blanks provided here, write a telephone message for the following calls received in the office today. Some of the information for the message will need to be obtained from the Lytec Medical 2001 software included with this text.

1. Maria Vasquez calls for results of her mammogram performed last Wednesday. She asks whether Dr. O'Brian or her nurse could call her back today after 4 PM at her home number with the results.

MESSAGE FROM								
For Dr.	Name of Caller	Rel. to pt.	Patient	Pt. Age	Pt. Temp.	Message Date	Message Time AM PM	Urgent ☐ Yes ☐ No
Message:						Allergies		
Respond to Phone #		Best Time To Call AM PM	Pharmacy Name/#		Patient's Chart Attached ☐ Yes ☐ No	Patient's Chart #		Initials

2. Gregory O'Henry has sprained his ankle and wants information on what he can do at home. He asks whether Dr. O'Brian can call him back at his home number as soon as possible.

MESSAGE FROM								
For Dr.	Name of Caller	Rel. to pt.	Patient	Pt. Age	Pt. Temp.	Message Date	Message Time AM PM	Urgent ☐ Yes ☐ No
Message:						Allergies		
Respond to Phone #		Best Time To Call AM PM	Pharmacy Name/#		Patient's Chart Attached ☐ Yes ☐ No	Patient's Chart #		Initials

3. Michelle Gibson calls to report that her daughter, Kirsten French has a fever and wants to know the correct amount of nonaspirin pain reliever to give for the fever. She asks that the doctor call her back as soon as possible at home.

MESSAGE FROM								
For Dr.	Name of Caller	Rel. to pt.	Patient	Pt. Age	Pt. Temp.	Message Date	Message Time AM PM	Urgent ☐ Yes ☐ No
Message:						Allergies		
Respond to Phone #		Best Time To Call AM PM	Pharmacy Name/#		Patient's Chart Attached ☐ Yes ☐ No	Patient's Chart #		Initials

To access patient information in the Lytec Medical 2001 program: (Follow Lytec software installation instructions before proceeding.)

1. Open Lytec Medical 2001. At the main menu, click *File,* then *Open Practice.*
2. In the open window, click *Horizons Healthcare Center,* then click *Open.* (Once the Horizons Healthcare Center practice is open, the practice name will appear on the title bar at the top of the window. You will also notice that the main menu selections have now expanded.)

3. On the main menu, click *Lists,* then click *Patients.* The patient list window will then open. To search for a patient, click the magnifying glass to the right of the *Patient Chart* box. The *Find Patient* window will open. The *Search By* box should read last name, first name. (If it does not, click the drop-down arrow on the right of the *Search By* box and choose that option.)

4. In the *Search For* box, begin typing the patient's last name. When the patient's name is located, double click the patient's entry and the patient's information will appear in the *Find Patient* window. Demographic information will be listed under the *Patient Information* tab in this window. When you have finished locating information in this list and no changes need to be made, click *Close.*

ACTIVITY 6–2   Establish a list of important telephone techniques for handling incoming calls. Call two places of business and evaluate their phone techniques based on the list you created.

ACTIVITY 6–3   As a class, take a personality style inventory. Compare your answers with those of others in the group.

ACTIVITY 6–4   Research e-mail etiquette on the Internet. Locate examples of at least 10 different emoticons.

ACTIVITY 6–5   Prepare the following letter in the letter formats as given in the text: block, modified block, and modified block with indented paragraphs. Insert paragraphs where appropriate, and consult an office reference manual if necessary. Locate the patient information in the Lytec software program using the instructions given in Lytec Software Activity 6–1. October 9, 200x letter from Kristine G. O'Brian, M.D. to Alice Shepard Chart #554148

Dear Mrs. Shepard–I have received the results of your hemoglobin A1C test that was done on September 25, and I am pleased to inform you that the test results were within normal limits. Your test result was 6.8%. Our desired results would be a value less than 7%. Your type II diabetes seems to be well under control, and your current dosage of Glucotrol XL of 5 mg/day is appropriate and should be continued. A prescription for Glucotrol is enclosed. I recommend that you repeat this test again in 6 months. Please contact me at my office if you have any questions. Sincerely, Kristine G. O'Brian, MD.

ACTIVITY 6–6   Prepare the following memo for Dr. Sanchez in the memo format given in the text. Use today's date. to: all employees, from: Mary M. Sanchez, MD, subject: employee parking

Next Monday, [insert date], resurfacing of our parking lot will begin. Construction will last for approximately 4 to 5 days. The construction will take place in two phases with each phase lasting 1 to 2 days. All employees are asked to not park in the lot during the construction to allow for ample parking for our patients. Temporary parking during the construction is available in the church lot on Midtown Avenue.

6

DISCUSSION

The following topics may be used for class discussion or for individual student essay.

DISCUSSION 6–1   As a patient is leaving the office, she turns to wish you a "Merry Christmas." You are Jewish. What should you say?

DISCUSSION 6–2   The telephone traffic at the office has been increasing to the point at which it is difficult to answer many calls within 3 to 4 rings. The office physician wants to purchase an automated system for the office that allows a computer to answer the phone. Calls will be answered by recorded voice that instructs the patient that his or her call will be handled by the next available assistant. How will you respond to the physician?

DISCUSSION 6–3   Read the quotation at the beginning of the chapter. How does this apply to working in the medical office and with patients?

CHAPTER OUTLINE

LEARNING OBJECTIVES

On successful completion of this chapter, the student will be able to

1. Describe the usage of computer and manual systems for scheduling appointments.
2. Identify types of scheduling methods used in offices today.
3. Identify the common components needed when recording an appointment.
4. Explain appointment scheduling procedures.
5. Schedule appointments on a computer and in a manual system.
6. Document no-shows and appointment cancellations.
7. Prepare written appointment reminders.
8. Deliver oral appointment reminders.
9. Explain proper handling of unexpected schedule interruptions.
10. Explain appropriate use of medical terminology on an appointment schedule.

CMA COMPETENCIES

1. Schedule and manage appointments.
2. Schedule inpatient and outpatient admissions and procedures.
3. Document appropriately.
4. Identify and respond to issues of confidentiality.

RMA COMPETENCIES

1. Know terminology associated with medical secretarial and receptionist duties.
2. Use appointment scheduling system (maintain appointment book, type daily schedule, review schedule with physician).
3. Use procedures for handling cancellations and missed appointments.

VOCABULARY

ancillary appointments
double booking
referral appointments
walk-in

APPOINTMENT SCHEDULING

There is no such thing in anyone's life as an unimportant day.
—*Alexander Woollcott, American author*

Appointment scheduling is the office activity that has, perhaps, the greatest influence on how a medical office functions. A well-managed schedule provides optimal availability of services for patients as well as maximal utilization of facility resources such as personnel, equipment, and buildings. A well-managed schedule avoids excessive downtimes and excessive hectic times. Downtimes are periods when equipment, personnel, or space are left idle or are unproductive for extended periods of time. Many offices prefer to use every available slot of appointment time that is available during the day. Proper use of appointment time will keep everyone in the office busy at a smooth pace throughout the day. A well-managed schedule reduces waiting time for patients and maximizes the number of patients the physician is able to serve.

COMPUTERIZED APPOINTMENT SCHEDULING

In most of today's medical offices, the most common piece of equipment used for appointment scheduling is the computer. Depending on the size of the organization, computers may be stand-alone personal computers or may be networked with a mainframe computer system.

The use of a computerized appointment scheduling system has many advantages for the medical office. First and foremost is the fact that most appointment scheduling programs allow more than one user at a time to enter appointments. This means that the office staff is able to assist more than one patient at a time and that office productivity is increased

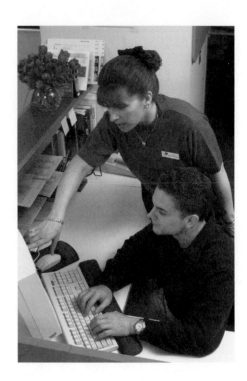

Figure 7–1. A computerized system in the medical office helps make appointment scheduling easy.

because more than one assistant at a time can schedule or modify appointments. Even while someone is entering appointments, other staff members can usually access scheduling information from the system (Fig. 7–1).

Most scheduling programs prompt the user for the essential information needed to schedule an appointment. Everyone

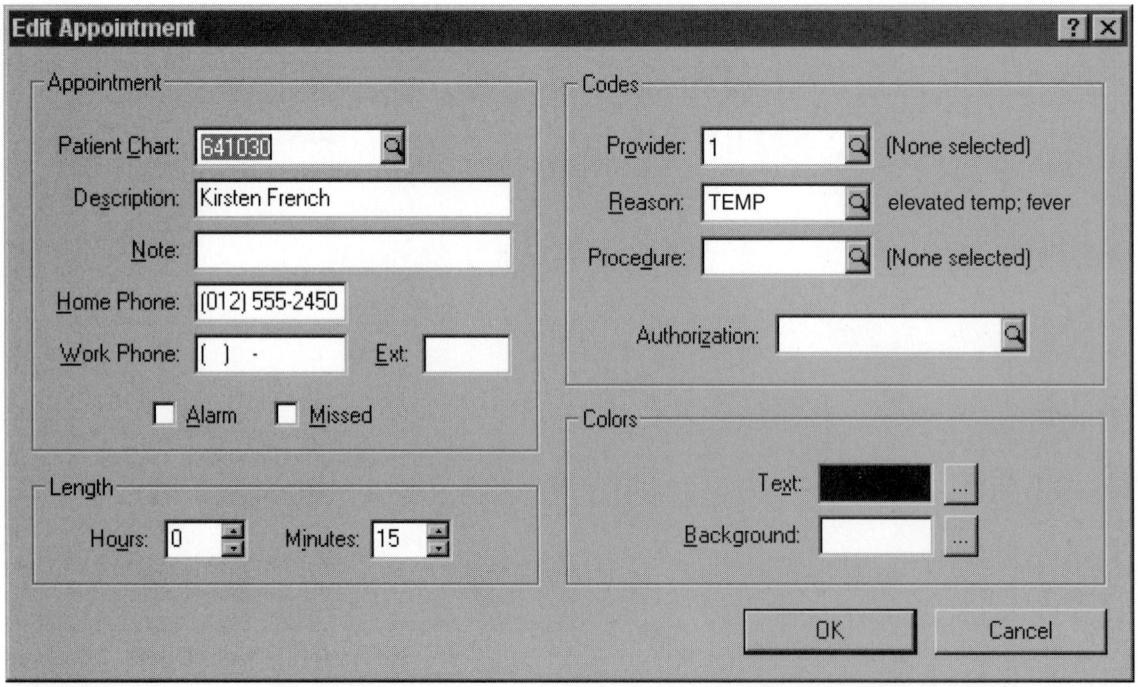

Figure 7–2. Information for a patient's medical appointment is entered on an appointment entry screen.

using the system is asked the same questions and responds to the same computer prompts. Therefore, the content of appointments entered into the computer is relatively uniform. The computer asks for information that a user might otherwise forget to enter if using a manual or handwritten system (Fig. 7–2).

Another advantage of using a computerized system is the ability to generate updated copies of the schedule quickly. Usually, just by entering a few simple commands, a copy of any day's schedule can be generated. Some offices even have computers at the nurses' station in the patient care area that enable the physicians or nurses to view or print, or both, the schedule at their command.

Appointment scheduling usually interfaces with a patient database. This means that when an appointment is made and a patient's name is entered into the schedule, other pertinent information—such as the patient's telephone number and the patient's chart number—is retrieved from the database and inserted into the schedule, as well. When the schedule is printed, the medical office assistant uses the schedule to pull charts for the day.

Also, appointment scheduling software may provide an interface with the patient billing system. With this interface, the chance of bills getting lost or misplaced is reduced because the software is able to identify patients that have been seen for an appointment but have not yet had charges entered for services rendered.

When scheduling an appointment, some programs allow the user to view several open appointment slots at one time (Fig 7–3). The user can specify that the program display openings for a specific provider or for a certain day. If the patient wants an appointment on a Wednesday or wants to see only Dr. Sanchez, the software will display only Wednesdays for Dr. Sanchez.

Computerized appointment scheduling enables an assistant to quickly access such information as

- The time of a patient's next appointment.
- A record of a patient's previous visits to the office.
- Identification of providers who have treated the patient.

Retrieving this type of information from a handwritten appointment book would be tedious and very time consuming.

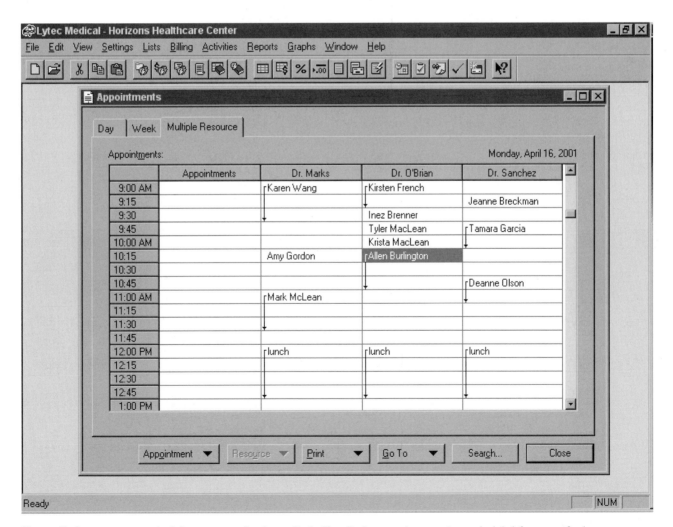

Figure 7–3. A computer scheduling program for the medical office displays appointment times scheduled for a specific day.

A computerized system can have this type of information available in a matter of seconds.

Software Packages for Appointment Scheduling

Several software programs have been developed for appointment scheduling specific to the medical office. The selection and implementation of a program may be a difficult and costly process.

Implementing appointment scheduling programs may cost several thousand dollars when the facility takes into account all the items necessary for implementation, such as
• The software itself.
• Computer hardware to run the software.
• Network cabling and other hardware necessary to connect and support the computer equipment.
• Training for personnel.

Although the implementation costs may seem high, computer implementation usually pays for itself by increasing the productivity of office personnel and by providing a detailed record of the office's activities.

Concerns when Using a Computerized Appointment System

Use of a computerized system is not without its drawbacks. Contingency plans must be developed to handle those times when the computer system is down. Schedules should be printed often throughout the workday (every 1 to 2 hours if the schedule changes frequently) and distributed to the physicians and nurses. Because appointment information is considered confidential, old copies of the schedule should be shredded when the new copies are printed.

If a patient calls for an appointment or information when the computer system is down, the medical office assistant should schedule an appointment manually on the computer printout. An assistant's response should *never* be "Our computers are down. You'll have to call back." Some patients may choose to never call back. If a patient desires an appointment for a day in the future, an assistant could offer to call the patient when the system is up and running.

MANUAL SYSTEM FOR APPOINTMENT SCHEDULING

Some of the smaller medical practices today have not yet "taken the plunge" and bought a computerized system. A few practices are using appointment books in which appointments are handwritten by the assistant (Fig. 7–4).

Open appointment times are easily spotted in Figure 7–4 because they are blank.

Appointments are entered under the appropriate physician's schedule by writing—in pencil—the patient's name, telephone number, chart number, and reason for the appointment in the appropriate blanks. An "X" is then placed in the corresponding square on the right. This allows anyone to view the weekly openings at a glance. If the patient requests an appointment at 9:30 PM sometime this week, open slots are easy to locate by looking at the grid on the right.

Pencil should always be used when entering appointments in manual systems. Cancellations and rescheduled appointments are frequent occurrences in a medical office, necessitating erasure of the originally scheduled appointment. Legible and accurate entries are essential so that personnel other than the assistant may also read the day's appointments. Books with entries that have been scribbled out or obliterated with

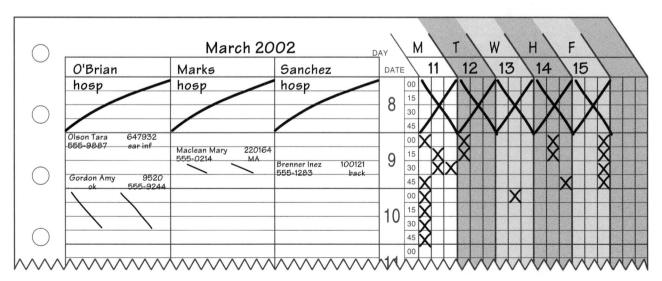

Figure 7–4. Appointment books are still used by some medical offices. Open appointment times are indicated by the blank boxes in the grid on the right of the schedule. (Form courtesy of Bibbero Systems, Inc., Petaluma, California, 800-242-2376. Fax 800-242-9330. www.bibbero.com.)

correction fluid are sloppy and sometimes even illegible. If ever subpoenaed, illegible records do not stand up well in court. It is a medical office assistant's duty to keep legible and accurate appointment records.

Concerns when Using a Manual Scheduling System

Although appointment books are relatively inexpensive to purchase, they do have some drawbacks.

Only one person at a time can schedule appointments for a specific physician. For example, you may be assisting a patient who wants to schedule an appointment with Dr. X, and another assistant is helping another patient who also wants to schedule an appointment with Dr. X. The second patient will need to wait to schedule an appointment because the appointment book is currently in use.

In a larger practice with several providers, more than one appointment book may be necessary. With several books on the desk, not only will the desk space be crowded, but the medical office assistant may need to thumb through all of the books to find an open appointment slot that meets the patient's needs. If more than one book is used, it is possible to write a patient's appointment on the wrong physician's schedule. If only one book is used for several providers, again, only one assistant can make an appointment at a given time for a patient.

A manual system for appointment scheduling can certainly get the job done, but, if at all possible, a computerized system should be used to increase the productivity in the office and, ultimately, to serve the patient in a more timely fashion.

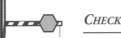

CHECKPOINT

The medical office where you are employed is evaluating two pieces of appointment scheduling software for implementation in the office. Software A is cheaper but allows only one user at a time to access the appointment system. Software B is twice as expensive but allows an unlimited number of users to access the appointment system at one time. There are three physicians, a nurse practitioner, three nurses, and three medical office assistants employed at the clinic. It is your job to recommend to the providers the appropriate software package for purchase. Which software package would you recommend? Defend your answer.

TYPES OF SCHEDULING METHODS AND APPOINTMENT PROCEDURES

Most of today's offices have an established system for scheduling appointments. One of the first things an office will determine for appointment scheduling is the type of increments that will be necessary for office appointments. Will appointments be scheduled every 10 or 15 minutes, or will appointments be scheduled every half hour or every hour? The type of practice and patients served will determine what increments are necessary. Family practice, internal medicine, pediatrics, and other providers involved in primary care will probably use 10- to 15-minute intervals for appointments. Examples of appointment times necessary for specific patient complaints are shown in Table 7–1. Note that the more complicated a presenting problem is, the more time is

---

Table 7–1. Horizons Healthcare Center Appointment Scheduling Guidelines

15 Minutes	Physicals (px) (schedule by age)	30 Minutes	45 Minutes	60 Minutes
Ear pain or infection	(Pap included for female patients over 18)	Postoperative visit	Lesion removal (2 or more)	Initial (new)
Burn	Sports px—30 minutes	Lump	Proctosigmoidoscopy	OB visit
Sinus pain	Under 18—15 minutes	Asthma	(procto)	Vasectomy
URI	18–39—30 minutes	Preop physical	Hearing check	
Cough	40 to 65—45 minutes	Depression, any psych	Colposcopy	
Pharyngitis	Over 65—60 minutes	(use 'personal')		
Ear wash	Preop px—30 minutes	Foreign body removal		
Wart treatment		(FB—location)		
Abdominal pain		Chest pain		
Rash/urticaria		Muscle strain		
Allergies		Back pain		
Rechecks		Sprain or suspected fracture		
Recheck Pap		Menstrual problems		
Conjunctivitis		Lesion removal (1)		
Elevated temp		Ingrown toenail		
OB recheck		Headache (HA)		
UTI		Eye injury		
HTN				
Diabetes				
Hemorrhoids				
Flu symptoms				

---

required. Specialists, such as neurosurgeons or psychiatrists, often require lengthy examinations or interviews to assess a patient and will schedule patients for longer appointments (30- to 60-minute intervals).

Some practices request that new patients be scheduled for an additional amount of time (usually 10 to 15 minutes) because the physician will need time to get acquainted with the patient. Some practices also request that new patients report for appointments 15 minutes early to allow for time to complete a medical history questionnaire.

Double Booking (Overbooking) Appointments

Some primary care physicians may allow the office staff to overbook their appointment schedules. This practice is known as **double booking.** Double booking involves scheduling an appointment at the same time that another appointment is scheduled. These types of appointments are usually quick, **urgent care**–type appointments similar to many of the 15-minute appointments that are shown in Table 7–1. The rationale for using double booking is to accommodate the patient's needs quickly. If a patient has a sore throat, he may not be able to wait a couple of days for the next available appointment. Double booking appointments allow patients to be served sooner.

When a patient is double booked for an appointment, the patient should be informed that there may be a slightly longer than usual waiting time to be seen by the physician. Double booking a physician's schedule should be done only with the physician's approval. Some physicians give blanket approval and always allow appointments to be double booked; other physicians give their approval on a case-by-case basis.

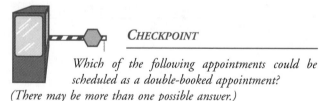

CHECKPOINT

Which of the following appointments could be scheduled as a double-booked appointment?
(There may be more than one possible answer.)

Wart treatment	Headache	Depression
Lump	Sinus pain	Cough
Ear infection	Hearing check	Burn

Walk-in Patients

Some providers may choose to leave occasional open spots in their schedule to accommodate acutely ill patients who walk into to the clinic to be seen (hence, the name "walk-in"). Most practices encourage patients to make appointments, but patients may occasionally elect to drop in to the physician's office with the hope of being seen.

Even if the schedule is full, it is extremely important to consult the physician about any walk-in patient to see whether the physician is able to see the patient. If the physician is unable to see the patient within a reasonable period, an appointment may need to be made for a later time. If the reason for the walk-in is a serious problem requiring immediate attention, the patient may need to be referred to an emergency room for treatment.

In some cases, the presenting problem is serious enough to warrant calling an ambulance to transport the patient from the clinic to the emergency room. Whatever the presenting problem, the referral of a patient to an emergency room should be the decision of the physician, not the medical office assistant, unless the assistant has been expressly instructed to do so by the physician. Imagine what could happen if a patient with severe indigestion is told to go to an emergency room. If the patient gets in a car, drives himself, and is actually experiencing a heart attack, the patient could die while driving the car. This, of course, could create potential liability on the part of the medical office and is not, obviously, serving the patient at all.

Walk-in Clinics

One of the latest trends in health care is the development of urgent care centers or **walk-in** clinics. These types of facilities are often open for extended hours to serve patients with health concerns that require immediate attention but that may not require the services of an emergency room. These facilities generally accept only walk-in patients, and patients are served in the order in which they arrive, with the exception of seriously ill patients who may receive top priority. Physicians should give the office front desk staff guidelines for identifying patients who need priority care. Examples of some symptoms that may indicate that a patient needs prompt medical attention are identified in Chapter 6, Box 6–1.

Group (Block) Scheduling

Sometimes, a practice will schedule several patients to come in at the same time, with the idea that patients will be served by different areas of the clinic at that time. This practice is known as group scheduling and suits some specialties very well.

For example, suppose you are working for an orthopedic practice. If four patients were scheduled at the same time, it is likely that one patient may be sent to x-ray, one patient may need cast removal and then x-ray, one patient may see the doctor for a recheck, and the remaining patient may see the doctor for a visit not requiring an x-ray. While the third and fourth patients are waiting in examination rooms to be seen by the physician, other office personnel attend to the first and second patients. Then, when the third and fourth patients' visits are completed, the first and second patients are ready to be seen by the physician.

Establishing Appointment Parameters

When setting up the schedule, it is important for the physician to communicate his or her scheduling preferences to the staff clearly and for the staff to understand what the physician likes and dislikes as regards the scheduling of patients.

Some providers prefer a very tight schedule to ensure that there are no downtimes, when no patient is being seen. Many providers view downtime as unproductive time. Other providers may prefer to be scheduled lightly because they do not like to keep patients waiting or they may feel pressured by several patients waiting in the lobby at once.

Many physicians prefer variety in scheduling and often restrict the repetition of similar appointments during the day. For example, a physician may allow only two physicals to be scheduled in the morning and two in the afternoon. Physicals are routine checks of a patient's health and can be planned weeks or months in advance. This restriction of the number of physicals per day allows the practice to keep appointment slots open for seeing acutely ill patients.

Multiphysician Practices

Scheduling gets tricky when an assistant is working in an office with several physicians. The assistant may need to remember that one physician does not see pediatric patients but that other physicians do see pediatric patients. Some physicians may prefer to be scheduled lightly, but others may prefer to be scheduled heavily.

Physicians in a larger office should try to have as much uniformity in their scheduling as possible in order to make scheduling appointments easier for their staff. The office staff must remember, however, that it is necessary to respect the physicians' preferences for scheduling.

Facility Limitations

A possible complication to the scheduling process is the availability of special facilities or equipment. Perhaps the clinic has only one minor surgery room or has only one piece of equipment that is used for a special procedure. In such a case, the room or equipment availability must be checked before the appointment is scheduled. If there are any room or equipment limitations, the office may choose to use a separate appointment schedule for the room or equipment to keep track of their usage.

Setting the Schedule

Whether using a computerized or manual appointment system, the first thing the assistant must do when setting the schedule is to block off days that the facility is not open (Procedure box 7–1). The facility may not be open on weekends or on certain holidays. These days must be clearly marked as closed or unavailable so that a staff member does not inadvertently schedule an appointment on a day that the clinic is closed. An assistant making an advance appointment may not realize that Monday, May 28, is Memorial Day that year.

Next, all vacation days and unavailable times need to be identified for every physician or provider in the office. If

PROCEDURE 7–1 *Prepare an Appointment Schedule for a Medical Office*

Materials Needed
- Appointment scheduling software on a computer system

or

- Appointment book and pencil

1. Identify and mark off the days that the office is closed.
2. Identify and mark off the time of each day that the office is closed.
3. Identify and mark off the time of each day that each physician is unavailable.

Dr. Marks does not work on Tuesday afternoons, then all Tuesday afternoons on his schedule need to be marked as unavailable (Fig. 7–5). If the clinic has some evening hours during the week, these slots must be made available for scheduling. And, of course, hours that the office is closed are marked on the schedule.

After the initial unavailable times and days are identified and marked on the schedule, other times the physician is unavailable must then be marked on the schedule. Hospital rounds, committee meetings, personal appointments, breaks such as lunch or dinner, and any other commitments that prevent the physician from seeing patients should be entered on the schedule. Some physicians prefer to have all commitments during the workday entered into the schedule. That way, when the physician checks the schedule, a clear picture of commitments and appointments is presented.

Advance Booking

Most offices have the schedule established well in advance. A typical schedule shows appointments scheduled and available for the next 6 months. Many appointments, such as physicals, will book far in advance. Physicians typically limit the number of such an appointment per day because this type of appointment is not urgent and physicians must leave part of their schedule available for patients with acute care needs. It is important to remember, however, that appointments made that far in advance will probably require a written reminder or a telephone reminder to the patient a short time before the appointment is scheduled. Reminders are discussed later in this chapter.

Components of an Appointment

There are four pieces of vital information in every appointment made in a medical facility. These are
- Name of patient.
- Reason for appointment.

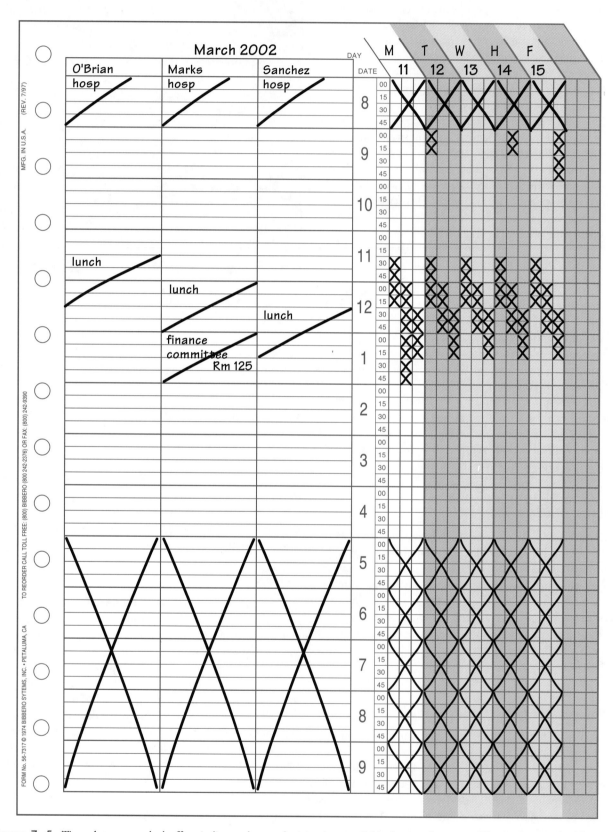

Figure 7–5. Time slots are marked off to indicate when a physician is unavailable for appointments. (Form courtesy of Bibbero Systems, Inc., Petaluma, California, 800-242-2376. Fax 800-242-9330. www.bibbero.com.)

- Telephone number to reach patient during the day.
- Chart number (if chart numbers are used). Date of birth (DOB) is required for new patients and in offices with alphabetical filing systems.

Name of Patient. The patient's name is needed, of course, to identify who is coming in to see the physician.

Reason for Appointment. The reason for the appointment helps the assistant determine the amount of time needed for the appointment and is necessary to enable the physician and nursing staff to prepare for what lies ahead that day. The assistant must be very careful when listing the reason for the appointment not to diagnose the patient's condition and not to enter anything on the schedule that might be potentially damaging or embarrassing to the patient.

If a patient calls and says that he thinks he has an ear infection, it is usually acceptable to write "ear infection" on the schedule. However, if a female patient calls and says that she has missed a period, the assistant should not enter "pregnant" on the schedule.

When scheduling appointments, a medical office assistant must constantly remember to avoid entering potentially damaging or embarrassing information (e.g., "STD," "venereal disease," "depression," "paranoid," or "nervous"). It is often best in these cases to list the reason for coming in as "personal," even if the patient states he thinks he may have a sexually transmitted disease. It is important to remember that appointment schedules are sensitive, confidential documents because of the nature of the information contained within.

If possible, use commonly accepted medical abbreviations when identifying the reason for the appointment. Not only will abbreviations save time and space, but they are also part of a language usually known only to medical personnel and will help keep some schedule information confidential. Definitions for commonly accepted abbreviations are listed in Box 7–1. Other definitions can be found in most medical dictionaries as well as in medical word books such as *Dorland's Medical Speller*.

Telephone Number. Listing the patient's daytime telephone number is useful in case the unexpected happens and the physician is unable to see that patient at the scheduled time. Situations such as a hospital emergency, weather cancellation, or physician illness may occur that will result in a large number of patients needing to be rescheduled owing to a physician's unavailability. The medical office assistant must then try to reach the patient by telephone before the appointment to reschedule. With the telephone numbers listed on the appointment schedule, patients can be called quickly about the schedule change.

Chart Number. For offices that use a numbering system for their medical records, the chart number is needed by the office personnel responsible for pulling the patients' charts for the day. Depending on the size of the facility, charts for a day's appointments are usually pulled a day or two in advance of the patient's appointment. In multiphysician offices, the charts for each day are usually grouped by physician and are kept near the registration desk. Many assistants who are in charge of registering patients for their appointments like to

Box 7–1 Common Abbreviations Used in Appointment Scheduling
AD — right ear
AS — left ear
AU — both ears
BCP — birth control pill
BP — blood pressure
bx — biopsy
Dx — diagnosis
FB — foreign body
flex or procto — proctosigmoidoscopy
Fx — fracture
HA — headache
HOH — hard of hearing
HTN — hypertension
LLQ — left lower quadrant
LOC — loss of consciousness
LUQ — left upper quadrant
OB — obstetric
OD — right eye
OS — left eye
OU — both eyes
pt — patient
px — physical
RLQ — right lower quadrant
RUQ — right upper quadrant
Rx — prescription, treatment, therapy
s/p — status post
SOB — shortness of breath
Stat — immediately
Sx — symptoms
tx — treatment
URI — upper respiratory infection
UTI — urinary tract infection
x — times

then place the charts for each physician in the order in which they have their appointment scheduled.

Date of Birth. If a patient is new to the facility, the patient's DOB should be obtained when booking the appointment. This will allow the medical office assistant to check the patient database to make sure a chart does not already exist for the patient.

In a facility that uses alphabetical filing for medical records, knowing the patient's DOB will allow an assistant to retrieve the correct chart for the patient. It is possible for a facility to have several patients with the same name (e.g., Robert Smith). Securing the patient's DOB enables the assistant to correctly identify the patient who has the appointment scheduled. A patient's address may not definitively identify a patient because an address may change—a birth date does not!

Offices using a computerized appointment system will have the patient's telephone number, chart number, and other necessary information inserted automatically on the printout of the schedule.

Once the appointment is secured for the patient, the medical office assistant should confirm the appointment by issuing a written reminder for the patient or, in the case of an appointment made over the telephone, the assistant should repeat all appointment information back to the caller and wait for acknowledgment of the appointment from the caller (Procedure box 7–2).

Prioritizing Appointments

It is often an assistant's job to decide who will get an appointment opening right away or who may need to wait to be seen. Of course, if the patient wants an appointment on the day he or she calls the office, an assistant should always try to accommodate the patient. Sometimes, accommodation may not be possible.

If a limited number of openings are left for the current day, the nature and duration of the problem will likely determine whether or not a patient is scheduled for one of the remaining appointments. A patient calling the office for treatment of warts could likely be accommodated some time later in the week when the schedule is not so heavily booked. If a patient calls with urinary frequency and burning, however, she may likely have a urinary tract infection (UTI) and cannot wait a few days to come in. A UTI left untreated could develop into a kidney infection, which can be a very serious medical condition.

In a busy primary care office, the assistant is not always able to accommodate all patients' needs for appointments. Sometimes, after a weekend or holiday, patients' needs for urgent care appointments are greater than on other days. Mondays can be particularly busy because patients may have had symptoms develop over the weekend and will call for appointments when the office opens on Monday morning. Some offices do not allow routine visits, such as physicals, to be scheduled on Mondays or the day after a holiday so that the office can accommodate patients who have become ill when the clinic is closed. Some offices allow acute care appointments only during evening or weekend hours.

It is important remember that because the mission of a medical office is to serve patients, a medical office assistant should ask a patient when he or she would like to come in for an appointment. An assistant should not begin suggesting appointment times without considering the patient's needs.

One technique that works well is to ask the patient what day of the week he or she would prefer and whether he or she would prefer a morning or an afternoon appointment. After listening to the patient's preference, the assistant can then let the patient know what time slots are available. Using this method, the patient's needs are more likely to be met. Remember, the patient is the office's number 1 priority!

If a medical office assistant is unsure whether the problem needs immediate attention, the assistant should consult the physician or nurse to determine when the patient should be placed on the schedule.

If there are no appointment openings and a patient calls with a problem that requires the attention of the physician that day, the medical office assistant should offer to take a message regarding the patient's call. The physician may then decide to overbook or, possibly, may recommend treatment for the patient over the telephone.

Sometimes, a patient with a severe complaint may call to request an appointment. If the medical office assistant determines that the patient's problem is a potentially life-threatening situation, it is important for the assistant to remain calm and not alarm the patient. Instead of scheduling the appointment, the assistant should say to the patient, "Before I schedule the appointment, I'd like to check something with the nurse." The assistant can then inform the nurse of the call. The nurse will likely screen the call and, if necessary, recommend appropriate action, possibly directing the patient to go to the nearest emergency room or instructing the patient to call an ambulance. By recognizing a potentially serious situation, the medical office assistant may help the patient avoid further harm and, perhaps, even save a life.

PROCEDURE 7–2 Schedule Appointments

Materials Needed
- Appointment scheduling software on a computer system

or

- Appointment book and pencil

1. Determine the reason for the appointment.*
2. Using scheduling guidelines, determine the length of the appointment.
3. Identify the patient's name.
4. Determine the preferences for a desired appointment time.
5. Identify the date and time for the appointment, and obtain approval for the date and time with the patient (or patient's representative).
6. Enter appointment on the schedule.
7. Confirm the appointment with the patient (or patient's representative).*

Optional

8. If patient is in the office, give the patient a written reminder of the appointment.

Denotes a crucial step in the procedure. This step must be completed satisfactorily for the procedure to be completed satisfactorily.

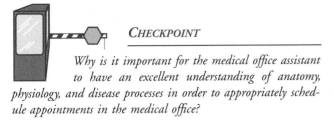

No-shows

Occasionally, a patient does not arrive for a scheduled appointment. This situation is known as a **no-show.** There may be many reasons why a patient does not show up for an appointment. Whatever the reason, it is important to give the patient the benefit of the doubt and to assume that the patient inadvertently missed the appointment. A medical office assistant should never assume that the patient missed the appointment intentionally.

The medical administrative assistant should give the patient sufficient time to arrive for the appointment before recording the appointment as a no-show. A simple traffic jam, stalled vehicle, or inclement weather could delay a patient for a few minutes. It is wise to wait at least 1 hour before documenting the appointment as a no-show.

Medical offices realize that from time to time patients may forget about an appointment that has been scheduled. Usually, patients are not billed for a no-show. An exception may be missed appointments at a mental health clinic, where many appointments are 1 hour in length. A missed 1-hour appointment may result in a substantial amount of unproductive time for the office. In that case, a no-show appointment may be billed to the patient. If the office has a policy of charging for missed appointments, the policy should be communicated clearly to patients.

Documentation of No-shows

Once it has been determined that the patient is a no-show for the appointment, it is important that the no-show be documented in the patient's chart. This documentation is done primarily to protect the physician or provider in case of any legal action. Suppose the patient is a diabetic and routinely misses appointments to monitor his or her disease. If the patient later develops complications and tries to place blame on the medical staff, the fact that the patient has neglected to monitor his or her disease appropriately with the physician's guidance may make the patient's claim difficult to prove in court.

When charting a no-show in the patient's record, a medical office assistant should document it on the date on which the no-show occurred. All chart documentation should be written in black ink. (Documentation is discussed further in Chapter 9.) Beginning at the left-hand margin of the patient's progress notes, the current date should be entered followed by a statement similar to "Patient failed to show for an appointment with Dr. X." The statement should then be signed at the right margin with the medical office assistant's name and job title. Any blank space between the statement and the signature should be marked out with a thin black line (Fig. 7–6).

Some offices may prefer to use a stamp or sticker that states "No-Show." Documentation with the stamp is similar to that in the preceding example. The assistant should enter the date, stamp "No-Show," write a statement comparable to "appointment with Dr. X," and then sign the entry as previously mentioned.

Some medical offices may request that the assistant telephone the patient and inform him or her of the no-show appointment. As mentioned previously, the patient may have a medical condition that warrants attention and may need to reschedule the appointment. This call should also be

---

Horizons Healthcare Center – Progress Notes

Patient Name: Brenner, Inez	Chart number: 100121

12-14-01 NO SHOW with Dr. Marks--B. Frost, med adm. asst.

Figure 7–6. No-show appointments must always be documented in the patient's chart to protect the health facility from possible litigation.

PROCEDURE 7-3 *Document Appointment Changes*

Materials Needed
- Patient's medical record
- Black ink pen

1. Identify appointment change (no-show, cancellation, reschedule, etc.)
2. Obtain patient's medical record.*
3. In appropriate location in the patient's record, enter the date and document the appointment change.
4. Sign the chart entry.*

Denotes a crucial step in the procedure. This step must be completed satisfactorily for the procedure to be completed satisfactorily.

documented in the patient's chart. The documentation explanation "Patient was called regarding no-show for 11-18-200x appointment with Dr. Martin" is sufficient. A notation should also be made as to whether or not the patient rescheduled the appointment (Procedure box 7–3).

Canceled and Rescheduled Appointments

A canceled appointment occurs when a patient has made an appointment and later requests that the appointment be deleted. If possible, an appointment cancellation should be documented in the chart, similar to the documentation for the no-show. The documentation should read "Patient canceled (date) appointment with Dr. X. Patient did not wish to reschedule" (Fig. 7–7).

Cancellations are documented for the same reason a no-show is documented. It is important to protect the physician and health care facility from any potential litigation whenever possible.

A rescheduled appointment occurs when a patient has made an appointment and later requests that the appointment time or, possibly, the physician be changed (Procedure box 7–4). Because the patient intends to meet the physician at the rescheduled appointment, there is no need at that time to document the rescheduling in the patient's chart.

When dealing with rescheduled appointments, it is important to remember to be sure to delete the first appointment from the schedule. When working in a busy office with a manual system, it is easy to forget to erase the first appointment. Many computerized systems have built-in rescheduling that automatically voids the first appointment when the second is made. It is important that the schedule be accurate to reflect open time slots for patients who need them.

Ancillary and Referral Appointments

Sometimes, it is necessary for the medical office assistant to schedule outside appointments for the practice's patients. Ancillary appointments are appointments made with departments, such as laboratory or x-ray, to have special diagnostic tests performed. Referral appointments are appointments made with a specialist to see the patient regarding medical concerns. Some insurance companies involved with managed care often require referrals to be approved first by the patient's primary care physician.

When scheduling any outside appointment, it is important to have all necessary information ready when calling the facility for the appointment. First, the medical office assistant should have already checked with the patient and obtained his or her preference for the day and time when the outside appointment could be scheduled. It is good practice also to have the patient's chart on hand. When the outside appointment is scheduled, it should be recorded in the patient's chart. The method of charting is similar to the previous examples in this chapter. A sample entry is shown in Figure 7–8. Any instructions for the referral appointment should be obtained for the patient.

Horizons Healthcare Center – Progress Notes	
Patient Name: Brenner, Inez	Chart number: 100121
11-08-01 Patient canceled appointment for post-operative recheck; did not reschedule. -------------------------------	
---B. Frost, med. adm. asst.	

Figure 7–7. Appointments that are canceled by the patient should be documented in the patient's chart to protect the health facility from possible litigation.

PROCEDURE 7–4 Reschedule Appointments

Materials Needed

- Appointment scheduling software

or

- Appointment book and pencil

1. Obtain the patient's name.*
2. Locate the original appointment.*
3. Verify the reason for the appointment. Using scheduling guidelines, determine whether the length of the appointment is correct.
4. Determine the preferences for a desired appointment time.
5. Identify the date and time for the appointment, and obtain approval for the date and time with the patient (or patient's representative).
6. Enter new appointment on the schedule.
7. Confirm the new appointment with the patient (or patient's representative).
8. Delete the original appointment.

Optional

9. Give the patient a written reminder of the new appointment.

Denotes crucial step in the procedure. This step must be completed satisfactorily for the procedure to be completed satisfactorily.

Surgical Appointments

If an assistant works for a surgeon, it will be the assistant's responsibility to schedule surgery for patients. A number of things are required for surgical appointments. First, and foremost, the assistant needs to obtain from the surgeon exactly what procedure or procedures the patient will have done. If the procedure is expected to be particularly difficult, the assistant may need to schedule additional time for the surgical procedure.

After identification of the procedure, the assistant needs to obtain the patient's current insurance information and should contact the insurance company for authorization for surgery. Because of requirements from most insurance companies today, authorization must be obtained or benefits will not be paid for the procedure. (Exceptions do exist in cases of emergency treatment.) Insurance coverage should be verified and authorization obtained or the patient may be responsible for the entire bill. At the time of authorization, the insurance company may issue an estimate of benefits that will be paid by insurance for the surgery.

Aside from insurance company requirements, patients scheduled for surgery almost always require a preoperative physical within a week before surgery. The preoperative physical may need to be scheduled with the patient's primary care physician. This physical helps ensure that the patient is able to undergo the surgical procedure. Of course, in emergency cases, surgery would be performed to save the life of the patient regardless of whether or not a physical was done.

At the time of the initial scheduling of the patient's surgery, the patient is given a tentative time for the surgery and instructions on when to report to the hospital or outpatient surgery center as well as instructions for preoperative care. Because surgical schedules can change often, the patient is usually instructed to telephone the surgeon's office the day before the surgery to obtain an update on the time the patient should report to the facility for surgery.

Pharmaceutical and Other Sales Representatives' Appointments

Many sales representatives selling pharmaceuticals, medical supplies, and office supplies often compete for the attention of the physician.

Pharmaceutical sales representatives meet with physicians and other clinical staff members to give them information on the medications their company produces, inform the staff about new products, and offer free samples of many

Horizons Healthcare Center – Progress Notes	
Patient Name: Brenner, Inez	Chart number: 100121

9-23-01 Appointment made on 9-24-01 with Dr. Gonzalez for surgical consult. --

--B. Frost, med. adm. asst.

Figure 7–8. Outside appointments scheduled by the medical office assistant should be recorded in the patient's chart.

of their products. Other sales representatives may request appointments to sell medical equipment or supplies. Some offices limit the number of sales visits per representative, and some offices may allow only a designated number of total appointments per week (e.g., two appointments available on Tuesday and two on Thursday). Appointments may be kept on the patients' schedule, but it is important that they not be recorded as medical appointments; rather, they should be recorded the way meetings are recorded. Pharmaceutical representatives are often allowed to check and replenish their sample stock in the office between visits.

It is important for the medical office assistant to recognize sales pitches and to require a representative to make an appointment to see the physician and office staff. Most offices are far too busy to handle drop-in sales people. Sales representatives often bring pens, pencils, notepads, and other office supplies to the medical office staff. The staff should be careful to not deviate from the office policy for handling pharmaceutical sales people, regardless of these "perks."

Posting the Schedule

Every day, the current day's appointment schedule is posted at or near the nurses' station for the use of the nurses and the physicians. As mentioned previously, new copies of the schedule are printed or copied throughout the day to keep the staff aware of changes in the schedule. It is extremely important to remember that the schedule should be posted out of the view of patients. The schedule should not be posted in examination rooms or in the hallway in the plain view of others. Remember, appointment information is considered to be confidential.

An additional copy of the schedule is sometimes posted at the front desk where patients check in for appointments. The front desk staff may elect to do this to keep a minute-by-minute check of who has and who has not arrived for an appointment. Most computer systems can also track such information.

Appointment Reminders

Written Reminders

When a patient makes an appointment in person, a written reminder is given to the patient before he or she leaves the office (Fig. 7–9). The written reminder serves as a "physical" reminder of the appointment. The patient may then use the reminder to transfer information to a calendar at home.

Reminders may look different in appearance from office to office, but they all contain the same basic information (1) patient's name, (2) date, (3) time of next appointment, and (4) provider's name. Reminder slips usually also contain office information, such as address and telephone number.

In completing a reminder, it is good practice to write only the patient's first name on the reminder slip. Although this slip is given directly to the patient, the medical office assistant must remember that the information contained on the slip is about a medical appointment that the patient has in the future. If the patient loses the reminder, the information on the reminder could potentially harm the patient. A patient's name on a reminder slip for an appointment at a local mental health facility would likely identify the patient as a client of the facility, and, because of existing social stigma connected with seeking some types of medical treatment, this could possibly harm the patient.

Telephone Reminders

Whenever the patient is present in the clinic, it is recommended that a written reminder always be given to the patient. Many appointments, however, are scheduled over the telephone. In those cases, a telephone call should be made to remind the patient of the appointment. These telephone reminders are usually done the day before the appointment to give the office staff enough time to reach the patient and to give the patient notice that the appointment time is near. Telephone reminders done too far in advance might give the patient too much time to forget the appointment.

When working in a primary care office, a good rule to follow is to give a telephone reminder to any patient who has an appointment for 30 minutes or more. Generally, if a primary care office is even moderately busy, a missed 15-minute appointment will not leave a huge gap in the schedule, but a missed 30- to 60-minute appointment might create a great deal of downtime. The office should establish a policy about which appointments are given telephone reminders.

The medical office assistant should use caution when leaving a telephone reminder. In no circumstance should the assistant leave the reminder with anyone but the patient unless he or she has been instructed otherwise by the patient. When telephoning the patient, the medical office assistant should first ask for the patient by name, to verify that the message is given to the individual for whom it is intended.

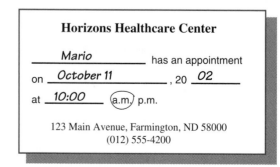

Figure 7–9. A written reminder will help the patient remember his or her next appointment.

A typical telephone reminder might sound like the following:

Assistant: Hello, may I speak with Amy, please?

Amy: This is Amy.

Assistant: Amy, this is Nancy calling from Horizons Healthcare. I'm calling to remind you of your 3:00 appointment tomorrow with Dr. Martin.

Amy: Oh, thank you for calling.

Assistant: You're welcome. We'll see you tomorrow. Good-bye.

Amy: Good-bye.

In this conversation, you will notice that the medical administrative assistant does not identify where she is calling from until she confirms that she is talking with the patient. It is important to keep the information about the appointment confidential and to not give that information to anyone else in the household. The patient may not want the information about the appointment to be shared with anyone. An exception is, of course, that parents will receive reminders for their children's appointments.

Planning for the Unexpected

Even the most organized, efficiently planned schedule may be ruined when the unexpected happens. A physician may be ill and be unable to see patients. The physician could be called away to the hospital for a delivery or to see a patient for a serious problem. An emergency patient may come to the clinic. Whatever the case may be, the medical office assistant and the rest of the office staff will need to minimize the impact of the unexpected on the appointment schedule.

The assistant should always notify patients when the physician has been delayed. Patients currently in the office when the unexpected occurs may be given the opportunity to perhaps see another provider in the office who can accommodate them. The patients may either wish to wait, or

they may want to reschedule. Try to accommodate patients whenever possible. Patients are usually very empathetic in these situations. Whatever the case may be, most patients understand that emergencies do arise, and they would want the physician to be available if they were to need emergency treatment.

SUMMARY

Efficient appointment scheduling is a critical element in any medical office. A large part of the office atmosphere is determined by the office schedule. Great care is needed in properly scheduling patients for appropriate appointment lengths and in managing no-shows, schedule changes, and unexpected occurrences. In addition, an assistant must continually try to accommodate a patient's needs when scheduling. The assistant who can successfully integrate these guidelines into everyday activities is an important asset to the medical office.

YOU ARE THE MEDICAL ADMINISTRATIVE ASSISTANT

You are working in a busy family practice office. It is midmorning, and there is only one appointment slot left for an appointment today. What options might be open for accommodating patients who need to be seen today?

Bibliography

Lytec Medical 2001 User's Manual. Lytec Systems, 2001.

REVIEW EXERCISES

Exercise 7–1 TRUE OR FALSE

Read each statement and determine whether the answer is true or false. Record your answer in the blank provided. T = true; F = false.

_____ 1. Most medical offices today use a manual system for scheduling appointments.

_____ 2. A computerized system can easily identify when a patient's next appointment is scheduled.

_____ 3. Offices with computerized appointment systems are often more productive than are offices with manual systems.

_____ 4. If the office computers are down, the medical administrative assistant should tell callers to call back in a few hours.

_____ 5. Appointment book entries in a manual system should be made in black ink to allow the schedule to photocopy well.

_____ 6. Computerized systems serve patients more quickly than a manual system.

_____ 7. The more complicated a patient's presenting problem, the less time required for the appointment.

_____ 8. Primary care providers will usually require short intervals for appointments, such as 10- to 15-minute intervals.

_____ 9. A double-booked appointment is an appointment that is scheduled in two different appointment books.

_____ 10. It is acceptable to leave a reminder for a patient's appointment with the patient's spouse.

_____ 11. It is critical to chart a no-show for an appointment to protect the facility in case of possible litigation.

_____ 12. Patients are usually billed for appointments missed.

_____ 13. If a medical administrative assistant suspects a patient is having symptoms of a heart attack, the assistant should not have the patient talk to the nurse but should instruct the patient to go directly to the emergency room.

_____ 14. In the absence of a chart number, the patient's DOB should be obtained when scheduling an appointment.

_____ 15. The medical administrative assistant should always list the patient's exact words as the reason for the appointment.

_____ 16. In nonemergency cases, failure to get an insurance authorization for a surgical procedure may mean the patient may have to pay the entire bill for the procedure.

Exercise 7–2 MATCHING

Using Table 7–1, match the length of time to schedule appointments with the following complaints of patients requesting appointments. Record your answer in the blank provided. Some answers may be used more than once; some answers may not be used.

(a) 15 minutes   (c) 45 minutes
(b) 30 minutes   (d) 60 minutes

_____ 1. Physical for 62-year-old

_____ 2. Abdominal pain

_____ 3. Ingrown toenail

_____ 4. Ear pain

_____ 5. Breast lump

_____ 6. Temperature of 103°

_____ 7. Plantar warts

_____ 8. Physical for 5-year-old

_____ 9. Rash

_____ 10. Two lesions to be removed

_____ 11. Sinus infection

_____ 12. Cough

_____ 13. Pulled muscle

_____ 14. Hearing check

_____ 15. Conjunctivitis

For a challenge, try the following:

_____ 19. A feeling of fullness in the ear

_____ 20. Pain when swallowing

_____ 21. Swelling of unknown cause

_____ 22. Severe sunburn

_____ 23. Twisted ankle

_____ 24. Red, mattery eyes

_____ 25. Feeling of pressure between eyes, stuffy nose

_____ 26. Toe is red, oozing pus, and painful to touch

_____ 27. FB eye

_____ 16. Procto

_____ 17. Urinary tract infection

_____ 18. Sprained ankle

_____ 28. Cold

_____ 29. px to play football

_____ 30. Med recheck

_____ 31. Migraine

_____ 32. wheezing

_____ 33. px before surgery

_____ 34. Irregular menstrual periods

_____ 35. Poison ivy

_____ 36. Dysuria

Exercise 7–3 PRIORITIZING

In each group, choose the symptom of the patient who should receive the first available appointment on the schedule today.

_____ 1. (a) Warts
 (b) UTI
 (c) Leg lump that has been present for 2 months

_____ 2. (a) Possible fx
 (b) px for 10-year-old
 (c) New OB visit

_____ 3. (a) Lesion removal
 (b) Sports px so student can practice this evening
 (c) Pain in the lower right quadrant of the abdomen

_____ 4. (a) Seasonal allergies
 (b) Recheck Pap
 (c) Asthma flare-up

_____ 5. (a) Proctosigmoidoscopy
 (b) Grease burn at work today
 (c) Recurrent cough

_____ 6. (a) Bleeding between menstrual periods
 (b) Ear wash
 (c) Pink eye

_____ 7. (a) Warts
 (b) Cough for past 2 weeks
 (c) Migraine

_____ 8. (a) Lump
 (b) FB—eye
 (c) Painful menses

Exercise 7–4 YES OR NO

Identify whether the following items should appear on the schedule as a reason for an appointment. Y = yes; N = no.

_____ 1. Abdominal discomfort

_____ 2. Recheck STD

_____ 3. HIV test

_____ 4. Pain with coughing

_____ 5. Feeling suicidal

_____ 6. Venereal warts

_____ 7. Lightheadedness

_____ 8. Recheck rash

_____ 9. Paranoid

_____ 10. Herpes

_____ 11. Rash

_____ 12. Nervous

_____ 13. Lump

_____ 14. Headache

_____ 15. Depressed

_____ 16. Genital warts

Exercise 7–5 ABBREVIATIONS

List the meaning of these common scheduling abbreviations.

1. fx _____	5. hx _____	9. UTI _____
2. tx _____	6. HA _____	10. OB _____
3. px _____	7. FB _____	11. SOB _____
4. bx _____	8. URI _____	12. HOH _____

7
ACTIVITIES

ACTIVITY 7–1 **Appointment Scheduling—Manual.** You are a medical administrative assistant working at Horizons Healthcare Center. Using the following guidelines, schedule the appointments listed below.

1. All patients should be scheduled for an appointment with the provider listed.
2. Establish appointment pages for an entire week beginning Monday, October 7, 2002, to Friday, October 11, 2002. Use the appointment pages provided in this text to establish your appointment book. Office hours are 9 AM to 5 PM Monday through Friday. Hours for each provider are listed below.

Provider	Monday	Tuesday	Wednesday	Thursday	Friday
Kristine G. O'Brian, MD	9–5	9–5	9–12	9–5	9–5
Timothy C. Marks, MD	9–5	9–5	9–5	9–12	9–5
Mary M. Sanchez, MD	9–5	9–12	9–5	9–5	9–5

Breaks for lunch are as follows:
- Dr. Marks, 11:30 to 12:30 (no lunch break on the day he works 9:00 to 12:00).
- Dr. O'Brian, 12:00 to 1:00.
- Dr. Sanchez, 12:30 to 1:30.

Dr. O'Brian has a board meeting every Thursday from 8 AM to 9:30 AM. Dr. Marks has a finance committee meeting this week at 5 PM on Tuesday. Dr. Sanchez has nursing home rounds scheduled from 1:00–3:00 PM on Tuesday this week.

3. Use the guidelines in Table 7–1 in your text to determine the appointment lengths for the following appointments. When referring to the appointment list here, schedule appointments for the day and time listed. Enter the patient's chart number as listed in the patient database in the appendix.

Patient	Reason	Appointment Time
Kirsten French	Fever	3:30 Monday
Timothy O'Malley	Lesion removal (2)	2:30 Thursday
Marge Armstrong	Procto	9:00 Tuesday
Deanne Olson	Sinus infection	4:45 Monday
Margaret Stein	px	3:00 Wednesday
Evan Stevens	Ear pain	4:15 Tuesday
Alice Shepard	UTI	10:30 Monday
Ann Walker	HA	2:30 Monday
Jose Garcia	FB eye	9:45 Monday
Amy Gordon	Hearing check	10:30 Friday
Adam St. Michael	Ingrown toenail	11:00 Wednesday
Tara Olson	Pinkeye	1:15 Monday
Susan Pearson	Personal	4:00 Wednesday
Christian Olsen	px	2:00 Wednesday
Tamara Garcia	Menses problem	11:15 Thursday
Inez Brenner	Pharyngitis	4:15 Monday
Mark McLean	Urticaria	10:45 Tuesday
Jeanne Breckman	Stomach upset	2:00 Monday

ACTIVITY 7–2 **Appointment Scheduling—Computerized.** Using Lytec Medical 2001 software provided with this text, schedule the appointments listed in Activity 7–1.

To begin scheduling computer appointments using Lytec Medical 2001

1. Open Lytec Medical 2001. At the main menu, click *file,* then *open practice.*
2. In the open window, click *Horizons Healthcare Center,* then click *open.* (Once the Horizons Healthcare Center practice is open, the practice name will appear on the title bar at the top of the window. You will also notice that the main menu selections have now expanded.)
3. On the main menu, click *activities,* then click *schedule appointments.* The appointment scheduling window will then open. Schedule the appointments listed in Activity 7–1. To determine the length of time needed for the appointment, refer to Table 7–1 in the chapter text. The first one is done for you.

To schedule an appointment

1. After performing step 3, click on the *multiple resource* tab near the top of the appointment window. Under this tab, you will view the schedule for all physicians employed by Horizons Healthcare Center, Drs. O'Brian, Marks, and Sanchez.
2. Click *Go To* at the bottom of the window, then click *specific day.* Insert 100702 in the blank provided and click *OK.* The schedule for 10-07-2002 should now be displayed. (Monday, October 7, 2002, will appear near the top of the window.)
3. Next, schedule Kirsten French's appointment with Dr. Marks. Her appointment is on Monday, 10-07-02 at 3:30 PM. Using the scroll bar on the right, find the 3:30 slot for Dr. Marks and double-click on that slot. The *edit appointment window* will open.
4. Click the magnifying glass on the right of the patient chart box. Locate Kirsten French's name by using the *search for* box or by using the scroll bar on the appointment list. If the practice has a large number of patients, the most expedient way to locate a patient would be to input the first three to four letters of the patient's last name in the *search for* box.
5. Click on Kirsten French's name to highlight her name and click *OK.* (You may also double-click on her name, and you will return to the *edit appointment* window.) You will note that the information for Kirsten that was listed in the database, such as chart number and telephone number, is now on the schedule.
6. To identify the reason the patient is seen, click the magnifying glass in the *reason* box. Select the reason that most closely identifies the reason for Kirsten's appointment. (She has a fever.) Click OK to select the reason for the appointment.
7. In the text box after *note,* any special comments about Kirsten's appointment may be entered.
8. Under the *length* portion of the window, specify the length of her appointment. Referring to Table 7-1, a patient with a fever would be scheduled for a 15-minute appointment.
9. Click *OK.* Kirsten's appointment should appear on Dr. Mark's schedule at 3:30 PM. The remainder of the information in the window is not required to be filled in for the appointment. (The patient's primary provider can be listed in the provider box. The procedure for the appointment is assigned during the billing process.)

To schedule breaks and meetings for the physicians

1. Double-click the beginning of the time slot to be blocked off. Be sure to select the time slot on the correct physician's schedule.
2. Do not specify a patient in the *edit appointment* window, but in the text box after *description,* insert the reason for the break or meeting the physician will be attending.
3. Specify the length of the break or meeting.
4. Click *OK.* The meeting should appear on the physician's schedule.

ACTIVITY 7–3 In the appointment schedules created in Activities 7–1 and 7–2, reschedule the following appointments:

Patient	Original Time	Rescheduled Time
Margaret Stein	3:00 Wednesday	3:00 Thursday
Timothy O'Malley	2:30 Thursday	4:00 Friday
Susan Pearson	4:00 Wednesday	10:00 Friday

To reschedule an appointment with the same provider in Lytec Medical 2001.

1. Locate the patient's appointment. Right-click on the appointment and click on *reschedule.*
2. In the window that appears, select the correct day for the appointment and change the

appointment time (if necessary). Click *OK.* The appointment should be moved from the old time slot to the new time slot.

To reschedule an appointment with a different provider in Lytec Medical 2001

1. The easiest way to move an appointment to another provider's schedule is to right-click on the appointment, click on *cut,* and click on *yes* when asked to delete the appointment.
2. To enter the appointment in a new time slot, simply locate the time slot (making sure you have the correct provider's schedule), right-click on the new time slot, and click on *paste.* The appointment should appear in the new time slot.

ACTIVITY 7–4 Using the progress notes sample pages here, document the following:
1. Today, Mrs. Webster calls to cancel an appointment scheduled for next Tuesday with Dr. Johnson.

Horizons Healthcare Center – Progress Notes

Patient Name: Chart Number:

2. Next Tuesday, Mr. Summerville fails to show for the appointment that was scheduled for that day with Dr. Marks.

Horizons Healthcare Center – Progress Notes

Patient Name: Chart Number:

3. You have scheduled an appointment for Miss Walker at Valley View Radiology Associates for an IVP next Monday at 8:00 AM.

Horizons Healthcare Center – Progress Notes

Patient Name: _____   Chart Number: _____

ACTIVITY 7–5 Read each situation and role play with a partner as to how the situation should be handled.

1. A patient's wife calls to request an appointment for her husband. They live out of town, and she would like the appointment for tomorrow because they have a trip to town planned. The patient's wife states that her husband is complaining of upper arm pain and a feeling of indigestion that is rather uncomfortable. What do you say?

2. Dr. Johnson has been called to the hospital to attend a delivery of one of her patients. She will be gone approximately 1 hour. No other providers are able to handle any of her appointments during the time she is gone. Explain the delay to her patient in the lobby, and offer alternatives to the patient.

3. A patient comes in at the wrong time for an appointment. The patient's appointment is a 15-minute appointment, but it is scheduled for tomorrow. What do you do?

4. Call your instructor or another student in the class, and practice giving a telephone reminder for an appointment scheduled with Dr. Sanchez at 9:30 AM tomorrow.

ACTIVITY 7–6 Complete the appointment reminders listed for Marge Armstrong and Margaret Stein as identified in Activity 7–1.

1.

Horizons Healthcare Center

_____ has an appointment

on _____ , 20 _____

at _____ a.m. p.m.

123 Main Avenue, Farmington, ND 58000
(012) 555-4200

2.

Horizons Healthcare Center

_____ has an appointment

on _____ , 20 _____

at _____ a.m. p.m.

123 Main Avenue, Farmington, ND 58000
(012) 555-4200

LEARNING OUTCOMES

On successful completion of this chapter, the student will be able to

1. Explain concept of exceptional patient service.
2. Describe activities involved in getting the office ready to receive patients.
3. Explain appropriate methods for welcoming a patient.
4. Explain registration procedures.
5. Identify considerations for office area layout.
6. Explain common medical emergencies and the use of protocol for those situations in the office.

CMA COMPETENCIES

1. Establish and maintain the medical record.
2. Identify and respond to issues of confidentiality.
3. Use computer software to maintain office systems.

RMA COMPETENCIES

1. Use appropriate interpersonal skills in the workplace.
2. Receive and greet patients and visitors under nonemergency conditions.
3. Screen visitors and salespersons requesting to see physician.
4. Obtain patient information.
5. Use computer for data entry and retrieval.

VOCABULARY

guarantor

PATIENT RECEPTION AND REGISTRATION

The reputation of a thousand years may be determined by the conduct of one hour.
—Japanese proverb

Aside from the telephone communication a patient has with the medical office staff, the moment at which the patient walks into the medical facility creates a lasting impression of the professionalism and competency of the staff members who work in the medical office. Providing exceptional patient service is essential to creating a good first impression and will communicate to the public the level of caring and concern to which the facility is committed. Not only are first impressions important, but patients deserve outstanding service at all times from all members of the health care team.

A good first impression and consistent quality customer service will help make patients more comfortable with and confident about the services provided in a medical office and will keep patients loyal to the medical office.

EXCEPTIONAL PATIENT SERVICE

The concept of exceptional patient service in health care has close ties to the concept of customer service in the business world. The business world has long known the importance of meeting the customer's needs, and the health care industry recognizes that patients expect their needs to be met, as well.

The health care industry has become extremely competitive, and it is increasingly apparent to health care providers that more is required of them than providing patients with the latest and greatest health care procedures. Today's patients are true consumers of health care and, as such, must be treated as other consumers in the marketplace are treated. Patients demand quality health care service and staff members who are genuinely concerned about their welfare, and the health care industry must be concerned about retaining their customers (patients) as would any other industry.

In the past 20 to 25 years, the health care industry has increased its focus on when and where services are provided. In the past, patients needing to see a physician did so according to the physician's schedule: usually 9 AM to 5 PM Monday through Friday. A patient needing immediate care at other times had to go to an emergency room. Now, many medical offices are open during the evenings and even on weekends. Also, large group clinics have extended their services to additional locations in the hope of attracting more patients. This shift in the offering of health care services has been in response to growing consumer demand for services outside the traditional method of delivery.

Today, the health care industry promotes its services to patients. Patients are targeted with advertisements and public relations materials in the hope that they will be persuaded to use a particular medical facility. These promotions rarely focus on price. The promotions usually focus on quality of care and the caring and concern of the staff, and they place a tremendous emphasis on serving patients' wants and needs. Promotions might also be targeted to a certain group of insurance policy holders. If patients are given exceptional service every time they enter a medical office, patients will be very loyal and will not be likely to switch health care providers; thus, a strong customer base is established for the office.

What, then, is exceptional patient service? It is providing the best possible assistance to or for the patient. Patient service becomes exceptional when staff members "go the extra mile," when they contribute above and beyond what is expected of them. A guiding concept in providing exceptional patient service might be to ask yourself how you would like to be treated or how you would like your loved ones to be treated. All activities of the medical office have an impact on the patient in some way, and even those staff members without direct patient contact are involved in patient service because their activities support the organization (Fig. 8–1).

To provide exceptional patient service, staff members must always focus on what is best for the patient. The patient is always number 1 and is the primary reason for the work of the office staff.

To illustrate this point, let's look at some examples of exceptional patient service.

1. A patient stops by the desk and asks where the nearest pay phone is located. Instead of answering the question by identifying the location of the pay phone, exceptional patient service would be to offer the office telephone for the patient's use.

2. An elderly patient is fumbling with her coat and having trouble putting it on. A simple offer to help ("May I help you with your coat?") might be greatly appreciated and will be long remembered.

For this type of service to be effective, *all* members of the health care team including the office staff, doctors, nurses, administrators, building services staff, and everyone in

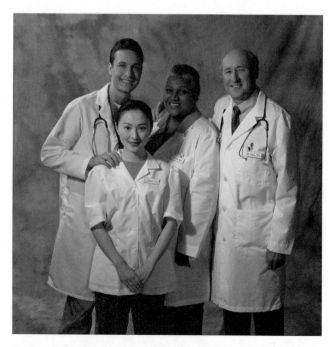

Figure 8–1. In a medical office that practices exceptional patient service, all staff members believe that the patient is always number 1.

between must be committed to participating in this concept of exceptional patient service. This concept should be the foundation for all activities of the medical office. If one group of employees does not believe in and adhere to this concept, the image of the facility will be diminished.

PATIENT HANDBOOK

Many medical offices develop promotional materials for distribution to patients. A patient handbook is a practical way of informing patients of the various services a medical facility has to offer. In addition to information about the services available, a patient handbook may provide a directory of addresses and telephone numbers and detailed maps to assist patients in locating specific areas of the facility.

A handbook is especially helpful for new patients of the practice who may not be familiar with the facility and may need a resource to obtain the information. Of course, a handbook is not a substitute for one-on-one interaction with a staff member of the office, but a handbook can supplement verbal information given to a patient.

GETTING THE OFFICE READY

Every day, even before the medical office is opened, certain activities must be performed to get the office ready for the day. Opening activities vary depending on the size of the office, but most practices have several activities that must be completed before the medical office is open to receive patients. Most of these activities must be done early, because once the office opens, patients will need your complete attention. Typical opening activities are the following:

Unlock the Door. This may seem rather obvious, but more is usually involved than simply turning a key.

To begin with, the office will probably have more than one entrance. Staff members responsible for opening activities will usually enter the office through a back entrance or an employee entrance—one not used by the general public. The front entrance may not be unlocked until the office is ready to receive patients for the day.

Most medical facilities are equipped with alarm systems to guard against vandalism and theft. After unlocking the door, the alarm system will need to be deactivated. Usually, there is only a short amount of time—typically 30 to 60 seconds—in which to turn off the alarm. Most alarm systems are deactivated by entering a numerical code on a keypad located inside the door. These systems are usually connected to the local police department, and if the alarm system is not deactivated in the necessary amount of time, the police may be summoned to the facility. If excessive false alarms are received, the medical office may have to reimburse the police department for expenses related to the false alarms.

Obtain Charts for the Day. Every day, a chart must be pulled for every patient with an appointment on that day. Usually, charts for one day will be gathered the day before, but, occasionally, an assistant may have had difficulty locating one or more of the charts. Each morning, the assistant will need to verify that all charts have been located for the day's appointments. Physicians and other providers dislike seeing a patient without the patient's chart because vital information needed for the office visit may be included in the chart. Ordinarily, new patients will have a chart started on the day of their first apointment.

Start and Check Office Equipment. A variety of equipment is used to support office activities and must be turned on early in the morning to be ready for use. Some large volume copiers require several minutes for warm-up in order to be ready for copying. Computer equipment will also need to be started to ensure that the equipment is working properly and is ready to conduct the day's work. E-mail and fax machines should be checked for transmissions that have been sent during the night.

Switch on Television or Music System. Most offices have some type of electronic media for entertainment. Television sets are generally present in the lobby, whereas music systems play throughout the facility. These systems provide a pleasant distraction for patients while they are waiting for an appointment. If these systems are not turned on right away in the morning, they are generally forgotten once the hectic pace of an office begins.

Count Cash Drawer. Most offices have a cash drawer for receiving payments for services on the day they are rendered. Patients may choose to write a check or use a credit card to charge visits to the doctor. Occasionally, patients may even pay with cash. For that reason, a small amount of change is needed in the office to handle cash payments. The change fund in the cash drawer should remain at a consistent amount and will need to be counted at regular intervals to verify that the money is still there.

WELCOMING PATIENTS

Once the opening activities have been completed, it is time to receive the day's patients. When a patient approaches the registration desk, the assistant should welcome the patient immediately. If the assistant is working with another patient, a simple acknowledgment, such as "I'll be right with you," conveys to the patient that you know the patient has arrived and that you will help the patient as soon as you are able. Patients should always be acknowledged on their arrival in the office because they are the chief focus of work every day.

An assistant can greet a patient with a cheerful remark, such as "Good morning" or "Hello, Mr. Smith." If at all possible, the patient's name should be used in the greeting. Most patients are pleased when the office staff can remember them by name. Even in some of the largest practices, many patients are repeat patients, and staff members are able to identify several patients by name.

When greeting patients, a medical administrative assistant must be careful to not comment personally on the patient's medical experiences. The following statements are examples of inappropriate and uncaring comments:

- "Oh, you're looking so much better compared to last week." (*A medical judgment should not be made about a patient's health.*)
- "It's nice to see you again." (*Are we really glad the patient is in the clinic again?*)
- "You don't look so good." (*This is a very personal comment about the patient's appearance.*)

If you are at a loss for words, it is best to simply welcome the patient with an acknowledgment such as "Hi, Mary. Let me verify your registration information for your appointment today," or "Good morning, Mr. Vasquez. Isn't the weather beautiful today?"

PATIENT REGISTRATION

The registration process involves gathering information about the patient to begin or update the patient's medical record and financial account. During registration, the medical administrative assistant asks the patient a series of questions to obtain information for inclusion in the patient's medical record and to accurately bill for the services rendered on that day.

The registration process is performed for all patients—existing patients (those who have been seen previously in the office) and new patients (those who have not been seen previously in the office). Registration for existing patients usually takes only a few minutes and involves updating the patient information by asking the patient whether certain registration information is still correct (Procedure 8–1). Registration for patients who are new to the clinic may take several minutes because a new patient record must be created (Procedures 8–2 and 8–3).

Registration Information

During the registration process, patients are asked for demographic information, including full legal name, address, telephone, place of employment, emergency contact information, and insurance coverage information. For established patients, the information is verified by reviewing a patient's information in a computer record or in the patient's medical record.

When patients are new to the medical office, patient registration information is usually gathered by asking the patient to complete a registration form, such as the one pictured in Figure 8–2. The information from the form is then transferred to the medical record and may also be entered into a computer database (Fig. 8–3).

The registration process is, perhaps, one of the most critical functions performed by the medical administrative assistant. It is at this point that current information about the patient is obtained. Registration information is used to gen-

PROCEDURE 8–1 *Update Existing Patient Registration Information*

Materials Needed

- Patient information
- Computer software for the medical office

1. Ask the patient for his or her full legal name, and locate the information in the patient database. Verify the patient's date of birth to ensure that the correct record is updated.*
2. Verify that the following information for the patient is current
   - Address
   - Telephone number
   - Employer
   - Insurance company name, address, policy number, and group number (copy insurance card if necessary)
   Record any changes given by the patient.
3. Thank the patient for the information, and ask the patient to be seated in the reception area.
4. Record any changes in registration information in the patient's medical record (as applicable).

Denotes crucial step in procedure. Student must complete this step satisfactorily to complete procedure satisfactorily.

erate computerized forms for the medical record, can be used to schedule appointments for the patient, and can also be used to process statements and insurance claims.

The patient registration information form (see Fig. 8–2) gathers the following information:

Patient's Personal Information

Patient information gathered in the registration process includes basic demographic data about the patient (e.g., name, address, telephone, date of birth [DOB], social security number). It is necessary to obtain the complete legal name of the patient to identify the medical record. No nicknames or abbreviations of names should be used because these can lead to confusion if at some point the patient uses a different form of his or her name. If the patient lists a nickname (e.g., Timmy, Sue, Butch) or an abbreviation (e.g., Wm., Chas.), the assistant should ask the patient for a complete legal name.

Information about where the patient works (e.g., name, address, and telephone number of employer) and about the patient's occupation is also obtained and may be used for

PROCEDURE 8-2 Obtain New Patient Registration Information

Materials Needed

- New patient registration form
- Patient medical history form
- Clipboard and pen or pencil
- Photocopier

1. Ask the patient for his or her full legal name, and check the patient database to determine whether the patient is new to the medical office.*
2. Attach a registration form and patient history form to the clipboard and give them to the patient, asking that he or she complete the forms and return them to you.
3. After the patient returns the forms, review each form to determine whether they are complete. Ask the patient for missing information if the forms are incomplete.
4. Ask the patient for his or her insurance card, and make a photocopy of it.
5. Thank the patient for the information, and ask the patient to be seated in the reception area.

Denotes crucial step in procedure. Student must complete this step satisfactorily to complete procedure satisfactorily.

Patient's Insurance Information

Complete information regarding the patient's insurance coverage is needed at the point of registration. The name and address of the insurance company as well as the name and address of the policy holder (the insured), policy number, group number, and relationship of the patient to the insured are gathered to be used for an insurance claim submission after the patient's visit. If the patient's insurance is new or changed, an assistant should copy both sides of the patient's insurance card for use at a later time should any billing questions arise.

Patient's Referral Information

Many physicians want to know who is referring a patient to their office. A patient may be referred by another patient of the medical office or by another health care professional. Physicians often make it a point to acknowledge their appreciation of referral patients to those who have referred patients.

Emergency Contact

From time to time, a medical facility will need to contact a patient's family member because of an emergency involving the patient. An emergency contact is included in the patient's registration information for use should an emergency situation arise.

Generally, the emergency contact requested is someone who does not live with the patient. This may seem odd at first, but imagine what would happen if the patient is in an accident along with a spouse. If the spouse is the patient's

various reasons. Occasionally, for such things as notification of a change in an appointment time or of results of tests, the patient may need to be contacted while at work. Some physicians make it a special point to know the occupation of a patient because the nature of the patient's employment may have an impact on the patient's health status.

Patient's or Responsible Party's Information

Sometimes, the patient and the person responsible for paying the medical bill are not the same person. A patient who is younger than 18 years of age, for example, can usually not be held responsible for a bill. Instead, the bill is sent to a responsible party, or **guarantor,** usually a parent. A guarantor is the individual responsible for a patient's bill and may be the patient or someone other than the patient.

During the registration process, demographic information about the guarantor is gathered for use at a later time in the billing process. All information requested about the guarantor *must* be gathered because, occasionally, the guarantor does not live at the same address as the patient. An example of such a situation is one in which a divorced parent pays for a child's health services but does not live with the child.

PROCEDURE 8-3 Record New Patient Registration Information

Materials Needed

- Completed new patient registration form
- Medical office management computer software

1. Check the computer database to determine whether a record of the patient exists.*
2. Once the patient has been verified as a new patient to the medical office, assign a medical record number to the patient.
3. Enter all pertinent data for the patient into the database.
4. Save the new record.

Denotes crucial step in procedure. Student must complete this step satisfactorily to complete procedure satisfactorily.

REGISTRATION
(PLEASE PRINT)

Timothy Marks, M.D.
123 Main Avenue
Farmington, ND 58000
TELEPHONE: (012) 555-4200

Home Phone: _____

Today's Date: _____

PATIENT INFORMATION

Name _____   Soc. Sec. # _____
      Last Name   First Name   Initial

Address _____

City _____   State _____   Zip _____

Single ___ Married ___ Widowed ___ Separated ___ Divorced ___   Sex M __ F__   Age ___   Birthdate _____

Patient Employed by _____   Occupation _____

Business Address _____   Business Phone _____

By whom were you referred? _____

In case of emergency who should be notified? _____   Phone _____
      Name   Relation to Patient

PRIMARY INSURANCE

Person Responsible for Account _____
      Last Name   First Name   Initial

Relation to Patient _____   Birthdate _____   Soc. Sec. # _____

Address (if different from patient's) _____   Phone _____

City _____   State _____   Zip _____

Person Responsible Employed by _____   Occupation _____

Business Address _____   Business Phone _____

Insurance Company _____

Contract # _____   Group # _____   Subscriber # _____

Name of other dependents covered under this plan _____

ADDITIONAL INSURANCE

Is patient covered by additional insurance? _____ Yes _____ No

Subscriber Name _____   Relation to Patient _____   Birthdate _____

Address (if different from patient's) _____   Phone _____

City _____   State _____   Zip _____

Subscriber Employed by _____   Business Phone _____

Insurance Company _____   Soc. Sec. # _____

Contract # _____   Group # _____   Subscriber # _____

Name of other dependents covered under this plan _____

ASSIGNMENT AND RELEASE

I, the undersigned, certify that I (or my dependent) have insurance coverage with _____ and assign
      Name of Insurance Company(ies)
directly to Dr. _____ insurance benefits, if any, otherwise payable to me for services rendered. I understand that I am
financially responsible for all charges whether or not paid by insurance. I hereby authorize the doctor to release all information
necessary to secure the payment of benefits. I authorize the use of this signature on all insurance submissions.

_____   _____   _____
Responsible Party Signature   Relationship   Date

ORDER # **58-8425** Σ © 1996 BIBBERO SYSTEMS, INC. Σ PETALUMA, CALIFORNIA Σ TO REORDER CALL TOLL FREE: (800) 242-2376 OR FAX: (800) 242-9330

Figure 8–2. The patient registration information form is used to gather information that is used for various activities in the medical office. (Courtesy of Bibbero Systems, Inc., Petaluma, California 94954; phone, 800-242-2376; fax, 800-242-9330; e-mail, info@bibberosystems.com; available at www.bibberosystems.com.)

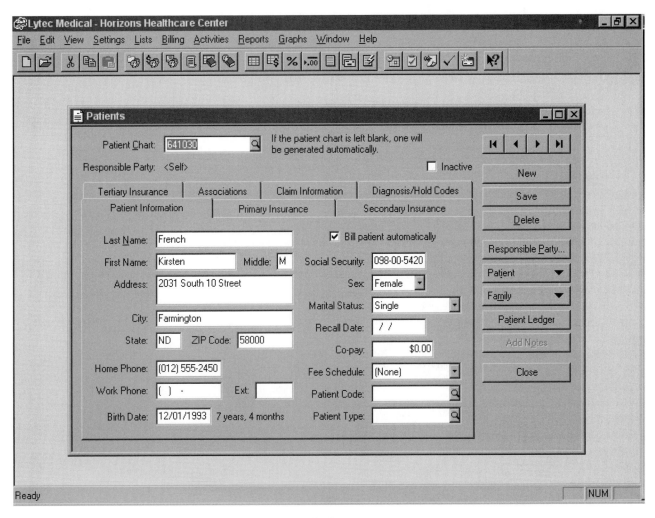

Figure 8–3. Patient information is often stored in a computer database.

emergency contact, there would not be anyone else listed in the registration information who could be notified. The spouse's name is usually already included in the patient information section.

If the patient is asked to identify someone not living with him or her as an emergency contact, family information is still included elsewhere in the form, and an additional contact is available in the emergency section of the form.

In case of an emergency involving only the patient, the patient's home is usually contacted first, and, if there is no answer, other contacts are attempted. Emergency contact information may also be used occasionally, if necessary, for account collection.

Authorizations

The registration form often contains statements near the bottom of the form that authorize the practice to release information to the patient's insurance company for billing and that authorize any payments of benefits to come directly to the practice. Also included in the authorization section may be a statement that the patient is ulti-

mately responsible for the charges that are incurred. If the patient's signature is not obtained in the authorization section, insurance claims cannot be filed directly from the medical office, and the responsibility for filing claims will rest with the patient. Failure to have these authorizations signed means the patient must file insurance claims, which will likely cause a delay in receiving payment for services rendered.

Patient History Form

At the time of registration, new patients are asked to complete a medical history form (Fig. 8–4) that asks for information regarding their past illnesses, surgeries, hospitalizations, drug allergies, family medical history, and other pertinent medical information. This form becomes a part of the patient's medical record and is reviewed by the physician when the patient is examined. Because of all the information that must be obtained from new patients, new patients take more time to register and should be asked to arrive 15 minutes earlier than a scheduled appointment to complete the registration process.

ADULT PATIENT'S CHECK LIST FOR MEDICAL HISTORY

NAME: _____ DATE OF BIRTH: __/__/__ DATE: _____

PAST SURGERIES: None ☐ — or, list here any past surgeries with approximate age at which performed.
_____

OTHER HOSPITALIZATIONS: List reason and date(s).
_____

ACCIDENTS: No injuries of consequence ☐ — or, list any serious type injuries, with approximate age.
_____

PAST MEDICAL ILLNESSES: List any serious illness, with approximate age: No serious past illnesses ☐
List any major childhood diseases:
Sexually Transmitted Diseases (past or current): ☐ Gonorrhea ☐ HIV/AIDS ☐ Herpes ☐ Chlamydia ☐ Syphilis ☐ Other
Any blood transfusions: ☐ Yes ☐ No

FAMILY HISTORY: If any of the following have run in your family, check appropriate block:
Allergies ☐;   Cancer ☐;   Tuberculosis ☐;   Diabetes ☐;   Heart Disease ☐;   Strokes ☐;   Hypertension ☐;
Any deaths below age of 55? ☐

CURRENT MEDICATIONS:
Please list all medications you are now taking, including those you buy without a doctor's prescription (such as aspirin, cold tablets or vitamin supplements) List name, dosage and times per day.

1. _____   4. _____   7. _____
2. _____   5. _____   8. _____
3. _____   6. _____   9. _____

CURRENT ALLERGIES, SENSITIVITIES AND INTOLERANCES:
List anything that you are allergic to such as foods, medications, dust, chemicals, household items, pollens, bee stings, etc., and indicate how each affects you:
_____

RECENT TRAVEL AND IMMUNIZATIONS:
Have you traveled out of the country in the last 2 years? ... ☐ No ☐ Yes, traveled in _____
Write in the dates for the shots you have had: Measles / Mumps / Rubella (MMR) _____ Polio _____
Tetanus / diphtheria (dt) _____ Typhoid _____ Flu _____ Pneumococcal/Pneumonia _____
Other _____
Have you had a tuberculin (TB) skin test: ☐ No ☐ Yes Date _____ Result ? ☐ Pos. ☐ Neg. ☐ BCG _____

OTHER MEDICAL CARE:
Living Will/Durable Power of Attorney: ☐ Yes ☐ No
If you are being treated for any other illness or medical problems by another physician or mental health practitioner, please describe the problems and write the name of the physician, health practitioner or medical facility treating you.

Illness or Medical Problem   Physician or Medical Facility   City
_____
_____
_____

REVIEW OF SYMPTOMS: Place a check mark in the appropriate blocks in the following list of <u>current</u> (within past 3 months) symptoms:

1. HEAD AND NECK

	YES	NO		YES	NO		YES	NO
Severe headaches	☐	☐	Severe hearing loss	☐	☐	Frequent colds	☐	☐
Dizzy spells	☐	☐	Ringing in ears	☐	☐	Sinus trouble or hayfever	☐	☐
Wear glasses	☐	☐	Pain in ears	☐	☐	Chronic nose obstruction	☐	☐
Failing vision	☐	☐	Discharge from ear	☐	☐	Persistent sore gums	☐	☐
Eye pain	☐	☐	Repeated nosebleeds	☐	☐	Prolonged hoarseness	☐	☐
Double vision	☐	☐	Teeth problems	☐	☐	Swelling in neck	☐	☐

2. HEART AND LUNGS

	YES	NO		YES	NO		YES	NO
Heart problems	☐	☐	Ankles swell	☐	☐	Smoking history	☐	☐
Chest pain on effort	☐	☐	Have chronic cough	☐	☐	Past ☐ Present ☐		
Skipping/irregular heart beats	☐	☐	Difficult breathing	☐	☐	Type ___ Qty ___		
Hypertension	☐	☐	Spit up blood	☐	☐	If currently smoking are you		
Cholesterol	☐	☐	Have night sweats	☐	☐	interested in quitting?	☐	☐

Continued on back page

Figure 8–4. All new patients complete a medical history form for inclusion in their medical record. (Courtesy of Bibbero Systems, Inc., Petaluma, California 94954; phone, 800-242-2376; fax, 800-242-9330; e-mail, info@bibberosystems.com; available at www.bibberosystems.com.)

2. HEART AND LUNGS (cont.)

	YES	NO		YES	NO		YES	NO
Cholesterol	☐	☐	Have night sweats	☐	☐	Wheezing	☐	☐
Lab test date _____			Frequent chest colds	☐	☐			
Results _____			Sit up to breathe easier	☐	☐			

3. STOMACH AND INTESTINES

	YES	NO		YES	NO		YES	NO
Chronic Abdominal Pain	☐	☐	Any chronic diarrhea	☐	☐	Sigmoidoscopy	☐	☐
Persistent nausea	☐	☐	Any black tarry stools	☐	☐	Date _____		
Heartburn	☐	☐	Any blood from rectum	☐	☐	Results _____		
Appetite loss	☐	☐	Clay colored stools	☐	☐	_____		
Vomit blood	☐	☐	Habitual constipation	☐	☐			
Skin turns yellow	☐	☐	Have hemorrhoids	☐	☐			

4. URINARY TRACT / GENITAL

	YES	NO		YES	NO		YES	NO
Frequent urination	☐	☐	Hard to start urinary flow	☐	☐	Weak stream/scanty urination	☐	☐
Any blood in urine	☐	☐	Frequent night urination	☐	☐	Pain with urination	☐	☐
Any leakage of urine	☐	☐	Passed any stones	☐	☐	Any bedwetting	☐	☐
Any retention of urine	☐	☐						

5. OB GYN (For Women Only)

Last menstrual period _____

If currently having periods
do you have:

	YES	NO		YES	NO		YES	NO
Painful menstruation	☐	☐	Previous Pap smear	☐	☐	Any breast lumps	☐	☐
			Date of most recent Pap			Mammography	☐	☐
Excess menstruation	☐	☐	_____			Date _____		
Bleed between periods	☐	☐	Results _____			Results _____		
Any missed periods	☐	☐	Current birth control	☐	☐	_____		
Any vaginal discharge	☐	☐	Type: _____					
			Number of pregnancies _____					
			Number of living children _____					

6. MUSCLES — JOINTS

	YES	NO		YES	NO		YES	NO
Physically handicapped/limited	☐	☐	Shoulder pain	☐	☐	Red or swollen joints	☐	☐
Joint or muscle problems	☐	☐	Back pain	☐	☐	Limitation of motion	☐	☐
Varicose veins	☐	☐						

7. NEUROLOGICAL

	YES	NO		YES	NO		YES	NO
Numbness	☐	☐	Any dizzy spells	☐	☐	Any shaking/tremors	☐	☐
Disturbance in walking	☐	☐	Any paralysis/weakness	☐	☐	Any falls	☐	☐
Trouble with balance			Any strokes	☐	☐	Speech disturbance	☐	☐
or coordination	☐	☐	Any seizures	☐	☐	Any memory loss	☐	☐

8. PSYCHOLOGICAL

	YES	NO		YES	NO		YES	NO
Psychological/emotional /			Excessive fears	☐	☐	History of:		
stress problems	☐	☐	Nervous breakdown	☐	☐	Alcohol problems	☐	☐
Psychotherapy/counseling	☐	☐	Depression	☐	☐	Total drinks consumed		
Currently	☐	☐	Sexual problems	☐	☐	for last week _____		
In past	☐	☐	Serious marital problems	☐	☐	Drug problems	☐	☐
						Any mood changes	☐	☐

GENERAL HEALTH .... Good ☐ .... Fair ☐ .... Poor ☐

Do you eat a balanced diet:	Yes ☐	No ☐	Explain _____
Do you have a lot of stress:	Yes ☐	No ☐	Explain _____
Do you get regular exercise:	Yes ☐	No ☐	Explain _____

Any exposure to environmental hazards such as chemicals, dust or fumes? ☐ Yes ☐ No

If yes, please explain:

IF THERE ARE ANY ADDITIONAL HEALTH FACTORS IN YOUR HISTORY
OR IF ANY OF THE ABOVE POINTS NEED CLARIFYING,
USE THIS SPACE FOR ADDITIONAL COMMENTS.

FORM # 25-8092 • 1974 BIBBERO SYSTEMS, INC. • PTETALUMA, CA. TO REORDER CALL TOLL FREE: (800) BIBBERO (800-242-2376) OR FAX (800) 242-9330   (REV 6/95)

Figure 8–4. (*Continued*)

Confidentiality When Registering Patients

When greeting patients, it is important to remember to keep your voice at a volume that cannot be heard by others who are seated in the lobby or elsewhere in the clinic. Protecting the confidentiality of the patient's visit is crucial, and the medical administrative assistant must pay special attention to protecting the confidentiality of all the information given by the patient.

When registering a patient, it is best not to repeat the reason for the patient's visit. Imagine the embarrassment if a patient were to be asked, "And you're being seen for genital warts today?" while others are standing behind the patient. If it is necessary for the assistant to conduct a question-and-answer interview with the patient to obtain information, it should be done in a private setting away from other patients. Some facilities have separate desks (apart from appointment check-in) that are used for registration interviews. To provide more privacy for patients, these desks may have multiple stations with glass or solid partitions that separate the area from the lobby and reception desk.

After a patient is registered, all paperwork related to that registration should be moved to another part of the desk so that the next patient in line does not see the previous patient's information.

CHECKPOINT

An assistant who is new to the office likes to help make new patients feel more welcomed to the practice by sitting next to the patient in the lobby to answer any questions the patient may have about completing the paperwork for registration. Is this a good idea?

RECEPTION AREA

The reception area (Fig. 8–5), or lobby, of the medical office is the area in which the patients are seated as they await their appointment. You will notice that the area is not called the "waiting room." The very use of the term "waiting room" has a negative connotation and implies that patients will need to *wait* to see the doctor.

Layout and Design of the Reception Area

Much thought and consideration is necessary to plan a functional and useful layout of the reception area of a medical office. This area is more than chairs and a few fixtures. Let's take a look at all of the items found in a well-planned reception area.

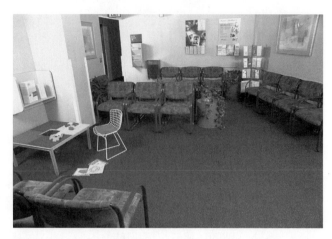

Figure 8–5. A well-planned reception area is an important component in a medical office.

Welcoming Atmosphere. The basic elements of the room—floor covering and wall treatments, for example—should be color coordinated and inviting. The services of an interior designer may be valuable in coordinating all of the basic elements of the room. Floors are usually covered in a multicolored, industrial carpet that is easy to clean and will not show wear too quickly. Walls are usually covered in a high-quality wallpaper or paint that is scrubbable. In addition, artwork, plants, and even an aquarium might be purchased to furnish the room.

When selecting colors for the reception area, keep in mind the structural components of the room. Are there windows to let in sunlight, or is this area enclosed? Deep, dark colors may be depressing to some patients, and bright, vivid colors can be nauseating and dizzying to others. A light- to medium-toned color palette is probably the best choice when decorating this area.

Traffic Patterns. The entire reception area should be planned to allow traffic to flow easily throughout. Tight spaces and areas that handle all of the traffic coming and going may cause problems if many patients are in the office at the same time.

Be sure to allow adequate space in all walkways and other areas to accommodate patients who use a wheelchair. Doors must have automatic openers, and all office accommodations such as restrooms and water fountains must be accessible to patients who have a disability. The Americans with Disabilities Act (ADA), a federal law, has mandated specific requirements for accessibility.

The reception desk should be located near the front entrance but aside from the main lobby (Fig. 8–6). This area needs to be private to ensure that patients cannot hear the activities of the office staff as well as the assistant's interactions with patients. When the assistant picks up the telephone at the front desk, patients sitting in the lobby should not hear the conversation.

Seating Arrangement. The best type of seating arrangement is a well-cushioned modular chair that can be rearranged in a variety of groupings. Patients should have a comfortable place to relax before an appointment. If a television set is present in the lobby, a group of chairs should be positioned around the set and a group positioned away from the set to provide a quiet space for patients.

Chairs should be covered with commercial-grade upholstery that is easy to clean in the event the furniture becomes soiled. Sofas are generally not used in a reception area because patients may not wish to sit near other patients. In addition, sofas can be very difficult to keep clean.

Television or Music System. As mentioned previously, most clinics have some type of electronic entertainment for their patients. Some facilities may have both television and music.

The type of music often heard in a health care facility is background music (frequently known as "elevator music") played at a very low volume. The music helps mask some of the noise of the office's everyday activities and is a nice addition to the office's atmosphere.

Television is common in many medical office reception areas. Even with background music playing, the music and television usually do not "compete" with each other.

If a television is present in the lobby, the assistant needs to pay close attention at all times to what is being shown on the television. Many pediatric reception areas post signs on television sets asking patients to consider the children present and to ask the front desk whether the channel may be changed. Many offices will not change the channel unless the programming is suitable for children. Even if you are working in a family practice or multispecialty clinic, chances are there may be children present, and it is wise to monitor what is appearing on the set. Many parents find soap operas, prime-time shows, and many talk shows unsuitable for children.

Reading Material. Nearly all physicians' offices have something available for patients to read. Magazines and medical pamphlets help patients pass the time. Professional medical journals, meant for physicians and nursing staff,

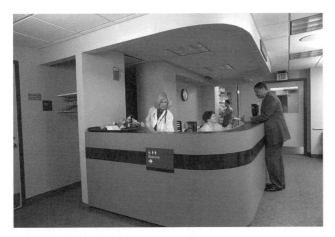

Figure 8–6. The front desk in a medical office should be positioned off to the side of the reception area to help protect the confidentiality of patient information.

are not placed in the lobby. Like the television situation mentioned earlier, some clinics are also very careful to supply only those magazines and pamphlets that are appropriate for all ages. Some materials, because of their content, are highly inappropriate for children.

Something for Kids. As mentioned previously, children may be present in the reception area. They may be patients or they may accompany a parent or grandparent to the clinic. Whatever the case, every lobby should have a few items available to keep children busy. Aquariums can help pass the time, as can children's magazines or books. Toys may be available but should not be a choking hazard. Sometimes, a small table and chairs with coloring books and crayons are available. In addition, an assistant should take special precautions to protect children who may visit the facility. Electrical outlets should be covered, and cords should be placed out of a young one's reach.

Refreshments. All offices should have a drinking fountain or water cooler available for anyone needing a drink of water. Some offices even supply coffee for patients and others in the reception area. If coffee is provided, the coffee machine should be located in an area not accessible to children.

Wheelchair. Every reception area should have a wheelchair located near the front door and easily accessible to the front desk staff. Patients entering the clinic with a variety of medical concerns may need transportation in a wheelchair. Wheelchairs should be used for many different emergency situations. These situations are discussed later in this chapter.

Other Reception Area Fixtures. No reception area is complete without a few more items.

- **Wastebasket.** Without a wastebasket, waste materials may be left on the furniture or floor.
- **Coat rack.** Without a coat rack, a coat may be left on a chair, taking up space while the patient is with the physician.
- **Clock.** Some offices are uncomfortable with a clock in the reception area. If the practice believes in and practices exceptional patient service, however, a clock should be almost a nonissue—patients will not be in the lobby long enough to watch it!
- **Restroom.** The restroom is usually positioned close to the front desk. When a patient asks the location of the restroom, the assistant should check the reason for the patient's appointment to determine whether a urine specimen may be necessary for the patient's visit. If a specimen is necessary, the assistant may need to direct the patient to the appropriate location in the office where a specimen can be left.

CHECKPOINT

Explain why music or television, or both, is an important addition to a reception area.

Reception Area Maintenance

Because the reception area has such heavy use during the day, it is the responsibility of the medical administrative assistant to make sure the area stays neat and tidy. The assistant will need to continually monitor the area and periodically walk through the lobby and straighten anything that is out of order.

EMERGENCY SITUATIONS

Chapter 6 discusses how to recognize some common emergency situations over the telephone, but what happens when an emergency presents itself in the medical office? The assistant must be able to recognize and react to common medical emergencies. How the medical administrative assistant responds to the situation may be critical to the health and welfare of the patient. To provide the patient with the best possible service, it is important for the medical administrative assistant to recognize a common emergency (Fig. 8–7) when it occurs in the reception area or when a patient in an emergency situation walks right through the front door!

Every office should prepare adequately for emergencies by establishing protocol for handling emergencies and by offering training in such things as cardiopulmonary resuscitation (CPR) for all staff in the medical office. Before implementing any emergency procedures, it is always necessary to obtain physician approval for any emergency procedures that will be used. It is not the medical administrative assistant's responsibility to treat the patient, but the assistant should be able to recognize signs and symptoms of common emergencies and must be able to get the patient to the medical staff as quickly as possible.

What Is an Emergency?

A situation is an emergency when a patient's health may be adversely affected if immediate action is not taken. Some emergency situations may even be life threatening. Heart attacks are obvious emergency situations. Other serious medical problems may be an emergency in that if action is not taken, the patient may be irreparably harmed. For example, a patient with a chemical splash to an eye may suffer permanent eye damage if immediate medical attention is not received.

Common Medical Emergencies

Following are examples of medical emergencies and common responses to these situations. All emergency protocol used in a medical office should be reviewed and approved by the physicians of the practice before being placed in use.

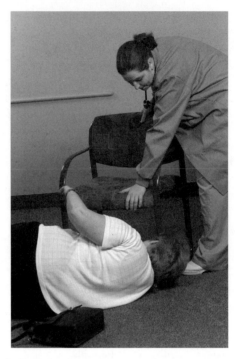

Figure 8–7. A medical administrative assistant must be able to recognize common medical emergencies and get help for the patient as quickly as possible.

Chest Pain

Chest pain may have various causes. Chest pain due to myocardial infarction, or heart attack, may have a predominant symptom of a painful crushing sensation or severe pressure to the chest. Pain may travel down arms, throat, or back and may persist for several hours. The patient may appear pale, diaphoretic (sweating profusely), nauseated, short of breath, and may complain of indigestion. It is important to note, however, that not all heart attack victims have the same symptoms. Only some of these symptoms may be present. Heart attack pain can be experienced quite differently from patient to patient.

If a patient enters the clinic with complaints of any of these symptoms, the patient should be placed in a wheelchair and immediately escorted to an examination area of the office. The medical staff can be notified via intercom that a patient is on the way to an examination room. A patient with heart attack symptoms should never be seated in the lobby. In any emergency situation, a patient's name can be obtained after the patient is in an examination room.

Seizure

Someone may experience a seizure while seated in the lobby. A grand mal seizure is evidenced by a sudden loss of consciousness and sudden involuntary movements of voluntary muscles. The patient's muscles may relax and contract in rapid succession. Some or all of the patient's body may jerk or twitch, or the patient may vomit or become incontinent.

When a seizure occurs, it is important to try to prevent further injury to the patient. Attempts should *not* be made to restrain the patient, however. If the patient is near any hard objects, such as furniture, the objects should be moved, if possible, out of the patient's way. If a hard object is struck repeatedly, the patient could awaken with multiple bruises and much discomfort over the injured region. Cushion the patient's head, if possible, with a pillow or other soft object.

Hard objects should *never* be inserted into the patient's mouth. Serious injury could occur if the object is broken by the patient's jaw and swallowed. The patient should be rolled onto one side to prevent aspiration of any vomitus that may occur. The assistant should summon the medical staff as quickly as possible.

The assistant should be ready to communicate to the physician any specific symptoms, if known, that occurred just before and at the time of the seizure, as well as the parts of the body involved.

Most grand mal seizures are short lived, lasting only about 5 minutes. On rare occasions, a grand mal seizure may not stop, and the patient may continue to convulse. This occurrence is known as status epilepticus and is a serious, life-threatening situation.

If a patient experiences a seizure while in the clinic, a physician should always be notified as quickly as possible, even if the patient has a known history of seizures.

Respiratory Distress

Respiratory distress may be caused by a wide variety of conditions, such as a cardiac problem, pulmonary problem, an allergic reaction, and even a panic disorder. A patient with respiratory distress exhibits dyspnea or wheezing and may even appear cyanotic.

Patients experiencing respiratory distress as a result of an allergic reaction may have urticaria or edema, or both, on the face, although that is always not apparent.

Occasionally, patients with asthma may experience an episode known as status asthmaticus. This type of asthma attack is ongoing and very severe and can result in respiratory arrest.

It is important for the assistant to obtain a wheelchair for a patient with respiratory distress because loss of consciousness may occur quickly. The medical staff should be alerted, and the patient should be escorted to the examination area of the office immediately.

Diabetic Emergencies

Two types of emergencies are related to a patient's blood sugar level—hyperglycemia and hypoglycemia. In both instances, a patient does not need to be a known diabetic to experience one of these occurrences.

Hyperglycemia is a blood sugar level that is too high. Patients with hyperglycemia have a rapid pulse, warm dry skin, and decreased perspiration.

In an episode of hypoglycemia (low blood sugar), the patient may appear confused, may hallucinate, or even go into a coma. The patient exhibits an increased pulse, rapid heart beat, and sweating and may appear anxious. The medical administrative assistant should obtain a wheelchair for any patient with a diabetic emergency and should escort the patient to the clinical area of the facility.

Both hypoglycemic and hyperglycemic patients may exhibit difficulty walking, may be irritable, and may complain of headache. The condition the patient is suffering from may not be readily apparent; thus, when a patient presents with a diabetic emergency, it is important for the assistant to not give the patient anything to eat or drink unless authorized by the physician. The physician should decide what treatment is appropriate for the patient's condition.

Profuse, Uncontrolled Bleeding

Sometimes, when injured, a person will grab the closest thing to wrap around the wound and head out the door to the nearest doctor's office. When the patient arrives at the clinic, his or her clothes may be soaked with blood, and the patient may need material to soak up additional blood.

To be ready for these emergencies, a clean supply of towels and rubber gloves should kept at the front desk. When a bleeding patient walks through the door, the assistant can grab a towel quickly and offer it to the patient to wrap around the wound. Be careful to hand the towel to the patient and let the patient apply it to the wound. Use the towels, if at all possible, to avoid a blood spill in the reception area.

When dealing with a patient who is bleeding profusely, it is important to realize that the patient could go into shock as a result of loss of blood. A patient with these types of wounds should be escorted immediately to the examination area via wheelchair to avoid harm to the patient in case of collapse.

Because of the potential hazardous nature of bodily fluids such as blood, any bloody cloths must be disposed of properly. Do not throw blood-stained cloths in the trashcan in the reception area. It is important to avoid any direct exposure to the patient's blood. If it is necessary to pick up bloody cloths that have fallen on the floor, it is absolutely essential to wear protective gloves before picking up any bloody materials. More information on dealing with bodily fluids is included in the "Standard Precautions" section of Chapter 12, Office Management.

Head Injury

All head injuries should be taken seriously. Patients with a head injury may appear dazed, may vomit, may have uneven pupils, or may be unable to move an extremity.

All head injuries are potentially dangerous because there is a chance that bleeding may occur in or around the brain. Patients reporting a head injury should be escorted via wheelchair to the examination area of the office immediately.

Syncope

Syncope (fainting) involves a sudden loss of consciousness. Syncope should be taken seriously because it may indicate a more serious problem occurring in the patient. If a patient faints while in the reception area of the clinic, it is important to summon the medical staff immediately to assess the situation.

Psychotic Episode

An individual experiencing a psychotic episode has a sudden break with reality and is not capable of rational thought at that time. It is important to realize that the individual is irrational and that attempts to reason with the individual may be futile. Psychotic individuals appear irritable and confused and may hallucinate, may have increased respirations, and may become violent. If confronted with a psychotic individual, it is important to be calm and to speak calmly. Be sure to consider the protection of yourself and others in the building. There is no need to be heroic to protect the physical contents of the office. Physical contents can be replaced—people cannot. If a psychotic individual makes demands for medical supplies, money, or other items in the office, comply with the individual's wishes. In such a situation, it is important to remember that a call to 911 may be warranted.

Eye Injury

Patients with eye injuries usually need immediate attention by the medical staff. The eye may need to be washed to remove an irritant. Patients with an eye injury should be escorted to an examination room as quickly as possible and should not be seated in the lobby.

Burns

Patients who have been burned also need the immediate attention of the medical staff. Treatment may need to be instituted immediately to diminish blistering and peeling of the wound. Treatment may range from immersing the area in cool water to applying either a moist or dry dressing. No treatment should be given without the permission of the physician.

What the Medical Administrative Assistant Should Do

When dealing with an emergency situation, the medical administrative assistant should always alert the medical staff (physician or nurse, or both) as soon as possible. In some cases, depending on the status of the patient, it may be necessary to assist the patient first to prevent further injury. For example, if a patient enters the office with some type of respiratory distress, the assistant may need to help the patient into a wheelchair before the patient collapses to the floor.

Whatever the emergency may be, it is imperative that the dignity and privacy of the patient be protected as much as possible and that the assistant try to avoid any further embarrassment to the patient.

Depending on the medical services available in the medical office, the medical administrative assistant may need to call 911 for an ambulance or may need to call a code team for an emergency situation. Sometimes, all physicians may be out of the office and it may be necessary to call 911 for emergency help.

The assistant's main goal in assisting patients with a medical emergency is to transfer the patient to the physician and nursing staff as quickly as possible.

After care of the emergency patient has been transferred to a member of the medical staff, the assistant is not finished dealing with the situation. It may be necessary to locate a family member for the patient. Family members are usually contacted by the nursing staff, who may be able to give more information about the patient's condition. It may be the medical administrative assistant's responsibility, however, to locate a family member by telephone and to transfer the call to the nurse. When contacting a family member for this reason, it is best to locate the individual and to choose a statement that will not alarm the family member (e.g., "This is Dr. Anderson's office calling. Could you hold for a moment to speak with the nurse?").

After an emergency situation has occurred in the lobby, patients who were present will be aware that appointment times are likely going to be delayed. Patients arriving for appointments after the situation has cleared the lobby, however, may need to be informed that there was an emergency situation and that an appointment may be delayed. These arrivals should be simply told that there was an emergency, but the assistant should keep the nature of the emergency confidential.

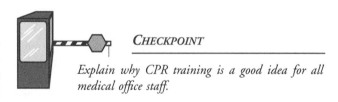

CHECKPOINT

Explain why CPR training is a good idea for all medical office staff.

Other Situations

Fractures

Although most patients with fractures who present to the clinic are not medical emergencies, the medical administrative assistant should be sure to provide special attention to the patient with a fracture. If at all possible, a patient with a fracture should be placed in a treatment room immediately and should not be expected to sit in the lobby. If a patient hobbles or "hops" in because of a leg injury, the assistant should insist that the patient sit in a wheelchair to allow for easier transfer to a treatment room. Nothing would be more embarrassing to a medical office than to have a patient fall and cause further injury because the patient was "hopping" to a treatment room.

Acutely Ill or Uncomfortable Patients

Whether or not a situation is a true emergency, no patient in distress should be left in the reception area. Patients who are acutely ill, vomiting, experiencing severe headache, or who are obviously uncomfortable should be transported to an examination room. Leaving the patient in the lobby conveys a feeling of uncaring and a lack of concern by members of the entire health care team. The assistant should pay attention to the overall appearance of all patients entering the office and, if necessary, should ask whether a patient needs to lie down.

Planning for Emergencies

No one ever really expects an emergency, but all medical offices must be prepared to handle emergencies that arrive. Sometimes, the only thing the staff will be able to do is to stabilize a patient while they wait for an ambulance to arrive.

Whatever the case, it is critical for the office staff to keep calm and to carry out the practice's approved protocol for emergencies.

SUMMARY

The moment a patient enters a medical office, a lasting impression of the office's commitment to patients is created. Providing exceptional service conveys a high level of commitment and caring toward patients.

Not only is exceptional service important, but the medical office's reception area should be well planned and accommodating for all of the practice's patients. Great care should be paid to the design of the room as well as to amenities necessary to serve the needs of patients.

An integral part of receiving patients each day is the patient registration process. The information gathered in this process supports many other important activities of the office. When registering patients, the medical administrative assistant should be aware of various symptoms that may indicate a potential emergency situation. If a patient enters the clinic with an alarming symptom, the assistant should be ready to act to prevent further injury to the patient.

Many things contribute to a patient's overall experience with a medical office, and how the patient is received by the practice contributes a great deal to the patient's experience.

YOU ARE THE MEDICAL ADMINISTRATIVE ASSISTANT

The medical office where you work is looking to trim operating costs. One of the physicians has suggested that the front desk staff come in 15 minutes before the first appointment instead of 1 hour before the first appointment. Is this a good idea?

Bibliography

Chester GA: Modern Medical Assisting. Philadelphia, WB Saunders, 1998.
Kinn ME, Woods MA: The Medical Assistant, Administrative and Clinical, 8th ed. Philadelphia, WB Saunders, 1999.
O'Toole M: Miller-Keane Encyclopedia & Dictionary of Medicine, Nursing, & Allied Health, 5th ed, Philadelphia, WB Saunders, 1992.

8

REVIEW EXERCISES

Exercise 8–1 TRUE or FALSE

Read each statement and determine whether the statement is true or false. Record the answer in the blank provided. T = true; F = false.

_____ 1. A patient's first impression of the medical office will be affected by the service given by the medical office staff.

_____ 2. Because many insurance companies specify which physician a patient must use, the medical office staff need not be concerned about customer service.

_____ 3. Medical offices have been responsive to patients' needs by offering extended office hours.

_____ 4. Medical offices advertise their services to patients.

_____ 5. An alarm system can be used to protect a medical office against vandalism and theft.

_____ 6. After the office is opened for the day, the assistant will pull the charts for patients who will be seen for an appointment that day.

_____ 7. If an alarm system has been accidentally set off, the assistant may need to notify the police department of the false alarm.

_____ 8. In order to make a patient feel more welcome to the office, a medical administrative assistant is encouraged to make personal comments about a patient's health.

_____ 9. An assistant should greet a patient by name, if possible.

_____ 10. A patient's full legal name is required during registration to prevent duplicate medical records from being created.

_____ 11. The chief reason a patient's employer's name and telephone number is obtained is to track the patient in case a bill is unpaid.

_____ 12. A guarantor is another name for insurance company.

_____ 13. Emergency information is sometimes used for account collection.

_____ 14. A medical history form asks questions about the health of the patient's family members.

_____ 15. If patients in the lobby can overhear the office staff discussing information about another patient's appointment, this would be a breach of confidentiality.

_____ 16. The physicians of the medical office must approve any emergency protocol used by the medical office staff.

_____ 17. An assistant should be prepared to call 911 if necessary to provide medical care for a patient in the office.

Exercise 8–2 CHAPTER CONCEPTS

Read each question and choose the answer that best completes the question. Record the answer in the blank provided.

_____ 1. Which of the following is not done by the assistant every day in the medical office?
(a) Pull medical records for the next day's appointments.
(b) Count cash drawer.
(c) Order supplies.
(d) Check fax for overnight transmissions.

_____ 2. Which of the following greetings would not be acceptable in the medical office?
(a) Good morning, Mr. Smith. Has there been any change in your address or insurance company?
(b) Hi, Lila. How can I help you this morning?
(c) Good afternoon, how may I help you today?
(d) Hello, Mrs. McDonald. I hope you're feeling better than yesterday.

_____ 3. What information is not required during registration?
    (a) Name of company.   (c) Policy number.
    (b) Amount of deductible.   (d) Address of company.

_____ 4. What does not apply to authorizations on a registration form?
    (a) Can authorize release of information to an insurance company.
    (b) If not signed, can delay receipt of payment for services.
    (c) If not signed, insurance claims can still be filed by medical office.
    (d) Can authorize payments from insurance companies to come directly to the medical office.

_____ 5. Why are new patients asked to arrive early for appointments?
    (a) The assistant must check the credit history of new patients with the local credit bureau.
    (b) Extra time is needed to complete the registration and medical history forms.
    (c) Extra time is needed for laboratory tests to be run.
    (d) None of the above.

_____ 6. Which of the following is usually not found in a reception area of a medical office?
    (a) Professional journals for physicians.   (c) Magazines for a general audience.
    (b) Television set.   (d) Wheelchair.

_____ 7. Which of the following is a concern when children are present in the reception area of a medical office?
    (a) Location of the coffee maker.
    (b) Large toys that do not present a choking hazard.
    (c) Children's books and magazines.
    (d) Television playing children's videos.

_____ 8. Which of the following should never be done for a patient who is having a seizure in the lobby?
    (a) Get help from the physician immediately.
    (b) Move hard objects out of the patient's way.
    (c) Insert a hard object in the patient's mouth.
    (d) Roll the patient to one side to prevent aspiration of vomitus.

_____ 9. Which of the following medical emergencies could be aided by the use of a wheelchair?
    (a) Chest pain.
    (b) Respiratory distress.
    (c) Profuse, uncontrolled bleeding.
    (d) All would be aided by the use of a wheelchair.
    (e) Only (a) and (b) would be aided by the use of a wheelchair.

_____ 10. Which of the following does not pertain to customer service in the medical office?
    (a) Patients are health care consumers.
    (b) The health care industry has been responsive to patient needs.
    (c) Health care promotions usually focus on price of services.
    (d) Exceptional customer service keeps patients loyal to the office.

Exercise 8–3 LEGAL NAMES

Read the following nicknames and write the legal names associated with them in the blank provided. Information on names can be found in the appendices of many collegiate English dictionaries.

1. Tim _____
2. Tony _____
3. Becky _____
4. Nate _____
5. Bill _____
6. Ned _____
7. Marge _____

8. Sue _____
9. Chris _____
10. Judy _____
11. Cindy _____
12. Jerry _____
13. Val _____
14. Dee _____

15. Kate _____
16. Chuck _____
17. Jack _____
18. Abby _____
19. Peggy _____

8

ACTIVITIES

ACTIVITY 8–1 *EXISTING PATIENT REGISTRATION—COMPUTERIZED (See Procedure 8–1)*

Using the Lytec Medical 2001 software provided with this text, record the following changes to the patient's registration information.

To enter changes to the registration information using Lytec Medical 2001

1. Open Lytec Medical 2001. At the main menu, click *file,* then click *open practice.*

2. In the open window, click *Horizons Healthcare Center,* then click *open.*

3. On the main menu, click *Horizons Healthcare Center,* then click *patients.* The *patients* window will open. The record for the first patient in the database will appear in the window. Click on the magnifying glass to the right of the patient chart box. The *find patient* window will open and display the entire list of registered patients. The search by box should read last name, first name. If not, click the drop-down arrow on the *search by* box and choose *the last* name option. Enter the patient's last name in the *search for* box, and the patient's record should appear highlighted below. Locate the patient records below by highlighting the patient's name and clicking *OK.* The correct patient information should appear in the *patient* window.

4. After necessary changes have been made to a patient's record, click *OK* to save the changes to the record.

   Update the following patient's records by entering the following changes:
   St. Michael, Adam. Change address to 1515 Roosevelt Avenue, Harvester, MN 55555 (same telephone number).
   Wang, Karen. Change last name to Stevens; do not change address or telephone; change marital status to married.
   Olsen, Christian. (DOB: 9-23-36) Change address to 354 Plentywood Road, Harvester, MN 55555, telephone number 010-555-1123.

ACTIVITY 8–2 *NEW PATIENT REGISTRATION—COMPUTERIZED (See Procedure 8–3)*

Using the Lytec Medical 2001 software provided with this text, enter the registration information for the following new patients. The registration information is below.

To enter registration information for a new patient using Lytec Medical 2001

1. Open Lytec Medical 2001. At the main menu, click *file,* then click *open practice.*

2. In the open window, click *Horizons Healthcare Center,* then click *open.*

3. On the main menu, click *lists,* then click *patients.* The patients window will open. The record for the first patient appearing in the database will appear in the window. From this window it is possible to enter a new patient by clicking *new* on the right side of the window. Whenever registering a new patient, however, it is extremely important to check the existing patient list to determine whether the patient has already been registered. Always begin a new patient registration by clicking the magnifying glass next to the patient chart box. The *find patient* window will open displaying the entire list of registered patients. The list can be sorted in a variety of ways by clicking on the drop-down arrow on the *search by* box. (Practice sorting the list by chart and ZIP code.)

4. Sort the patient list by last name, first name. Search for the names below to be sure the patient is new to the office.

5. Enter the registration information as listed for each patient. When a patient record is completed, click *OK* to save the changes to the record.

Record registration information for the following new patients:

William C. Frost
Chart # 691123
1764 Vermont Avenue, Farmington, ND 58000
Home phone: (012) 555-1234
Work phone: (012) 555-9019
SSN: 121-XX-0012
Patient is a married male whose birthdate is 08-04-40.
Primary insurance: Best Kind Insurance (enrolled through his employer).
Insurance policy number: 121XX0012.
Patient is the policyholder (insured = self).

Erin D. Olson
Chart # 691124
1452 Pleasant View Road, Harvester, MN 55555
Home phone: (010) 555-9887
SSN: 321-XX-2222
Patient is a single female whose birthdate is 04-01-01.
Primary insurance: Healthy Insurance (available through her father's employer).
Insurance policy number: 123XX6791.
Patient is the child of Christian B. Olson (insured = child. Choose *set insured* to another patient, Christian B. Olson.)

ACTIVITY 8–3 Locate information about two to three health care facilities (local or national) on the Internet. Compare the information that is presented for patients.

ACTIVITY 8–4 Using the blank registration information form (see Fig. 8–2), perform Procedure 8–2 identified in the chapter.

ACTIVITY 8–5 Consider the following situations. What is the appropriate response to the situation given?

1. A patient enters the office with acute respiratory distress. You immediately transport the patient to an examination room. When you return to the front desk, a patient approaches the desk inquiring about what happened. How do you respond?

2. Explain the authorizations on a registration form to a patient.

3. Design a sign that might be placed near a television set alerting patients to consider young children who may be present. Be sure to communicate in a polite, considerate manner.

8

DISCUSSION

The following topics can be used for class discussion or for individual student essay.

DISCUSSION 8–1 Read the quotation at the beginning of the chapter. How does this quotation apply to customer service in the medical office?

DISCUSSION 8–2 A medical office has decided to streamline registration for patients and has placed a sign-up sheet at the front desk for patients to sign in as they arrive. Is this a good idea?

DISCUSSION 8–3 Discuss the importance of keeping the reception area of a medical office tidy.

DISCUSSION 8–4 The physicians of a medical office have decided that all employees should take a course in CPR. Is this a good idea?

Providing Patient Services

CHAPTER OUTLINE

LEARNING OUTCOMES

On successful completion of this chapter, the student will be able to

1. Explain the role of health information management.
2. Explain confidentiality and the importance of protecting patient confidentiality.
3. Explain the role of computers in health information management.
4. Identify the components of the medical record.
5. Describe quantitative analysis.
6. Describe medical transcription.
7. Describe the necessary filing supplies and filing equipment.
8. Use methods of filing and locating medical charts.
9. Demonstrate color coding.
10. Describe the concerns about retention and disposal of medical records.
11. Explain the procedures for releasing medical information.
12. Discuss the legal and ethical issues surrounding medical records.

CMA COMPETENCIES

1. Perform medical transcription.
2. Organize a patient's medical record.
3. File medical records.
4. Identify and respond to issues of confidentiality.
5. Perform within legal and ethical boundaries.
6. Document appropriately.
7. Establish and maintain the medical record.
8. Use computer software to maintain office systems.

RMA COMPETENCIES

1. Know disclosure laws, what constitutes confidential information, and what information may be disclosed under certain circumstances.
2. Manage complete patient medical records system.
3. File records according to appropriate system.
4. Transfer files.
5. Protect, store, and retain medical records according to appropriate conventions.
6. Arrange contents of patient charts in appropriate order and perform audits for accuracy.

HEALTH INFORMATION MANAGEMENT

What you do is as important as anything government does.

—*George W. Bush*

RMA COMPETENCIES *(Continued)*

7. Record patient communication in charts.
8. Maintain confidentiality of medical records and test results.
9. Observe special regulations regarding the confidentiality of human immunodeficiency virus test results.
10. Transcribe notes from dictaphone or tape recorder.
11. Use computer for data entry and retrieval.
12. Use procedures for ensuring the integrity and confidentiality of computer-stored information.

VOCABULARY

accession ledger
assessment
breach of confidentiality
chart entries
chart notes
chief complaint
color coding
consecutive number filing
consultation
continuation sheets
cross-referenced
diagnosis
discharge summary
face sheet
health information management
history and physical
identification sheet
impression
laboratory report
master patient index
medical history
medical transcription
objective
operative report
outguide
pathology report
problem-oriented medical record
progress notes
quantitative analysis
radiology report
release of information
shingling
SOAP method
source-oriented medical record
subjective
summary sheet
terminal digit filing
tickler file

WHAT IS HEALTH INFORMATION MANAGEMENT?

Health information management involves directing and organizing all activities related to keeping and caring for information concerning health care provided for patients. All aspects of every patient's care are documented for future use. Health information management personnel are responsible for maintaining the medical record, preparing medical reports, releasing appropriate medical information, compiling statistics related to health care services, and coding for billing and insurance purposes.

Individuals responsible for health information management activities in the medical office ensure that patient information is documented properly and that it is used appropriately in the business of health care. These individuals are chiefly responsible for maintaining every patient's medical record and ensuring that the record is complete and accurate.

Purpose of Recordkeeping

Medical records are kept in a health care facility for a variety of reasons. One of the most important uses of a medical record is to document the care given to a patient. Without the record to chronicle the various treatments administered to a patient, health care providers would not be able to treat the patient in the most effective manner. The record also contains documentation of the patient's health status and history. It would be impossible for the physician or any other health care provider to remember everything that had been done for a patient. Even patients themselves would likely not be able to remember absolutely everything in their medical history. The medical record is an essential document needed by every health care provider to supply the best possible care to a patient.

Medical records are also used for legal purposes. If a patient suffers an injury due to an accident and makes a claim against a third party, the patient would seek a medical professional's advice for treatment for that injury. The medical record would then contain documentation as to the extent of the patient's injury. In this type of case, the health care provider would testify as to the patient's injuries, and the patient's medical record would be entered as evidence in court. Sometimes, a health care provider is the defendant in a malpractice suit. The medical record then shows proof of the treatments and advice the patient was given and may actually be used as evidence in support of or against the provider.

The medical record serves as documentation for insurance claims that are filed on behalf of the patient. An insurance company may require a copy of a patient's record to determine whether charges were medically necessary or whether services provided were a covered benefit. Workers' compensation agencies require periodic reporting about a claimant's condition, and the medical record authenticates a patient's condition and treatment.

Data from medical records may also be used in a variety of ways for planning. Many of the following examples do not require identification of a patient's name, but the information contained in a patient's medical record can lead to various improvements in providing health care. The gathering of treatment data from medical records enables health care providers to offer better and more effective treatments for their patients.

Medical information might be used for business planning when a health care facility is considering future expansion of services offered. Records are also reviewed to ensure that treatment provided by a physician or other health care professional meets the facility's standards of quality. Students involved in medical education routinely review case histories to learn more about the practice of medicine. Medical research also requires the use of medical records to track the progress of diseases or injuries and patients' responses to treatment.

CONFIDENTIALITY

Many treatments in the office are of a highly personal nature, and confidentiality is a "must" for all employees of the office. Patients need to be able to trust that their medical histories and treatments will be held in the deepest confidence. Day after day in the medical office, an assistant deals with this personal information about patients. All information received in the process of working in the medical office should be kept private unless the patient or someone with the proper authority has approved disclosure of the information. Everything that is seen, heard, or done in the medical office should be considered confidential. A patient's name, diagnoses, procedures, bills, laboratory tests—essentially everything about the patient's interaction with the office is confidential.

Information about a patient's medical treatment should not be released unless the release is authorized. Releasing medical information that should *not* be released is known as a **breach of confidentiality,** and anyone involved in breaching confidentiality may be subject to termination of employment, legal penalties, or both. A medical administrative assistant must do everything possible to protect all patients' medical information.

The United States Department of Health and Human Services developed national medical record privacy standards as part of the Health Insurance Portability and Accountability Act of 1996 (HIPAA). These standards will be in full effect in April 2003 and apply to all personal health care information. These regulations (as mentioned in Chapter 3) include
● The right to know how personal health information is used.
● A patient's right to obtain a copy of his or her medical record.
● Restrictions on how health information can be used.
● Civil and criminal penalties for violating a patient's privacy.
● Requirements for protecting patients' medical records.

Confidentiality Agreements

Individuals beginning employment in any type of health care facility should be asked to sign a confidentiality agreement. No matter where employees may work within a health care facility, they may come into contact with a patient's medical information. Front desk and nursing staff are privy to a patient's diagnoses and procedures. Even building maintenance staff may be responsible for proper disposal of medical information. To emphasize the importance of confidentiality, all employees as well as volunteers should be asked to sign a confidentiality agreement. An agreement should include a definition of confidential information and the expectation of keeping information confidential, as well as the consequences of breaching confidentiality. Consequences often include termination of employment. A sample of a typical confidentiality agreement appears in Figure 4–3 in Chapter 4, Medical Ethics.

Confidentiality and Computerized Medical Records

A computer is present in almost every medical office. It assists the staff in a variety of office tasks, one of which is health information management. A computer system contains health information about patients, their appointments, and the diagnoses and procedures that will appear on insurance claims. Results of diagnostic studies such as laboratory tests and x-rays can be entered into a computer system in one location and retrieved by a physician in another location. Computers allow for easy retrieval of medical information. Portions of a medical record can be placed in a computer system, or an entire medical record can be stored in a computer system. With the growth of computers in our society, the latter is likely to be commonplace within the next several years.

Protecting the confidentiality of the health information contained in a medical record is one of the chief concerns about computerized medical records or electronic patient records (EPR). Computer systems must be secure and must not be prone to break-in. Most employees should not need access to an entire system; they should have access only to those parts of a system needed to do their job. As the use of computers in health care continues to grow, medical offices will need to be increasingly vigilant in ensuring the confidentiality of medical information.

COMPONENTS OF THE MEDICAL RECORD IN A MEDICAL OFFICE

In a health care facility that provides any type of care for a patient, information related to the patient's condition or treatment is kept in some form of medical record. A patient's record in a medical office would contain documentation related to the patient's office visits, medical tests, and correspondence pertaining to the patient's treatment. A home health agency keeps a record of physicians' orders for patients, services, and even equipment supplied to a patient. A medical record is a written record of *all* aspects of a patient's care in a health care facility.

The medical record in the medical office contains information about a patient's office visits; medical history; immunizations; laboratory, radiology, and other diagnostic testing; and any correspondence sent or received by the office. The record chronicles the history of medical treatment in the physician's office. If a patient is hospitalized, copies of hospital reports are sent from the hospital to the office for inclusion in the patient's medical record.

The basic medical record, medical chart, or patient chart may contain some or all of the following: (1) summary sheet, (2) medical history, (3) progress notes, (4) immunizations, (5) laboratory and pathology reports, (6) radiology reports, (7) other specialized reports, (8) correspondence, and (9) hospital reports.

Summary Sheet

This form is the first page or top sheet that appears in the chart. The **summary sheet** (sometimes called the **identification sheet** or **face sheet**) (Fig. 9–1) contains the patient's insurance information and basic demographic data such as the patient's complete name, address, date of birth, telephone number, employer, and next of kin. The summary sheet may also contain a brief section for recording significant diagnoses, and it may contain a release-of-information statement or other necessary medical information.

Medical History

When establishing a relationship with a health care provider, every patient should be asked to complete a **medical history** form (Fig. 9–2). This form includes questions about the patient's history of disease and injury, questions about the family medical history, and, perhaps, even a summary of any current symptoms. If a patient cannot complete the history form, a family member or caretaker may be asked to complete the form for the patient. If an individual other than the patient completes the history form, that individual's name should be noted on the form.

Progress Notes

Information regarding the patient's visits to the health care provider is listed on the **progress notes** page (Fig. 9–3). Every time the patient sees a physician for an appointment, the patient's condition and treatment are documented on a chart note or progress notes page. Progress notes pages are sometimes referred to as **continuation sheets,** because when one sheet is completed, the progress notes are "continued" onto the next page. All activity regarding the patient—office visits, telephone calls, and

documentation of outside appointments—is documented on a progress notes page. To identify the patient and the date of the office visit, every chart note includes some required information, such as patient name (last, first), medical record number, or date of birth.

One of the most common methods of documenting patient visits in a chart note involves the use of the **SOAP method** (Fig. 9–4). This is an easy method to learn and practice. Each letter stands for the type of information that is included in that section of the chart note.

S = **Subjective.** This portion of the chart note is the patient's account of the reason for the visit. **Subjective** information is the patient's account of his or her illness. In the subjective section, the physician identifies the patient's chief reason for the office visit. This reason is known as the **chief complaint.** This *does not* mean that the patient is a "complainer;" the term "complaint" is used to describe the patient's primary reason for seeing the physician.

Subjective information includes such things as how the patient describes his or her illness (e.g., "I can't sleep at night" or "I feel a sharp stabbing pain in my lower back when I bend over") and also includes a patient's review of body systems. In subjective review of body systems, the physician asks whether the patient is experiencing any problems with vision, hearing, bowels, stomach, muscles, or any portion of the body that may be related to the complaint. The physician then makes a note of any comments the patient makes, such as complaints about coughing at night or about excessive urination.

Although subjective information sometimes cannot be proved by the physician, it is very important to the physician because subjective information describes the history of the patient's illness. The history (subjective) combined with the following physical examination (objective) allows the physician to arrive at a diagnosis.

O = **Objective.** After interviewing the patient, the physician conducts a physical examination to investigate the patient's complaint. This is known as the **objective** portion of the examination. The objective portion of a SOAP note is often the largest portion of the note.

In this portion of a chart note, factual information about the patient is recorded. In other words, information that can be proved or demonstrated by the physician is recorded in this section.

Objective information can include some or all of the following items:

- The patient's sex.
- Observations about the patient's general appearance.
- Vital signs, including temperature, blood pressure, and respiration.
- A review of systems with physician observations of each body system. This objective review differs from the subjective review, because here, the physician's observations (e.g., "There is a moderate swelling over the patellar tendon" or "Chest is clear to auscultation and percussion") are noted. These are statements that can be verified by the physician or by diagnostic studies.
- Results of laboratory and radiologic tests.

A = Assessment. In this part of the chart note, the physician, having considered the subjective and objective information gathered during the examination, arrives at a conclusion. This conclusion is known as the **diagnosis, assessment,** or **impression.** If the patient has more than one condition, each diagnosis is listed in order of significance, with the most significant diagnosis mentioned first.

P = Plan. Once the physician has determined a diagnosis, he or she recommends a treatment plan. Instructions are given to the patient as to actions the patient should take, such as "Call me if you're not feeling better in 3 days or if symptoms worsen" or "Apply warm moist pack to the affected area three times a day." Any medications prescribed for the patient are also listed in this section with the name of the medication, strength, dosage, and duration of treatment. Further tests or even hospitalization may also be part of the plan.

Sometimes, the physician may document information about the patient that does not fit into the SOAP format. In this instance, the physician dictates the essential information about the visit but does not use a clearly defined format. Instead, the chart note is written in paragraph form (Fig. 9–5).

Handwritten entries are sometimes made in the chart by the physician, nurse, assistant, or other medical office staff members. These entries are also known as **chart notes** or **chart entries** (Fig. 9–6) and are included in the progress notes section of the medical record. Only those persons authorized to make entries should make entries. Entries regarding telephone calls, outside appointments, or other information related to the patient's medical care is recorded in the chart and is done so in an appropriate manner (Box 9–1).

The record of an office visit does not always use an entire page. When entries are made in a patient's chart, the medical office staff should be careful to not skip lines or to leave any large gaps on the progress notes page. Any extra space should be crossed out so as to not allow information to be inserted in an incorrect order.

Persons making handwritten entries in a patient's chart should write with black ink only. Blue ink is not an appropriate substitute. Black ink is preferred because it will appear darker than will any other color when photocopied. Pencils, colored pens, markers, and the like are inappropriate for use in a medical record. Pencil marks could be erased, ink from colored pens may not copy well, and markers may smear if a page becomes damp (Procedure box 9–1).

Occasionally, a mistake may be made in the process of recording information in a patient's chart. The person making the mistake must correct the entry. When correcting an erroneous entry in a chart, the assistant should be careful to never obliterate the previous information. If the previous information becomes unreadable when crossed out, a court of law would not look favorably on the medical office: the action may be interpreted that someone in the office wished to hide something.

The proper way to correct an error is to draw a single line through the incorrect information with black ink, write the correct information above it, and date and sign the entry (Fig. 9–7).

No attempt should ever be made to erase an entry or to block it out with correction fluid. There should never be a question about what information was in the chart previously. An honest mistake will probably be forgiven—but not if it looks as though an attempt was made to hide something.

Immunizations

Information regarding a patient's immunization history may be present on the medical history form or may be included on a separate page in the chart. The immunization form often includes a place for the patient's signature for consent to receive the vaccine. This section of the chart also includes information about the manufacturer's lot number of the vaccine.

Laboratory and Pathology Reports

The laboratory section of a medical record contains written results of a patient's laboratory tests and pathologic analysis. The pathology department is concerned with the study of disease, and the laboratory is the place in which that study takes place. A medical laboratory tests blood, urine, and biologic specimens that are removed from the body. A urinalysis and complete blood cell count (CBC) are examples of tests typically referred to as **laboratory reports** or laboratory tests. **Pathology reports** contain descriptions of body tissue that has been sent to a medical laboratory for study. Both of these types of reports are placed in the laboratory section of a medical record. The pathology department is also responsible for conducting autopsies and for verifying specimens that are removed from the body (e.g., the vas deferens removed during a vasectomy). Basically, anytime anything is removed from the body, a specimen is usually sent to the laboratory to be reviewed by the pathology department.

To save space in a patient's chart, the office may place laboratory test results in this section of the chart by using a **shingling** method. If laboratory reports measure less than a full page, shingling the reports allows more reports to fit on one page. Shingling of reports involves placing the oldest laboratory report near the bottom of the page and laying new reports slightly above and overlapping the top of the previously placed report, with the reports thereby appearing in the chart in chronological order (Fig. 9–8). This method allows the physician to quickly flip through the reports to find the desired test results. Reports are often color coded to make them easier to locate in the laboratory section. The lower portion of the report that is visible contains information about when the test was performed. Although shingling saves space, a disadvantage of using shingling is that reports must be removed for photocopying (because they are overlapping) when releasing information.

Thank you for selecting our healthcare team! We will strive to provide you with the best possible healthcare. To help us meet all your healthcare needs, please fill out this form completely in ink. If you have any questions or need assistance, please ask us - we will be happy to help.

Personal Information

Date _____

Birthdate _____

Soc. Sec. # _____

Name _____

Wishes to be called _____

☐ Male   ☐ Female   ☐ Minor   ☐ Single   ☐ Married   ☐ Divorced   ☐ Widowed   ☐ Separated

Address _____

City, State, Zip _____

Employer _____ Occupation _____

Referred by _____

Contact Information

Home Phone _____ Pharmacy Phone # _____

Work Phone _____ Ext. # _____

Car Phone _____ E-Mail: _____

Where do you prefer to receive calls?   ☐ Home   ☐ Work   ☐ Car

When is the best time to reach you?   Time _____ Days _____

In the event of an emergency, who should we contact?

Name _____ Relationship _____ Work # _____ Home # _____

Insurance Information

Primary Insurance

Name of Insured _____

Relationship to patient _____

Insured's birthdate _____

Soc. Sec. # _____

Employer _____

Date Employed _____

Occupation _____

Insurance Company _____

Group # _____

Employee/Cert. # _____

Ins. Co. Address _____

Deductible _____

Amount already used _____

Max. annual benefit _____

Additional Insurance

Name of Insured _____

Relationship to patient _____

Insured's birthdate _____

Soc. Sec. # _____

Employer _____

Date Employed _____

Occupation _____

Insurance Company _____

Group # _____

Employee/Cert. # _____

Ins. Co. Address _____

Deductible _____

Amount already used _____

Max. annual benefit _____

WELCOME

Figure 9–1. A summary sheet, or identification sheet, lists important information about the patient. (Courtesy of Colwell Systems, St. Paul, Minnesota.)

Responsible Party

Who is responsible for the account?

Name _____

Relationship to patient _____

Birthdate _____ Driver's License # _____

Soc. Sec. # _____

Address _____

City, State, Zip _____

Employer _____

Occupation _____

Work Phone _____ Ext. # _____

Home Phone _____

Authorization and Release

I authorize the release of any information including the diagnosis and the records of any treatment or examination rendered to me or my child during the period of such care to third party payors and/or other health practitioners.

I authorize and request my insurance company to pay directly to the doctor or doctor's group insurance benefits otherwise payable to me.

I understand that my insurance carrier may pay less than the actual bill for services. I agree to be responsible for payment of all services rendered on my behalf or my dependents.

Any outstanding balance may be charged to my credit card. ☐ Visa   ☐ Mastercard   ☐ American Express

Card Number _____ Expiration Date _____

X _____

Signature of patient or parent if minor   Date

Financial Arrangements

For your convenience, we offer the following methods of payment.
Please check the option which you prefer.
Payment in full at each appointment.

_____ Cash

_____ Personal Check

_____ Credit Card ____ Visa ____ MC ____ AE

_____ I wish to discuss the office's payment policy.

Thank you for filling out this form completely. The information you have provided will help us serve your healthcare needs more effectively and efficiently. If you have any questions at anytime, please ask- we are always happy to help.

ITEM 29010

WELCOME

Figure 9–1. (*Continued*)

Welcome to our practice. As a new patient, please fill out the information found below to the best of your ability.

Date: _____

Patient Name _____ Birthdate _____ Patient # _____

Chief Complaint: _____

History of present illness:

Location: _____
(Where is the pain/problem?)

Quality _____
(Example: normal versus abnormal color, activity, etc.)

Severity _____
(How severe is the pain/problem on a scale of 1-5 with 5 being the most severe?)

Duration _____
(How long have you had this pain/problem?, or, When did it start?)

Timing _____
(Does the pain/problem occur at a specific time?)

Context _____
(Where were you at the onset of this pain/problem?)

Associated signs/symptoms _____
(What other associated problems have you been having?)

Modifying factors _____
(What makes the pain/problem worse or better?, or, Have you had previous episodes?)

Past Medical History

Have you ever had the following: (Circle "no" or "yes", leave blank if uncertain)

Measles	no yes	Anemia	no yes	Back trouble	no yes	Hepatitis	no yes
Mumps	no yes	Bladder Infections	no yes	High Blood Pressure	no yes	Ulcer	no yes
Chickenpox	no yes	Epilepsy	no yes	Low Blood Pressure	no yes	Kidney Disease	no yes
Whooping Cough	no yes	Migraine Headaches	no yes	Hemorrhoids	no yes	Thyroid Disease	no yes
Scarlet Fever	no yes	Tuberculosis	no yes	Date of last chest x-ray ____		Bleeding Tendency	no yes
Diphtheria	no yes	Diabetes	no yes	Asthma	no yes	Any other disease	no yes
Smallpox	no yes	Cancer	no yes	Hives or Eczema	no yes	(please list):	
Pneumonia	no yes	Polio	no yes	AIDS or HIV+	no yes		
Rheumatic Fever	no yes	Glaucoma	no yes	Infectious Mono	no yes		
Heart Disease	no yes	Hernia	no yes	Bronchitis	no yes		
Arthritis	no yes	Blood or Plasma		Mitral Valve Prolapse	no yes		
Venereal Disease	no yes	Transfusions	no yes	Stroke	no		

Previous Hospitalizations/Surgeries/Serious Illnesses   When?   Hospital, City, State

_____   _____   _____
_____   _____   _____
_____   _____   _____

Medications: (Include nonprescription) _____

Patient social history:

Marital status   Single:_____   Married:_____   Separated:_____   Divorced:_____   Widowed:_____
Use of alcohol: Never:_____   Rarely:_____   Moderate:_____   Daily:_____
Use of tobacco: Never:_____   Previously, but quit:_____   Current packs / day:_____
Use of drugs: Never:_____   Type/Frequency: _____
Excessive exposure   Air-borne
at home or work to: Fumes:_____   Dust:_____   Solvents:_____   Particles:_____   Noise:_____

Family medical history:

	Age	Diseases	If Deceased, Cause of Death
Father	____	_____	_____
Mother	____	_____	_____
Siblings	____	_____	_____
	____	_____	_____
	____	_____	_____
Spouse	____	_____	_____
Children	____	_____	_____
	____	_____	_____
	____	_____	_____

ITEM 29011

HEALTH HISTORY

Figure 9–2. A patient's medical history plays an important role in treating the patient. (Courtesy of Colwell Systems, St. Paul, Minnesota.)

Radiology Reports

Radiology reports contain results of a patient's radiologic study. Some examples of radiologic studies include x-ray, magnetic resonance imaging (MRI), computed to-mographic (CT) scanning, and nuclear medicine. Radiology reports (Fig. 9–9) include the name of the film or procedure that was performed along with the findings of the radiologist, a physician trained in the use of radiology to diagnose and treat disease. Although there is no

Review of Systems: Please indicate any personal history below:

☐ **Constitutional Symptoms**
Good general health lately . . . . . No   Yes
Recent weight change . . . . No   Yes
Fever . . . . No   Yes
Fatigue . . . . No   Yes
Headaches . . . . No   Yes

☐ **Eyes**
Eye disease or injury . . . . No   Yes
Wear glasses/contact lenses . . . . No   Yes
Blurred or double vision . . . . . . No   Yes

☐ **Ears/Nose/Mouth/Throat**
Hearing loss or ringing . . . . No   Yes
Earaches or drainage . . . . No   Yes
Chronic sinus problem or rhinitis . No   Yes
Nose bleeds . . . . No   Yes
Mouth sores . . . . No   Yes
Bleeding gums . . . . No   Yes
Bad breath or bad taste . . . . . . No   Yes
Sore throat or voice change . . . . No   Yes
Swollen glands in neck . . . . No   Yes

☐ **Cardiovascular**
Heart trouble . . . . No   Yes
Chest pain or angina pectoris . . . No   Yes
Palpitation . . . . No   Yes
Shortness of breath w/walking
or lying flat . . . . No   Yes
Swelling of feet, ankles or hands   No   Yes

☐ **Respiratory**
Chronic or frequent coughs . . . . No   Yes
Spitting up blood . . . . No   Yes
Shortness of breath . . . . No   Yes
Wheezing . . . . No   Yes

☐ **Gastrointestinal**
Loss of appetite . . . . No   Yes
Change in bowel movements . . . No   Yes
Nausea or vomiting . . . . No   Yes
Frequent diarrhea . . . . No   Yes
Painful bowel movements
or constipation . . . . No   Yes
Rectal bleeding or blood in stool   No   Yes
Abdominal pain . . . . No   Yes

☐ **Genitourinary**
Frequent urination . . . . No   Yes
Burning or painful urination . . . No   Yes
Blood in urine . . . . No   Yes
Change in force of strain
when urinating . . . . No   Yes
Incontinence or dribbling . . . . . No   Yes
Kidney stones . . . . No   Yes
Sexual difficulty . . . . No   Yes
Male - testicle pain . . . . No   Yes
Female - pain with periods . . . . No   Yes
Female - irregular periods . . . . . No   Yes
Female - vaginal discharge . . . . No   Yes
Female - # of pregnancies . . . . _____
Female - # of miscarriages . . . . _____
Female - date of last pap smear. _____

☐ **Musculoskeletal**
Joint pain . . . . No   Yes
Joint stiffness or swelling . . . . . No   Yes
Weakness of muscles or joints . . No   Yes
Muscle pain or cramps . . . . No   Yes
Back pain . . . . No   Yes
Cold extremities . . . . No   Yes
Difficulty in walking . . . . No   Yes

☐ **Integumentary (skin, breast)**
Rash or itching . . . . No   Yes
Change in skin color . . . . No   Yes
Change in hair or nails . . . . No   Yes
Varicose veins . . . . No   Yes
Breast pain . . . . No   Yes
Breast lump . . . . No   Yes
Breast discharge . . . . No   Yes

☐ **Neurological**
Frequent or recurring headaches   No   Yes
Light headed or dizzy . . . . No   Yes
Convulsions or seizures . . . . . . No   Yes
Numbness or tingling sensations   No   Yes
Tremors . . . . No   Yes
Paralysis . . . . No   Yes
Head injury . . . . No   Yes

☐ **Psychiatric**
Memory loss or confusion . . . . . No   Yes
Nervousness . . . . No   Yes
Depression . . . . No   Yes
Insomnia . . . . No   Yes
Suicidal Thoughts . . . . No   Yes
Violent or Unusual Thoughts . . . No   Yes

☐ **Endocrine**
Glandular or hormone problem . No   Yes
Excessive thirst or urination . . . . No   Yes
Heat or cold intolerance . . . . . . No   Yes
Skin becoming drier . . . . No   Yes
Change in hat or glove size . . . . No   Yes

☐ **Hematologic/Lymphatic**
Slow to heal after cuts . . . . No   Yes
Bleeding or bruising tendency . . No   Yes
Anemia . . . . No   Yes
Phlebitis . . . . No   Yes
Past transfusion . . . . No   Yes
Enlarged glands . . . . No   Yes

☐ **Allergic/Immunologic**
History of skin reaction or other adverse
reaction to:
Penicillin or other antibiotics . . No   Yes
Morphine, Demerol,
or other narcotics . . . . No   Yes
Novocain or other anesthetics . No   Yes
Aspirin or other pain remedies   No   Yes
Tetanus antitoxin
or other serums . . . . No   Yes
Iodine, Merthiolate or
other antiseptic . . . . No   Yes
Other drugs/medications: _____

_____

Known food allergies: _____

_____

Environmental allergies: _____

_____

To the best of my knowledge, the questions on this form have been accurately answered. I understand that providing incorrect information can be dangerous to my health. It is my responsibility to inform the doctor's office of any changes in my medical status. I also authorize the healthcare staff to perform the necessary services I may need.

_____   _____
Signature of Parent or Guardian   Date

Doctor's Review

_____   _____
Signature of Doctor   Date

HEALTH HISTORY

Figure 9–2. (*Continued*)

standard size for a radiology report, x-ray and other radiology reports may be done on a special radiology form, usually 8 1/2" wide × 5 1/2" high, or may be done on a standard 8 1/2" × 11" sheet of paper. Radiology reports can also be shingled to save space in the chart.

Other Specialized Reports

Sections may also be included in a medical record for other specialized types of studies. A miscellaneous section may be used for medical reports that would not be filed elsewhere. In

---

Horizons Healthcare Center – Progress Notes

Patient Name: *Pearson, Steven*   Chart number: *230184*

1-5-02 Patient calls in today regarding three-day history of 102°F temp, congestion and

cough. Patient to make an appointment for sometime later today. ----- J. Mason, R.N.

Pearson, Steven #230184

Visit Date: 1-5-02

Chief complaint: Three-day history of elevated temp, congestion and cough.

S: Patient reports to the office today with a three-day history of temperature ranging from 100-102º, sinus congestion and

cough. Review of systems: Patient reports the above-mentioned symptoms and mild frontal headache. Remainder of

review of systems is unremarkable.

O: Patient is a well-developed, well-nourished 39-year-old male in no acute distress, appearing his stated age. Ht: 5'10",

Wt: 170 lbs. HEENT: Head is normocephalic. Eyes: Pupils equal, round react to light and accommodate. Ears: TMs are

clear. Nose: Nasal passages are boggy with purulent yellowish discharge. Throat is erythematous with thick PND.

Chest: Clear to percussion and auscultation.

A: Sinusitis.

P: Amoxicillin 250 tid for 10 days. Patient also instructed to use an OTC decongestant as per package instructions.

Return to clinic if condition does not resolve.

T.I. Marks, M.D.

Timothy I. Marks, M.D.

D: 1-5-02/TM

T: 1-6-02/mt

Figure 9–3. Office visits, telephone calls, and other interactions with a patient are documented in the progress notes section of a medical chart.

medicine, there are many different types of specialty reports, some of which include electroencephalograms (EEGs), electrocardiograms (EKGs), and electromyograms (EMGs).

Correspondence

The correspondence section of a medical record may contain a variety of documents. Medical records that have been received from a hospital or from other offices may be included in this section. Copies of medical record releases, consent forms, letters the patient writes to the physician or that the physician writes to the patient are also kept in this section. Copies of a patient's advance directives may be included here.

Occasionally, a patient may need to be referred to a specialist for a **consultation** regarding treatment for a medical condition. For example, if a patient's physician is a family practice physician and the physician suspects that the patient has heart disease, the physician will refer the patient to a cardiologist for a consultation. After examining the patient, the cardiologist will document the findings of the examination in a consultation report. A consultation report may be filed in the correspondence section of the medical record.

Hospital Reports

When a patient is admitted to the hospital, certain reports document the treatment given while the patient is hospitalized.

Patient name: Smith, Alice
Chart #483920
Date: 10-17-01

Chief complaint: Pain, left elbow.

S: The patient is a 28-year-old female who has a two-week history of tenderness over the lateral aspect of the left elbow. Patient is left-hand dominant. She has had lateral epicondylitis in the past, approximately five years ago. At that time she reports receiving injections for pain relief.

O: Examination of the left elbow reveals full range of motion with a mild amount of swelling, no erythema and elbow is slightly warm to the touch. She has a negative Tinel's. There is tenderness to palpation over the lateral epicondyle and mild tenderness with resisted wrist dorsiflexion.

A: Left lateral epicondylitis.

P: Patient will be sent to Physical Therapy for ultrasound with hydrocortisone treatments and should return to the clinic if pain does not resolve or worsens.

Brian H. Anderson, M.D.

D: 10-17-01/BA
T: 10-19-01/mt

Figure 9–4. SOAP notes document a patient's office visit. Each of the letters in the word *SOAP* represents the type of information included in the report.

History and Physical

A report known as a **History and Physical** (H&P) documents the patient's condition on admission to the hospital. This report must be completed for every patient within 24 hours of admission.

The content of an H&P (Fig. 9–10) is much like the SOAP notes described previously. The sections of the H&P are identified in the following list:

- **History.** This section is similar to the subjective section of a SOAP note. The reason for admission is listed along with the patient's account of his or her condition. A subjective review of body systems, the patient's medical history, and the family medical history are recorded in this section of an H&P.

- **Physical Examination.** Objective information that the physician has observed during examination of the patient

Patient name: Olsen, Amy
Chart #: 110878
Date: 4-12-01

Patient is progressing nicely. There is still a small amount of swelling in the left knee. Patient will continue anti-inflammatory medication and we will continue with physical therapy. Return in one week.

Brian H. Anderson, M.D.
D: 4-12-01/WS
T: 4-14-01/mt

Figure 9–5. A patient's treatment may also be documented in a chart note written in paragraph form.

Horizons Healthcare Center – Progress Notes	
Patient Name: Stevens, Evan D.	Chart number: 689723
5-8-xx Patient's mother phones in today regarding patient's immunization status. Told	
mother that patient is up-to-date with immunizations and should return to the clinic in one	
year for additional immunizations. --J. Mason, R.N.	

Figure 9–6. A handwritten chart note is used by the medical office staff to document the details of interactions with the patient or other activities performed on behalf of the patient.

is listed in this section. Results of laboratory, radiology, and other testing are recorded under the physical examination information.

- **Impression.** This section identifies the physician's assessment, impression, or diagnosis of the patient's ailment.
- **Plan.** The treatment plan is identified. This will include a comment about admission to the hospital as well as diagnostic tests, procedures, or medications ordered for the patient.

Operative Report

An **operative report** (Fig. 9–11) is a detailed account of a patient's surgical procedure. The preoperative and postoperative diagnosis is listed along with a step-by-step description of the surgical procedure itself. Information is also included in this report about how the patient was placed on the operating table, what type of incision was made, and what instruments and techniques were used.

Discharge Summary

The **discharge summary** (Fig. 9–12) provides a synopsis of the patient's hospital treatment. Information is included about the patient's condition when admitted as well as information about treatments and procedures performed during hospitalization. The discharge summary also contains details about the instructions given to the patient when he or she is discharged from the hospital.

MEDICAL TRANSCRIPTION

Many of the reports contained in a medical record are dictated by the physician and then transcribed by a medical transcriptionist for inclusion in the patient's medical record. The process of **medical transcription** involves the production of a typewritten medical report from physician dictation for placement in a patient's medical record.

Transcribing of reports is preferred over handwritten reports mainly because of concerns about legibility. Typewritten

reports allow information to be easily understood by all members of the health care team as well as by others who may review the record at other facilities. Dictation is also a timesaver for the physician. It takes far less time to dictate a patient's report than to write it out by hand.

Skills Needed

Individuals who do medical transcription need to be highly skilled in several areas. They must be experts in medical language and grammar—able to decipher the physician's dictation and to produce a readable medical report. Transcriptionists must also have a high level of understanding of human anatomy, physiology, and pathophysiology to be sure that the medical reports they type are, indeed, what the physician dictated. They must possess exceptional hardware and software computer skills, because virtually all transcription today is done using some type of computer system. Their keyboarding skills must be exceptional as well: accuracy and speed are expected in the field of medical transcription.

Box 9–1 Guidelines for Handwritten Chart Entries

- Write legibly. No one should have to guess at what was written.
- Use black ink only. No colored markers, pens, or pencils should be used in a chart.
- Every entry in the record should be signed and dated by the individual making the entry. Never make, sign, or date an entry for someone else.
- Make entries promptly.
- Leave no gaps or empty lines when making an entry.
- Make any necessary corrections in an appropriate manner.
- Be objective, specific, and complete when making entries.

PROCEDURE 9–1 Document an Event in a Patient's Chart

Materials Needed
- Patient's medical record
- Black-ink pen

1. Obtain the patient's medical record. Locate the next available place for documentation in the progress notes (continuation sheet).*
2. Determine the information to be written in the patient's chart. Be sure you are authorized to enter such information.
3. With black ink, record the date and the information regarding the patient.*
4. Sign the entry with your first initial, last name, and employment position in the medical office.*

Denotes crucial step in procedure. The student must complete this step satisfactorily in order to complete the procedure satisfactorily.

Equipment Used

Medical transcription involves a transcriptionist listening to the physician's dictation and keying the reports (Fig. 9–13). The physician may use small cassette tapes (minicassettes) that fit in a palm-sized tape recorder that can easily fit in a laboratory coat pocket. After seeing a patient, the physician dictates the details of the patient's visit by stating the patient's name, chart number, and the contents of the medical report. Cassette tapes are then given to the transcriptionist (usually at the end of the day) to transcribe (Procedure box 9–2).

Dictation may also be done using a telephone system that can hold several hundred reports from various physicians throughout the facility. The physician enters patient information by pressing buttons on the telephone, and the dicta-

tion is deposited in a digital system. The transcriptionist then accesses the reports using a hookup with the digital system that enables the transcriptionist to type reports for a specific physician or patient. These systems often make it easy to locate one report for transcription in a matter of seconds.

Medical chart notes are commonly typed on an adhesive-backed paper that reveals a sticky coating when the backing is peeled off. The note can then be adhered to the progress notes page in the patient's chart.

Signature

All physician dictation—whether chart notes or any report dictated by the physician—requires a space for the physician to sign the report. Dates of dictation and the initials of the person dictating, along with transcription dates and the transcriptionist's initials, are included at the bottom of every report.

After any dictated medical report is complete, the report is sent to the physician for signature. In a medical office setting, each patient's report may be attached to the outside of his or her chart when it is sent for signature (Fig. 9–14). This can be very useful if the physician needs the chart to verify any information included in the report.

ORGANIZING THE MEDICAL RECORD

Charting Methods

Charts in many medical offices are arranged in what is known as a **source-oriented medical record.** In this type of arrangement, similar information is kept together or information from like sources is grouped together. In other words, all office visits are together, all laboratory reports are together, all radiology reports are together, and so on. This method makes it easy for the physician to review a particular section of the patient's chart. In a source-oriented format, each section in the chart is arranged in chronological order, with the earliest document placed first on the page and the most recent placed last.

Horizons Healthcare Center – Progress Notes	
Patient Name: Breckman, Jeanne N.	Chart number: 75600

10-24-xx Appointment made for consultation regarding menometrorrhagia with Dr. J. Martino

11-3-xx (BF 10-24-xx)
on 11-1-xx at 11:30. --B. Frost, med. admin. asst.

Figure 9–7. When correcting a chart entry, specific guidelines should be followed.

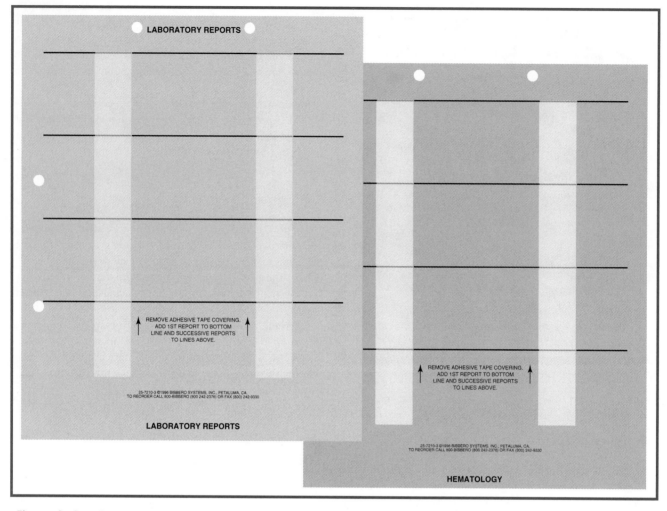

Figure 9–8. Laboratory reports may be shingled to save space in a medical record. (Courtesy of Bibbero Systems, Inc., Petaluma, California, 800-242-2376. Fax, 800-242-9330; www.bibbero.com.)

A few practices choose to arrange the patient's chart in a **problem-oriented medical record** (POMR). This method involves grouping together all the information relating to each problem. If a patient is seen for a broken leg, all information relating to the leg is placed in the same section. The problem-oriented format sometimes makes it difficult to compare like items in the chart, such as laboratory reports or even progress notes, because they may not be grouped together.

record allows for speedy recovery of needed information (Box 9–2 and Procedure box 9–3).

Occasionally, depending on the setup of the health care facility, one common medical record is used for both the office and the hospital. A central health information department oversees the content of a combined record. In the case of a combined record, more than one volume may be necessary to hold all of the patient's medical information.

Chart Order

To make it easy to locate items in a medical record, dividers that section off portions of the chart can be used. Chart dividers are a heavyweight, tabbed paper used to separate different parts of the record. When using dividers and organizing the medical record, all records within a medical office should be organized the same way; that is, all dividers are placed in the same order in every record and all documents are placed in the chart in a specific order within the appropriate divider. Maintaining the same order in every

What Does Not Belong in the Record

The medical record is a compilation of data collected during the course of the patient's medical treatment. Items that contain any type of medical information about the patient should be included in the chart. Some items, however, definitely do not belong in the patient's chart.

First and foremost, no report of any kind should be added to a patient's medical record until the patient's physician has reviewed the report. Even if results of a laboratory study are normal, the physician must review the

HORIZONS MEDICAL CENTER
123 Main Ave.
Farmington, ND 58000

RADIOLOGY REPORT

PATIENT NAME: Webster, Elsie

CHART NO. 352645

DATE: 5-7-2001

PHYSICIAN: Timothy M. Miller, M.D.

DESCRIPTION OF FILM: Upper GI and small bowel

FINDINGS: Swallowing mechanism and esophagus were normal. The stomach filled and emptied in a normal manner, showing only normal gastric mucosa. The duodenal bulb and duodenal loop were normal. Barium meal was followed until it reached the colon in one hour. All small bowel loops including the terminal ileum were normal. There was no evidence of Crohn's disease.

Jennifer E. Braun, M.D.

D: 5-7-01/KS
T: 5-8-01/MT

Figure 9–9. Results of radiologic studies are reported in a radiology report.

report. A transcribed SOAP note or other documentation of a patient's treatment must be authenticated by the patient's physician. If an abnormal test result were to be filed away without the physician's knowledge, a patient might suffer serious medical consequences. Litigation is quite possible if a report does not receive physician review. Failure to obtain appropriate signatures demonstrates sloppy recordkeeping.

Information regarding the patient's financial status with the health care facility does not belong in the patient's medical record. Copies of collection letters or credit arrangements, for example, or references about the patient's ability to pay should **never** be placed in the patient's chart. In the event a patient were to pursue litigation against the physician or the health care facility, it could be absolutely devastating to the case if the patient alleges that certain necessary treatments were not done because of the patient's financial situation. Information regarding a patient's financial arrangements should be kept in a separate account folder in the business office of the health care facility.

Offensive, insulting, callous comments about the patient, another health care provider, or medical office also have no place in the medical record. If such comments appear in the record, the supervisor of health information should be notified.

Records Flow

When a patient makes an appointment, a medical record number or chart number is entered into the appointment schedule. Each day, a printout of the next day's schedule is obtained, and the assistant uses the schedule to pull the patients' medical records for the next day.

When a patient arrives at the office for an appointment, information such as the patient's address and insurance is verified in the front of the chart as well as in any computer records. The chart and computer records are updated if necessary. When an examination room is open, the chart is taken along with the patient to the examination room. The nurse or clinical medical assistant then conducts a brief interview and takes vital signs such as temperature and blood pressure. The nurse or clinical medical assistant records the vital signs in the patient's record.

The chart is then closed and placed outside the examination room door, usually in a plastic holder located on the wall. When the physician is ready to see the patient, he or she brings the chart into the examination room and begins collecting data from the patient. Although the patient is entitled to know the contents of his or her medical record, the record is removed to avoid alarming the patient with something in the record that may be misunderstood.

Horizons Healthcare Center
123 Main Ave.
Farmington, ND 58000
(012) 555-1234

HISTORY & PHYSICAL EXAMINATION

Patient Name: Wang, Karen
Chart # 230192
Date: 6-3-02

HISTORY OF PRESENT ILLNESS: Patient is a 28-year-old Caucasian female with a history of asthma resulting in multiple hospital admissions. She had a recent upper respiratory infection that lasted approximately 10 days. She has complained of cough, chest congestion and blood-tinged sputum for the past three days. She was started on oral erythromycin without improvement. She presents today with increasing shortness of breath and chest discomfort. She uses only a Proventil inhaler and erythromycin at home.

PAST MEDICAL HISTORY: Noncontributory. **ALLERGIES: Aspirin**.

FAMILY HISTORY: Unremarkable.

REVIEW OF SYSTEMS: Her last normal menstrual period was approximately one month ago, but she denies the possibility of intrauterine pregnancy.

PHYSICAL EXAMINATION: Patient is a well-developed, well-nourished female appearing her stated age. She is in moderate distress.

VITAL SIGNS: Temp: 100.4°F. She had a sinus tachycardia of 110/ BP: 110/60. Respirations: 24. HEENT: Sclerae are clear. Conjunctivae are pink and dry. Nasopharynx and TMs are clear. Oropharynx is clear. NECK: Supple without masses or lymphadenopathy. LUNGS: Coarse rales and rhonchi were heard in the right upper and left lower lobe region. There were a few scattered expiratory wheezes. HEART: Sinus tachycardia without murmur or S3. ABDOMEN: Soft with mild suprapubic tenderness without rebound, rigidity or mass. Bowel sounds were active. EXTREMITIES: No edema; calves are benign. NEUROLOGIC: Grossly intact.

DIAGNOSTIC TESTING: Chest x-ray reveals infiltrates and atelectasis in the right upper lobe with right middle lobe and left lower lobe infiltrates.

IMPRESSION: 1. Trilobed pneumonia. 2. History of asthma with intermittent steroid use.

PLAN: Admit the patient and place her on aerosol bronchodilator, IV steroids, IV antibiotics and oral erythromycin pending sputum gram stain C&S. Obtain arterial blood gases, WBC, and hematocrit. We will also gently hydrate her over the next 24 hours and get a follow-up chest x-ray after 24 hours.

T.I. Marks, M.D.

Timothy I. Marks, M.D.

D:6-3-02/TM
T:6-3-02/mt

Figure 9–10. A history and physical documents the details of a patient's condition on admission to a hospital.

Of course, if an electronic patient record is used, the record will be accessible by means of a computer in the examination room or at the nurse's station. At the completion of the visit, the physician may write or dictate office notes of the patient's visit, and the chart is returned to the records room and reviewed in a process known as quantitative analysis.

Quantitative Analysis

After a patient has seen a physician, the patient's chart is returned to the records room. At this point, an assistant reviews the record to ensure that all necessary components are included in the chart. This process is known as **quantitative analysis,** as Edna Huffman describes in *Health Information Management*. The main purpose of quantitative analysis is to verify that all essential pieces of the record are in place. If some portions of the record are not completed or not included in the chart, the assistant should make sure the items are done or located.

A typical analysis of a record might reveal the following:
- Chart notes are not yet completed by transcription.
- A signature on a report is missing.
- A chart entry has not been dated.
- A laboratory or x-ray report is missing.

Records that are missing components may be returned to the health care professional responsible for completion,

Horizons Healthcare Center
123 Main Ave.
Farmington, ND 58000
(012) 555-1234

OPERATIVE REPORT

Patient Name: Walker, Ann
Chart # 152634
Date: 9-7-02

PREOPERATIVE DIAGNOSIS: Sterile pyuria.

POSTOPERATIVE DIAGNOSIS: Normal bladder.

OPERATION PERFORMED: Cystoscopy.

PROCEDURE: The patient was taken to the urology suite and placed in the lithotomy position. The perineum was prepped with Betadine and draped in a sterile manner. Xylocaine jelly was injected into the urethra. Subsequently, the rigid cystoscope was inserted and the cystoscopy was performed. The urethra appeared normal. The bladder showed a normal trigone with normal orifices bilaterally. There was clear urine effluxing from both orifices. The mucosal pattern of the bladder was normal. No foreign bodies or stones in the bladder were seen. The bladder was drained and the cystoscope was removed.

IMPRESSION: Normal examination of the bladder.

Mary Sanchez, MD
Mary Sanchez, M.D.
D:9-8-02/MS
T:9-9-02/mt

Figure 9–11. An operative report gives a step-by-step account of a patient's surgical procedure.

or the assistant may be required to locate documents necessary to complete the file. Incomplete records should be kept in a separate holding place apart from the complete records.

It is extremely important for the medical record to be complete because

- Delays in processing and filing reports and other information in patients' records do not serve patients well. Reliable, complete information is necessary to provide quality patient health care services.
- Accreditation standards for health care organizations require complete and accurate records be kept on every patient.
- Records are required by many governmental agencies.
- Medical record information is necessary to obtain reimbursement from insurance companies.
- The record is essential to a physician's defense. If something is not recorded or included in a chart, it is assumed it was never done. A complete and accurate record is perhaps the best defense in court.

After all necessary information has been included in the record, it may be filed with the completed records in the records room.

FILING SUPPLIES

Charts

A durable heavystock folder is essential to protect the contents of the medical record. Folders may be ordered in a variety of colors, or manila folders may be used with colored numbers along an edge of the folder (Fig. 9–15). The folder should be identified in some way with a color to expedite locating files in the medical office. Color coding is discussed later in this chapter.

The folders must also allow for a fastener of some type to hold the pages of the chart together. The fasteners may be located at the top of a page to allow for a flip-style chart, or fasteners may be located on the side to allow the pages to open like a book. Fasteners should be durable, because pages will be added continually to the chart.

Horizons Healthcare Center
123 Main Ave.
Farmington, ND 58000
(012) 555-1234

DISCHARGE SUMMARY

Patient Name: Armstrong, Marge
Chart # 100120
ADMISSION DATE: 10-5-02
DISCHARGE DATE: 10-10-02
ADMITTING DIAGNOSIS:

1. Pneumonia.

2. Hypertension.

3. History of congestive heart failure.

4. Menopause.

HISTORY: The patient is an 80-year-old female with a complaint of chest tightness. She was seen at the emergency room at Horizons Hospital, was found to have bilateral pneumonia and hypoxemia and was admitted.

HOSPITAL COURSE: Upon admission, the patient was placed on IV antibiotics and oxgyen supplement. She improved and demonstrated gradual resolution of the hypoxemia. She was discharged in stable condition.

DISCHARGE DIAGNOSES:

1. Pneumonia.

2. Hypertension.

3. History of congestive heart failure.

4. Menopause.

PLAN: The patient was discharged in stable condition. She was placed on Ceftin 100 mg bid for seven days. The patient is to see me for a follow-up appointment in one week.

Kristine G. O'Brian, M.D.

Kristine G. O'Brian, M.D.

D: 10-11-02/KO
T: 10-11-02/mt

Figure 9–12. A discharge summary reviews significant events of a patient's hospitalization.

Labels

Several different kinds of labels may be used on the exterior of a patient's chart (Fig. 9–16). Numeric labels that correspond to one or more of the chart numbers may be used on the side of the chart to facilitate filing. Labels identifying important information about a patient might be placed on the outside of a patient's chart. This may be done when the information may be critical to the health care provider. An example of this type of label is an allergy label. Allergy labels may be a bright color to attract attention to the fact that the patient has an allergy to a certain type of medication.

Outguides

When removing a medical record from the records room, an **outguide** is used to hold the place of the record. An outguide is a plastic envelope with two pockets (Fig. 9–17), one of which is about 3 1/2" by 5" and can be used to hold a note indicating from where the chart was taken. The

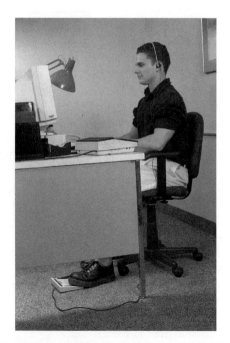

Figure 9–13. A medical transcriptionist prepares medical reports from physician dictation.

PROCEDURE 9–2 *Transcribe a Medical Report*

Materials Needed
- Dictated medical report
- Equipment to play report (digital or transcriber)
- Computer with word processing software
- Printer

1. Locate the beginning of the report dictation.
2. Adjust the volume and speed of the dictation as necessary.
3. Choose the appropriate report format.
4. Type the dictated report.
5. Proofread the report and make any necessary corrections.*
6. Print the report for physician signature and insertion in the patient's medical record.

Denotes crucial step in procedure. The student must complete this step satisfactorily in order to complete the procedure satisfactorily.

Box 9–2 Sample Chart Order

Identification sheet (summary or face sheet)
Medical history
Progress notes
Laboratory/pathology reports
Radiology reports
Other specialty reports
Correspondence

---

time when charts are returned to filing because the chart's original location is marked and any newly received documents can be waiting in the outguide for inclusion in the patient's chart.

FILING METHODS

Filing of medical records is a very important activity in the medical office. Filing should be kept up-to-date to allow for more expedient retrieval of records (Procedure box 9–4). It is much easier to locate a chart when it is where it belongs. A wide variety of filing methods can be used in medical offices. Probably the most preferred methods are numerical systems, because a number provides some degree of confidentiality for a patient. (When it pertains to records in the medical office, it may be good to be just a number!) The use of a numerical filing system does provide some anonymity for the patient.

---

larger pocket is big enough to hold reports pertaining to the patient. When the chart is returned to the records room, the reports held in the outguide can be placed in the patient's record. Outguides are available in a variety of colors, and colors can be assigned to indicate the department or provider who has the chart. Using outguides will save

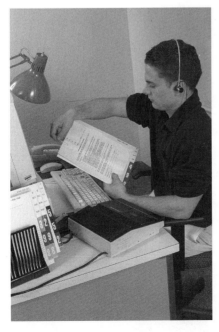

Figure 9–14. All medical reports must be reviewed and signed by the dictating physician before the report can be permanently added to a patient's medical record.

PROCEDURE 9–3 *Organize a Patient's Medical Record*

Materials Needed
- Patient's medical record
- Medical reports

1. Verify the patient's name on the reports and on the medical record.*
2. Determine where the reports should be inserted in the medical record.
3. Open fasteners holding the chart documents together.
4. Insert the reports in the appropriate location in the patient's medical record.
5. Close the fasteners to secure chart documents.

Denotes crucial step in procedure. The student must complete this step satisfactorily in order to complete the procedure satisfactorily.

Numerical Filing Systems

When beginning a chart numbering system, whether consecutive or terminal digit, it is common to start at a number higher than 1, such as 1000. An **accession ledger** is used to keep track of each number as it is assigned to a patient (Fig. 9–18). In today's medical office, accession ledgers are usually accessible by means of a computerized system. The assistant has merely to type in a number, and the system will display to whom the chart is assigned.

Sometimes, numbers are automatically assigned by a computer system. No matter how the charts are filed, the numbers should be assigned in consecutive order because this avoids missing or skipping any available numbers. Even when numbers are assigned consecutively, the records may be filed in the records room using a different method. Two of the most commonly used numerical filing systems are consecutive number and terminal digit filing.

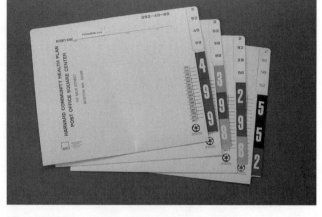

Figure 9–15. The folder for a patient's medical record may be color coded to expedite filing. The year grid on the lower right of the chart is used to identify an active record.

Consecutive Number Filing

Consecutive number filing is probably the easiest of all the filing systems. Charts are filed in the order of lowest to highest number.

If chart numbers consist of a varying number of digits (e.g., 1342 and 145365), zeros can be mentally added to a number with fewer digits, if necessary, to assist with filing. Thus, 1342 becomes 001342.

Use of the consecutive number filing method would place this list of chart numbers in the following order from first to last:

005365
045265
135365
145365
830308
850508

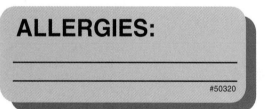

ALLERGIES:

_____
_____

#50320

ADVANCE
DIRECTIVES

#50378

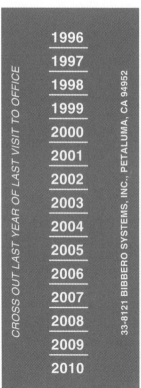

CROSS OUT LAST YEAR OF LAST VISIT TO OFFICE

1996
1997
1998
1999
2000
2001
2002
2003
2004
2005
2006
2007
2008
2009
2010

33-8121 BIBBERO SYSTEMS, INC., PETALUMA, CA 94952

Figure 9–16. Labels may be affixed to the outside of a patient's chart to alert the medical staff about important information.

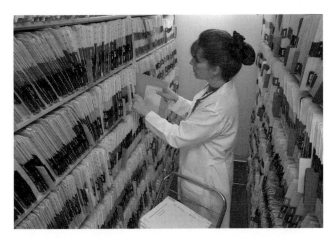

Figure 9–17. When a chart is removed from the records room, an outguide marks a chart's location and can be used to hold documents that may need to be filed with the chart.

A consecutive number filing system is quite easy to learn. A drawback to the system, however, is that it is sometimes very easy to transpose numbers when looking at a large group of digits.

Although everyone knows how to count, mistakes may be made in consecutive filing. A common mistake is transposing a number. A transposition involves reversing the order of some of the digits. For example, 48732 becomes 47832. To avoid transposing numbers when filing, the numbers of the records before and after the record to be filed should be checked to be sure the record is placed in the proper sequence.

Terminal Digit Filing

The **terminal digit filing** method involves breaking a chart number into a series of groups and filing within each group.

PROCEDURE 9–4 Index and File Medical Records

Materials Needed
- Medical records

1. Place the medical records in indexing order following the guidelines for the filing system adopted by the medical office.
2. Determine where the record will be filed.*
3. Verify that the filing location is correct by checking the record in front and in back of the record to be filed.
4. Complete the filing by repeating steps 2 and 3 for each record.

Denotes crucial step in procedure. The student must complete this step satisfactorily in order to complete the procedure satisfactorily.

A chart with the number 145365 becomes 14 53 65. The assistant determines the filing order by looking at the chart number from right to left. Chart number 145365 would be indexed as follows:

primary unit—65
secondary unit—53
tertiary unit—14

The primary unit, 65, indicates that the assistant will file the chart in section 65 of the records room. Once the assistant arrives at section 65, he or she will look for the number 53 grouping in section 65. After that grouping is located, the assistant will place the chart between the numbers 13 and 15 in that grouping.

Horizons Healthcare Center Accession Ledger		
Date	**Chart Number**	**Patient Name**
04-15-02	712536	Smith, Robert M.
04-15-02	712537	Smith, Tyler R.
04-15-02	712538	Jones, Kyle B.
04-16-02	712539	Carpenter, Janet T.
04-18-02	712540	Maxwell, Tana J.
04-18-02	712541	Warren, Jamie Z.

Figure 9–18. An accession ledger is a log that keeps track of chart numbers assigned and to whom and when the chart number was assigned.

Using the chart numbers previously mentioned under consecutive filing, the terminal digit filing method would place the numbers in the following order from first to last:

83 03 08

85 05 08

04 52 65

00 53 65

13 53 65

14 53 65

Of course, there will be many charts between those numbers, but this clearly illustrates that terminal digit filing would probably be a bit confusing for an untrained person who is trying to locate a chart. Although some extra training may be needed for new personnel, use of the terminal digit filing system usually reduces the chances of misfiles because the filing personnel file the records using only two digits at a time. An added benefit of terminal digit filing is that confidentiality is increased: it might be very difficult for someone not familiar with this filing method to locate a patient's record.

Alphabetical Filing

Although most medical offices prefer numerical systems, many offices continue to use alphabetical filing systems. Even if a numerical system is used for filing charts, alphabetical filing may be used in other areas of the office. One example of an alphabetical system is a **master patient index.**

The master patient index is an alphabetical file of all office patients and their chart numbers. The master patient index contains the name of every patient that has ever been treated in the office. If a patient's name changes because of marriage or for another reason, the patient's previous name is **cross-referenced** to the patient's new name and vice versa (Fig. 9–19). Cross-referencing allows a patient's medical record to be easily located if a name change occurs.

Although everyone knows the letters of the alphabet and in what order the letters appear, the medical office should adopt—and strictly follow—a specific set of rules when filing alphabetically to avoid misplacing records and making them difficult to locate.

National organizations have recommended guidelines to use when filing alphabetically, but recommendations can differ among the various organizations. The most important thing to remember about alphabetical filing is that everyone in the office must adhere to one set of guidelines established for that office, otherwise it could be very difficult to locate even a seemingly simple name.

To create an easy-to-use alphabetical filing system, the following guidelines are *recommended*:

- Every name should be arranged in the following order for filing: last name, first name, middle or maiden name or initial. The last name (surname) is known as the primary unit, the first name (given name) becomes the secondary unit, and the middle name or middle initial is the tertiary unit. The names are then placed in alphabetical order. The name *Gordon Michael Smith* should be indexed as *Smith Gordon Michael.*

- Every patient's complete legal name should be obtained. Nicknames (*Butch*) or shortened versions of a name (*Sue*) should not be used. Names such as these can lead to duplicate records in the medical office. If a patient comes in one day and gives the first name *Charles* and on a subsequent day gives the name *Chuck,* a duplicate record may be created if the patient's full legal name is not obtained. The patient should be asked for a complete legal name.

- Abbreviations of names should be filed as though they were spelled out (e.g., *Geo.* = *George; St. Michael* = *Saint Michael*). Here, again, the possibility exists for creation of duplicate records if a patient registers under different forms of a first name.

- In the instance of identical names, the files should be arranged by patient's date of birth (DOB), oldest first. Some filing guidelines state that the address should be used to determine filing order in the case of identical names. When filing in the medical office, however, date of birth should be used because a date of birth never changes, but an address does.

- When initials appear as part of the patient's name, the initial should be considered a complete name (e.g., *Smith, M. Gordon* is filed before *Smith, Mark G*). The rule "nothing comes before something" applies in this case.

- Prefixes of names should be included with the name (e.g., *Van Buren* is filed as *VanBuren; Mac Lean* is filed as *MacLean*).

- Punctuation, such as apostrophes and hyphens, should be ignored. The last name *Johnson-Smith* becomes *JohnsonSmith* when filing.

- Professional (*Dr.*) and religious titles (*Rev., Father, Sister*) should be disregarded when filing. Patients should be listed by last name. Filing patients under the title *Sister,* for example, would be of no benefit.

Even if an office is computerized, information should be entered into the computer program in a consistent manner. A computer software program will have a specific way of recognizing all characters that are entered into the program. It is important that everyone in a computerized medical office enter every patient's information in a consistent manner. If someone enters a punctuation mark or space in a patient's name, a computer system will identify those spaces and punctuation marks. It may be extremely difficult to search for a patient's name if it is entered correctly at a later date but had been entered incorrectly initially (see Procedure box 9–4).

Color Coding

Adding color coding to a filing system is an enormous timesaver. Proper use of a color-coding system can save hours looking for charts. **Color coding** involves assigning

Vasquez, Maria T.
See Gonzales, Maria T.
725 West 42 Avenue
Harvester, MN 55555
010-555-9429

#621348
DOB: 10-3-77

Figure 9–19. Cross-references help track patients who have had a name change.

colors to represent letters and numbers in order to aid in record filing and retrieval (Fig. 9–20).

One of the main reasons for using color to identify charts is to reduce the number of misfiles that occur in the records room. An orange chart would look conspicuously out of place in the midst of hundreds of green charts. If specific colors are assigned to certain charts, it is necessary to look only for a chart assigned a particular color.

An example of how a color-coding system could be arranged appears in Table 9–1. A color-coding system for numerical filing works well if 10 different colors are chosen. Each digit from 0 to 9 is assigned a different color. A specific digit of the medical record number (100ths or 1000ths) is used to determine the chart color. To make color coding work, specific characters are assigned to a color, and that assignment determines the color of the patient's chart.

If an office using a consecutive filing system were to assign the colors listed in Table 9–1 based on the 1000th place in the chart number, the charts identified here would be assigned the following colors:

Chart Number	Chart Color
194356	tan
030383	blue
122113	orange
079936	gray
173402	brown

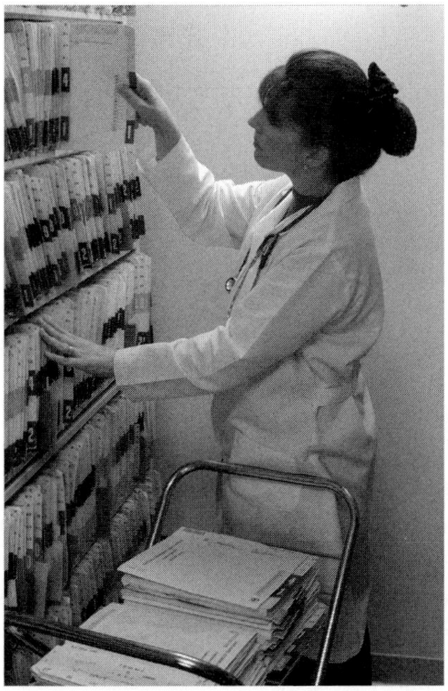

With use of such a color scheme in a consecutive filing system, the color would change every 1000 charts.

If the office is using a terminal digit filing system, the last two numbers in the chart number would identify the section of the records room in which the chart will be located. These two numbers may be represented by colored labels that are placed on the outside edge of the chart.

If the labels for each chart were chosen using the colors listed in Table 9–1, the colors of the chart labels would be listed as follows:

Chart Number	Chart Label Color
194356	red, green
030383	pink, white
122113	yellow, white
079936	white, green
173402	blue, orange

This assignment would be logical, because all charts with 56 as the first unit would be filed together. Therefore, all charts in section 56 would have a red label and a green label. If a chart with a pink label and green label were brought to that section, it would be identified as being out of place.

If color coding is adopted for alphabetical filing, an assistant may choose to assign the color by using the first letter of the patient's last name. Using color coding with an

Figure 9–20. Color coding of medical records can save time when filing and retrieving records.

Table 9–1. Example of a Color-Coding System

Number	Color	Letter
0	Blue	A, K, U
1	Yellow	B, L, V
2	Orange	C, M, W
3	White	D, N, X
4	Tan	E, O, Y
5	Red	F, P, Z
6	Green	G, Q
7	Purple	H, R
8	Pink	I, S
9	Grey	J, T

alphabetical filing system will create a pattern in that for each successive letter of the alphabet, the chart color will change. The charts would have the colors identified as follows:

Patient's Last Name	Chart Color
MacLean	orange
Dale	white
Pearson	red
Rodriguez	purple
Steinberg	pink

Why Use Color Coding?

The use of color coding has several advantages for the medical office. The chief advantage is that if 10 colors are used and an assistant is looking for a chart of a specific color, the search is reduced by approximately 90%, because the 9 other colors can be ignored. In other words, if an assistant is looking for a blue chart, he or she can ignore any color that is not blue. This can save a great deal of time when looking for a patient's chart.

Another advantage is that a color-coding system can be learned easily. Let's take another look at the consecutive number filing system in which a color is assigned to the 1000th digit. The assistant will quickly learn each color and its associated number just by retrieving and filing charts each day. Then, when the assistant sees chart numbers such as 131003, 841835, 471384, and 281867, the assistant will know that all of those charts are yellow because yellow represents the number 1.

A color-coding system should be strictly followed. Improper use of color coding can defeat the purpose of the system. The use of color coding should streamline the filing of records (Procedure box 9–5).

CHECKPOINT

1. A medical office is using a terminal digit filing system in its records room. All chart numbers are composed of at least six digits. Charts are marked with labels corresponding to the first unit used for filing. Should the medical office also use colored chart folders in addition to the colored labels, or will manila folders suffice?
2. The credit department of the medical office has asked that the assistant place a colored label on the front of a patient's chart if the patient's account has a large balance that is grossly overdue. Is this a good idea? Why?

Locating Missing Files

Although it is a rare occurrence, a missing chart is a serious problem in the medical office. Careful attention should be paid to the records when filing to be sure they are placed in the proper location. Much time can be wasted looking

PROCEDURE 9–5 Color Code Medical Records

Materials Needed
- Medical records
- Color-coding scheme
- Labels compatible with color-coding scheme

1. Obtain the color scheme for color coding medical records.
2. Affix the appropriate label to each medical record that corresponds to the filing system and associated color scheme.*
   - Alphabetical filing—use a label corresponding to the first letter of the patient's last name.
   - Consecutive number filing—use a label corresponding to the 1000th digit of the chart number.
   - Terminal digit filing—use labels corresponding to the two digits in the primary indexing unit.
3. Verify that the color coding is correct by placing the records in order for filing. Colors will appear together.

Denotes crucial step in procedure. Student must complete this step satisfactorily in order to complete the procedure satisfactorily.

for a misplaced or misfiled record. When a chart is missing, it is extremely important that it be found. A number of things can be done and a number of places can be checked, as shown in the following list:
- An assistant should look in the few charts preceding and after the spot in which the chart should be filed. Occasionally, the chart may be misplaced by only a few files.
- An assistant should double- and triple-check the physician's office, nurse's station, business office, manager's office, laboratory, and radiology areas for the file.
- If a color-coding system is in place in the records room, an assistant should scan all shelves or drawers for a color that is out of place.
- An assistant should check areas behind the shelving or drawers that hold the charts. The chart may have fallen behind or below a drawer or shelf.
- An assistant should check areas holding charts that are no longer active.
- An assistant should check to see whether the chart has been inadvertently placed inside another chart near where it should have been filed.
- If using an alphabetical filing system, an assistant should identify another possible spelling of the patient's last name (e.g., *Larson* or *Larsen*).

The medical office should have a policy regarding removal of charts from the office. It is generally recommended that no one—not even the physician—should ever remove a chart from the office, because the chance exists that it may never come back.

Records Retention and Disposal

Requirements for the retention of records vary from state to state. An assistant should verify the state requirement for medical records retention. The statute of limitations for malpractice suits generally dictates the minimum amount of time a record must be kept.

The statute of limitations for a minor's record may not even begin until the minor is an adult. Therefore, if the statute of limitations for litigation is 7 years, a minor could have until age 25 to sue for something that occurred when the minor was 4 years old.

Records of Medicare patients are required to be kept for a minimum of 5 years after the patient's last treatment. Some states have enacted laws specifying the length of time a record should be kept. Some facilities have adopted policies that say no medical records be destroyed. Each state chapter of the American Health Information Management Association (AHIMA) should have information on requirements for retention of records.

The medical office should establish a retention schedule that specifies the parameters for retaining records. Records are usually divided into three basic categories: active, inactive, and closed.

Active records are records of patients who are currently undergoing or have recently undergone treatment. Inactive records are records of patients who have not received treatment in a specified period of time, perhaps 6 months or 1 year. Closed records are records of patients who have died, moved from the area, or who will likely not return for treatment in the future. Closed records are usually moved to a storage location in the medical office or off the premises. If storage space for closed records is limited, the medical office must make arrangements for additional space or have an alternative for storing the records. Electronic media, such as CD-ROM or microfilm, make possible compact storage of medical information, so that space to retain records is not a problem.

On a weekly or monthly basis, names from obituaries in the local newspaper should be cross-checked with the patient database in the medical office. Every name that appears in the obituaries should be checked; do not rely on memory. If a name is found in the database, the outer cover of the chart should be marked with the word *deceased* and the patient's date of death. A deceased record is then filed in the closed files.

On a yearly basis, the medical office should purge from the active files in the records room any charts that are no longer used. Each chart should be marked on the outside with the last year the patient received treatment. A check mark on a grid located on the front of the chart can indicate the last year of treatment (see Fig. 9–15). The assistant can then quickly look at the cover of each chart to discern the most recent treatment of the patient.

If the current date is January 1, 2002, then any record without a check mark in 2001 can be assumed to be inactive.

If medical records are to be destroyed, the records should be shredded or incinerated. If incinerated, signed agreements should be obtained with the disposal company to ensure that confidential information is not released. If at all possible, all records should be kept.

Tickler File

Occasionally, for certain tasks, an assistant needs a reminder to do a specific activity in the office. Charts may need to be purged at a specific time, billing statements may need to be run, government reports may need to be filed, or patients may need to be reminded to set up an appointment. A **tickler file** can be used to provide these reminders for office staff.

A tickler file can be easily set up in a file drawer with a separate folder for each month of the year. If a patient needs an appointment in December and it is currently only February, a reminder could be entered in October's file to call the patient to arrange an appointment. Then, at the beginning of each month, the tickler file for that month is opened and the activities completed as necessary.

Electronic office systems often have features available that allow electronic reminders to be created in a computer system. Task lists can be created to identify necessary timelines for task completion. Reminders can be inserted into appointment schedules. Calendaring features allow office activities to be scheduled far in advance. Often, these programs are interconnected and create one large electronic tickler file that can remind an assistant about what needs to be done daily. The ability to have the office computer system electronically track necessary tasks helps ensure that nothing is forgotten.

FILE STORAGE AND PROTECTION

Many types of units may be purchased to hold records. Open shelving units, shelving units that have pullout drawers, and four-drawer file cabinets may be used to hold medical records.

Whatever type of storage is used, the units should be easily accessible to all staff members. Shelves must not be too high because staff members may have trouble reaching the top shelf. The use of stepstools should be discouraged in the records room because of the hazard of falling or tripping over a stool.

If shelving is used, there must be sufficient space between the charts on the top shelf and the ceiling. Local fire departments have strict fire codes concerning the space that is required between an object such as the top of a shelf or a chart and a fire extinguishing system. Sprinkler systems are generally discouraged in a records room because water and paper do not mix. Even if there is never a fire, sprinkler systems may malfunction, or a pipe may break and destroy the records. Systems that emit a gas substance to extinguish a fire are available to use in areas in which records preservation is vital. Necessary steps should be taken to protect all records from damage. A record that is destroyed will provide no support for a physician involved in litigation.

Furthermore, medical records should not be kept in the basement, although it is a common place to store records in many facilities. In the event of a flood, water main break, or other catastrophic occurrence, the unintentional destruction of a record is no defense in a court of law. It is the responsibility of everyone in the office to safeguard the medical records.

Medical Offices with Multiple Locations

A trend in some areas of the United States today is for large health care organizations to have several branches or locations of outpatient clinics. Multiple branches or locations present a special problem in the area of medical records.

Suppose a health care organization in a large metropolitan area has a central multispecialty clinic and five branch clinics within a 30-mile radius of one another. Patients are seen at a primary care branch clinic, and, when a specialist is needed, patients are seen at the central clinic. How will medical records be coordinated? Will one record be transferred back and forth to where a patient receives medical services? This would create a comprehensive medical chart for the patient but would necessitate physically moving records from one building to another. Or would each clinic keep its own record for the patient? The concern that comes with transferring records would be minimized, but it may be difficult for a comprehensive medical chart to be developed for the patient.

Each health care facility faced with this decision will need to determine what works best in its organization. This dilemma will not be solved easily but could be addressed with the increasing use of computers in the medical office.

LEGAL AND ETHICAL ISSUES

Because there are so many legal and ethical issues that pertain to medical records, they would constitute an entire text or an entire course. Some of the more prominent issues are identified here.

Release of Information

Medical record information contains sensitive, personal details of a patient's life. It is extremely important for an assistant to remember that these details are private and should not be released to anyone without the expressed written consent of the patient. In most cases, it is up to patients to decide who has access to their medical information and to authorize the disclosure of medical information.

If a patient requests information to be released to a third party, such as to another medical office, hospital, or an insurance company, a **release of information** form (Fig. 9–21) is necessary. The release specifies in writing what medical information regarding the patient should be released. The release must be signed by the patient, unless the patient is a minor or is not capable of granting permission. In those cases, the patient's guardian is responsible for authorizing release of medical information. If a patient is deceased, the patient's personal representative (as appointed by the court) may request a release of medical records for the deceased.

A copy of the release should be filed in the correspondence section of the medical record, and the fact that the release was done should be noted by the assistant in the progress notes section of the patient's chart. (Fig. 9–22). The chart notation should be dated and signed by the individual who released the information. Patients who are seen by different providers within the same health care facility usually do not have to sign a release of information for records to be transferred within the facility. For a step-by-step guide for releasing information and for requesting information to be released from another facility, refer to Box 9–3 and Procedure box 9–6.

When releasing information for a patient, an assistant should be careful to release only that information that has been requested. Occasionally, nonrequested information may be located near requested information, and the assistant should carefully review the information requested to be sure that only authorized information is released.

Methods of Releasing Medical Information

A patient's medical information may be released in a variety of ways. If a patient requests a copy of the medical record, the assistant photocopies the records that are requested. After photocopying information for release, the photocopies—not the original records—are always sent. Because of the importance of the medical record, the original record should never leave the health care facility in which it originated. The record is the physician's and medical office's only protection if they should ever be involved in litigation with a patient.

Currently, the use of outside photocopying services are common. A copy service is contracted, and companies are paid by the amount of work that is done. The photocopying services actually send people directly to the medical office to copy requested records. With this type of arrangement, the original records never leave the office.

In the case of a patient's health care emergency, critical information may be released over the telephone. The physician or nurse may ask the caller for some verification of information about the patient, such as mother's maiden

HORIZONS MEDICAL CENTER
123 Main Ave.
Farmington, ND 58000

REQUEST TO RELEASE MEDICAL INFORMATION

To: _____

Name of facility releasing medical information

_____

Address

_____

City, state, ZIP

I hereby request that the following information be released from my medical record:

(Circle items requested)

complete medical record	psychiatric records (initial)
progress notes	HIV/AIDS related records (initial)
lab/x-ray studies	other _____

Dates of Treatment _____ to _____
                              mo/day/yr   mo/day/yr

The above-requested information should be sent to:

_____

Name of facility to receive medical information

_____

Address

_____

City, state, ZIP

_____

Please print patient name (last, first, MI)

_____

DOB (mo/day/yr)   chart number

_____

Signature of patient or authorized representative

_____

Date of request

1-00

Figure 9–21. A release of information form specifies what should be done with a patient's medical information.

Horizons Healthcare Center – Progress Notes	
Patient Name: St. Michael, Adam C.	Chart number: 200123
7-9-xx Request for release of medical records sent to Peaceful Valley Medical Center,	
Farmington, ND. ---B. Frost, med. admin. asst.	

Figure 9–22. When a release of information has been done for a patient, the release should be noted in the progress notes section of the patient's chart.

name. The decision to release this information over the phone should be made by the physician.

Fax Machines

The use of a fax machine to send medical information is not recommended. A chance always exists that a fax could be sent to an incorrect telephone number. Fax machines should be used only if the record is needed quickly and there is no other way to get the information to the requesting party. Information could be mailed, if possible, or could be given directly to a patient.

Redisclosure of Medical Information

Information or records received from another health care provider may not be re-released or redisclosed to a third party. In other words, if Clinic A receives records from Clinic B, and a patient then requests information to be released from Clinic A, the assistant may send only the part of the record that originated in Clinic A. The assistant should not photocopy the information received from Clinic B. The patient must request the release of Clinic B's information from Clinic B, which has the original record.

When a Release Is Not Required

A release of information from the patient is not required if the law requires the information to be released. As mentioned in Chapter 3, public health laws often require the reporting of certain diseases and medical occurrences, such as births, deaths, or gunshot or stab wounds. Such reporting does not require an authorization from the patient. It is also generally held that another health care provider who is treating the patient has a right to the patient's record.

If the record is being used for purposes of research or for medical education, release of information is usually not required. Because use of such records does not require

identification of the patient, the patient's identity is protected. Records can be used for such purposes only as long as their use is consistent with the health facility's policy on such use.

Records may also be reviewed for quality assurance purposes. This practice allows the health facility to monitor the quality of care provided to patients in their facility.

Attorneys for a plaintiff or a defendant do not have the right to a patient's medical record without the patient's permission. Records should not be released unless the patient authorizes the release or unless a subpoena duces tecum (as mentioned in Chapter 3) is served.

An exception to this rule is that legal counsel for a medical office may review a patient's record if litigation commences regarding one of the office's patients. In the case of a subpoena duces tecum, a medical administrative assistant or a health information employee from the medical office will likely be required to testify as to the completeness of a patient's record when it is submitted to the court. Once a record becomes involved in litigation, it is recommended that the record be removed from the active file and be kept in a locked cabinet until the entire record has been photocopied and submitted. This action will help avoid any possible accusations of tampering with a record.

A physician may also release medical information if the physician believes that the patient may harm himself or herself or another individual or if the patient is a serious threat to society (See Box 3–2). In this case, the provider is allowed to inform the proper authorities to protect the patient or society as a whole.

Ownership

It is generally held that the medical office or physician owns the physical medical record—the medical office or physician is responsible for taking care of the record. The patient owns the right to release the information. In other words, the patient controls who gets access to the information. The patient must authorize information to be released

Box 9-3 Release of Medical Information

Requesting Medical Records for a Patient from Another Health Care Facility

1. Patient expresses desire to obtain records from another facility.
2. Medical administrative assistant completes release of information form and obtains patient's signature on form. If patient is a minor, a parent's or guardian's signature is obtained.
3. Release of information form is photocopied, copy is placed in the patient's record, and original form is mailed. Assistant notes request for records in progress notes of patient's medical record.
4. Facility receiving the request photocopies the records that are requested and mails the records to the requesting facility.
5. Requesting facility receives the records.
6. Assistant sends the patient's chart and records received to the physician for review.
7. After the physician reviews the records, the physician initials the records and returns the chart and records to the assistant.
8. Assistant places the records in the designated section of the medical record.

Processing a Request to Send a Patient's Medical Record to Another Health Care Facility

1. Patient expresses desire for medical records to be transferred to another facility.
2. Release of information form is completed and patient's signature is obtained on form. If patient is a minor, a parent's or guardian's signature is obtained.
3. Assistant photocopies records requested to be released.
4. Copy of release form is attached to the photocopied record.
5. Original of release form is placed in the correspondence section of the medical record.
6. Assistant makes a notation in the progress notes of patient's medical record that the information was released.
7. Copy of release of information and patient's medical record is sent to the other health care facility.

record. The patient may want to review the information in the record with a trained medical professional, or the patient may request that the record be photocopied for the patient's personal use. If the records are reviewed with a health care professional, the professional should remain in the room with the patient to be sure that no parts of the record are removed.

If the patient is to receive a photocopy of the record, charging the patient a nominal fee for photocopying is appropriate. Charging a fee is not appropriate for viewing the record. A photocopying charge should not be made if the patient is transferring to another facility; the photocopying is usually done as a courtesy to the patient.

A physician, psychiatrist, or psychologist may decide that psychiatric records, because of the sensitive nature of such records, may not be released to the patient. Because of the great potential for damage to the patient if the records should accidentally become public while in the patient's hands, patients have been discouraged from obtaining copies of psychiatric records. There has also been case law that supports patients' restricted access to mental health records.

PROCEDURE 9-6 Process a Request to Release Medical Information

Materials Needed
- Release of Information form
- Black-ink pen
- Patient's medical record

1. If needed, help the patient complete the release request.
2. Verify that all necessary information is included on the release.
3. Obtain the patient's medical record and confirm that the patient's name on the release is the same as the name on the medical record.*
4. Photocopy the requested information to be released.
5. Arrange the information in logical order.
6. Attach a copy of the release of information request on top of the release.
7. Place the original release request in the correspondence section of the patient's medical record.
8. Send the information to the medical facility identified on the release.*
9. In a chart entry, document that the release was processed.*

Denotes crucial step in procedure. Student must complete this step satisfactorily in order to complete the procedure satisfactorily.

in order for information to go to a third party. Attorneys and private insurance companies are not entitled to a patient's medical information without the patient's consent.

The AHIMA's position is that patients have the right to have access to information in their medical record. Occasionally, a patient may request information from his or her

Human Immunodeficiency Virus and Acquired Immunodeficiency Syndrome Records

Many states enact laws that protect the confidentiality of patients who have a diagnosis related to the human immunodeficiency virus (HIV) or the acquired immunodeficiency syndrome (AIDS). A patient who requests an HIV test may be asked to sign a consent form that stipulates to whom test results will be sent if the results are positive. Because of the social implications of HIV and AIDS, great care should be taken to protect a patient's identity when involved in HIV testing.

The AHIMA's position on handling insurance claims for patients with an HIV- or AIDS-related diagnoses is to require the patients' written consent for listing the diagnosis on the insurance claim form. Because of the sensitive nature of this type of diagnosis, it is important for patients to understand that information will be sent to an insurance company about the specific cause of their treatment.

SUMMARY

Patients' medical records are the most important documents in the medical office. The ultimate purpose of maintaining medical records is to have a record that enables the physician to deliver to the patient the best possible care. Medical records are necessary for continuity of patient care and are used to gather information for statistics. They may be used in a legal case and may be reviewed to monitor quality of care and to provide documentation for billing and insurance statements. Complete, accurate records are essential to support all of these activities.

The medical administrative assistant may be chiefly responsible for maintaining the medical records in the office. A thorough understanding of the support activities, such as transcription, filing, and quantitative analysis, is necessary to ensure a complete and accurate record. Health information management is an ingredient that is essential for providing patients with quality health care services.

YOU ARE THE MEDICAL ADMINISTRATIVE ASSISTANT

You are the office supervisor, and the medical office in which you are working has gotten far behind in quantitative analysis of the office's medical records. One of your colleagues suggests that she take 50 to 100 charts home each night to review. If she reviews the charts at home, she estimates that it should take only a week to bring the records completely up to date. Should you allow her to do this?

Bibliography

Huffman EK: Health Information Management. Berwyn, Ill, Physician's Record, 1994.

Judson K, Blesie S: Law and Ethics for Health Occupations. New York, Glencoe McGraw-Hill, 1994.

Lewis MA, Tamparo CD: Medical Law, Ethics and Bioethics for Ambulatory Care. Philadelphia, FA Davis, 1998.

Internet Resources

American Health Information Management Association

Joint Commission on Accreditation of Healthcare Organizations

Exercise 9–1 TRUE OR FALSE

Read each statement and determine whether the statement is true or false. Record the answer in the blank provided. T = true; F = false.

_____ 1. Statistics gathered from medical records might be used in planning for future health care services.

_____ 2. It is acceptable to begin destroying all inactive and closed medical records if the records room runs out of space.

_____ 3. HIPAA is a federal law that protects the confidentiality of medical information and will be in full effect in April 2003.

_____ 4. Anyone who can type fast can be a medical transcriptionist.

_____ 5. A consistent chart order makes it easy to locate items quickly in the patient's chart.

_____ 6. Once a patient is deceased, there is no need for the patient's medical record and it can be destroyed.

_____ 7. A surname with a prefix is indexed and filed as if it were spelled as one word.

_____ 8. White correction fluid should be used when correcting errors in the medical record to ensure that the correction is done neatly.

_____ 9. All medical reports must be reviewed and initialed (or signed) by the physician before permanently adding the reports to a patient's chart.

_____ 10. A patient's medical record may be reviewed to ensure that care was properly given.

_____ 11. Copies of medical records are necessary for all claims filed to insurance.

_____ 12. Use of a number system for filing medical records could provide more confidentiality than could alphabetical filing.

_____ 13. Medical facilities must absorb the cost of photocopying records for legal cases.

_____ 14. A written consent is nice to have, but a telephone consent for release of information is acceptable.

_____ 15. Hyphenated names are considered as two units when filing.

_____ 16. Abbreviated names, such as *Chas.* and *Geo.,* are indexed as they are written.

_____ 17. All medical records should be saved if at all possible, but if the medical records room runs out of space, it is acceptable to begin destroying records that have not been active for at least 4 or 5 years.

_____ 18. An insurance company may request a patient's medical record to determine whether the services provided to a patient were covered by insurance.

_____ 19. Medical records are reviewed to determine whether care given to patients meets the quality standards of the health care facility.

_____ 20. As of April 2003, federal law prohibits the unauthorized release of all patients' private medical information.

_____ 21. An employee who releases medical information that should not be released may be subject to termination of employment.

_____ 22. A problem-oriented medical record involves grouping together all like information in a chart. For example, all laboratory reports or all office visits are in their own individual section.

_____ 23. An outguide is used to mark the location of a record that has been removed from the records room.

_____ 24. Local obituary listings should be checked with the medical office's database to identify patients who have died.

_____ 25. A tickler file reminds an assistant of activities that must be completed at a certain time.

_____ 26. Redisclosure of medical information refers to the patient allowing medical information to be released on an as-needed basis without the patient's signature.

_____ 27. Public health laws may necessitate the release of certain medical information.

_____ 28. A patient's attorney has the right to view a patient's record without the patient's permission.

_____ 29. A patient may not be able to obtain a personal copy of psychiatric records.

_____ 30. Whenever copies of a patient's medical record are made, the patient should be billed.

Exercise 9–2 CHAPTER CONCEPTS

Read each statement or question and choose the answer that best completes the statement or question. Record the answer in the blank provided.

_____ 1. Health information management personnel are responsible for all of the following except
(a) Releasing medical records.
(b) Dictating medical reports.
(c) Compiling health care related statistics.
(d) Reviewing medical records for completeness.

_____ 2. A medical record can be used for all of the following except
(a) Publication in a medical journal.
(b) Planning for future health care services.
(c) Documentation in a legal case.
(d) Documentation for an insurance claim.

_____ 3. All of the following are found in a medical record except
(a) Results of laboratory tests.
(b) Patient's medical history.
(c) Copy of the patient's monthly bill.
(d) A letter from the physician to the patient.

_____ 4. Which of the following is not a use of the medical record?
(a) Documentation of care given to a patient.
(b) Review of patient care for quality assurance standards.
(c) Medical education and research.
(d) All are uses of a medical record.

_____ 5. In which of the following circumstances should medical information be released?
(a) Attorney involved in litigation regarding a patient requests the patient's medical record.
(b) An employer requests an employee's medical record.
(c) Patient's spouse requests results of a patient's laboratory testing.
(d) Patient completes release of information form requesting information to be sent to another medical facility.

_____ 6. What is the purpose of quantitative analysis?
(a) To determine whether the medical record is complete.
(b) To identify health care procedures that need to be improved.
(c) To tally errors made by physicians and nurses when documenting patient care.
(d) To penalize office staff who need to improve.

_____ 7. Which of the following does not belong?
(a) Diagnosis.
(b) Assessment.
(c) Impression.
(d) Examination.

_____ 8. Which of the following is synonymous with face sheet?
(a) SOAP note.
(b) Assessment.
(c) Summary.
(d) Consultation.

_____ 9. Color coding of medical records will
(a) Eliminate the need to perform quantitative analysis on medical records.
(b) Increase the time required to file records.
(c) Reduce the number of medical records required.
(d) Make it easier to locate records.

_____ 10. The proper way to correct an entry in a medical record is to
(a) Use correction fluid to ensure that the previous information is obliterated.
(b) Draw a single line through the incorrect entry.
(c) Erase previous entry.
(d) Have the physician initial every correction made in a chart.

Exercise 9–3 SOAP NOTES

Information found in a SOAP note is listed here. Identify the part of the note in which the information would be found. Match the information with the answers listed. Record the answer in the blank provided. Each answer may be used more than once.

(a) Subjective
(b) Objective

(c) Assessment
(d) Plan

_____ 1. Patient's description of illness.

_____ 2. Results of a urinalysis.

_____ 3. Instructions on wound care.

_____ 4. Patient's diagnosis.

_____ 5. Information on prescription given to patient.

_____ 6. Vital signs.

_____ 7. Chief complaint.

_____ 8. Observations on patient's appearance.

_____ 9. Patient's answers to review of body systems.

_____ 10. Physician's observation of body systems.

Exercise 9–4 RELEASE OF INFORMATION

Read each statement and determine whether the medical information requested should be released. Record the answer in the blank provided.
Y = Yes, the information should be released.
N = No, the information should not be released.

_____ 1. A mother is requesting a release of her minor son's medical records to an orthopedic specialist in another city.

_____ 2. A 28-year-old man is requesting information about his father's medical history because a hereditary disease is expected.

_____ 3. A mother is requesting information about her 15-year-old daughter's strep test results.

_____ 4. A father calls requesting information about his 18-year-old son's psychiatric treatment.

_____ 5. A son requests copies of his late father's medical records. He has a legal document that names him the personal representative of his father's estate.

_____ 6. Wife calls to request the results of her husband's postvasectomy sperm count.

_____ 7. A news reporter calls for information regarding a rumor about a patient with tuberculosis. He is calling to confirm the rumor and, if it is true, wants the patient to be identified.

Exercise 9–5 CONSECUTIVE NUMBER FILING

Using the guidelines presented in the chapter, identify which number in each group would be first when using a consecutive number filing system. Write the letter identifying the first number in the blank provided.

_____ 1.
(a) 126342
(b) 145632
(c) 126432
(d) 123642

_____ 2.
(a) 123642
(b) 1236
(c) 145632
(d) 142364

_____ 3.
(a) 81562
(b) 631795
(c) 6587
(d) 76142

_____ 4.
(a) 531200
(b) 62100
(c) 181200
(d) 882200

_____ 5.
(a) 73355
(b) 183245
(c) 93165
(d) 263054

_____ 6.
(a) 145177
(b) 415177
(c) 25177
(d) 235177

_____ 7.
(a) 432588
(b) 342588
(c) 345288
(d) 435288

_____ 8.
(a) 40801
(b) 10804
(c) 80201
(d) 10208

Exercise 9–6 TERMINAL DIGIT FILING

Using the guidelines presented in the chapter, identify which number in each group would be first when using a terminal digit filing system. Write the letter identifying the first number in the blank provided.

_____ 1.
- (a) 126342
- (b) 145632
- (c) 126432
- (d) 123642

_____ 2.
- (a) 123642
- (b) 1236
- (c) 145632
- (d) 142364

_____ 3.
- (a) 81562
- (b) 631795
- (c) 6587
- (d) 76142

_____ 4.
- (a) 531200
- (b) 62100
- (c) 181200
- (d) 882200

_____ 5.
- (a) 73355
- (b) 183245
- (c) 93165
- (d) 263054

_____ 6.
- (a) 145177
- (b) 415177
- (c) 25177
- (d) 235177

_____ 7.
- (a) 432588
- (b) 342588
- (c) 345288
- (d) 435288

_____ 8.
- (a) 40801
- (b) 10804
- (c) 80201
- (d) 10208

Exercise 9–7 ALPHABETICAL FILING

Using the alphabetic filing guidelines presented in the chapter, identify which name in each group would be first when indexed. Write the letter identifying the first name in the blank provided.

_____ 1.
- (a) Andrew R. McKay
- (b) Georgia McNeely
- (c) Harvey MacKay
- (d) Karen S. Martin

_____ 2.
- (a) Maxwell Stevens
- (b) Herbert Stephens
- (c) Martha Stevenson
- (d) Alice I. Steen

_____ 3.
- (a) Hunter Johnson
- (b) Amy Johnston
- (c) Mitchell Johnson
- (d) Jeanette Johnson

_____ 4.
- (a) Louis Demarco
- (b) Marco D'Leone
- (c) Debra Smith-Deane
- (d) Cristine Dennis-DeJong

_____ 5.
- (a) Matthew St. Andrew
- (b) Olivia St. Marie
- (c) Myrtle Sandborn
- (d) Dora Saint James

_____ 6.
- (a) Donald A. Meyer
- (b) Donald A. Myer
- (c) Donald G. Meier
- (d) Donald B. Meiers

_____ 7.
- (a) Barbara A. Nelson; DOB, 5-23-81
- (b) Barbara A. Nelson; DOB, 3-4-45
- (c) Barbara A. Nelson; DOB, 2-4-60
- (d) Barbara A. Nelson; DOB, 10-17-92

_____ 8.
- (a) Robert D. Smith
- (b) R. David Smith
- (c) Robert David Smith
- (d) Robert G. Smith

_____ 9.
- (a) Dr. Sharon T. Rose
- (b) Rev. Nancy West-Richman
- (c) Father Martin Turner
- (d) Kelly L. St. Claire

_____ 10.
- (a) Aaron Williams
- (b) Davis Thomas
- (c) Todd Weber
- (d) Linda Lee

Exercise 9–8 ALPHABETICAL FILING

Place the following names in alphabetical order in the blanks provided. Identify the primary, secondary, and tertiary units for each name.

Sandi J. Schmid

Dawn L. Johnson-Greene

Aubrey I. Schmit

Angela R. Berlin

Monica T. Olsen

Marcos L. Shmidt

Julie A. Johnson

Michelle R. Schimtke

James I. Bergquist

Gretchen K. Olson

Harriet G. Schmitt

Tamara A. Gregor

Stanley R. Olsson

Mark C. Schmidt

Laura S. St. Marie

Gary R. Olson

Elaine D. Berg

Mark T. Schmidt

Steve R. Bergman

Dr. Donna M. Snow

	Primary Unit	Secondary Unit	Tertiary Unit
1.			
2.			
3.			
4.			
5.			
6.			
7.			
8.			
9.			
10.			
11.			
12.			
13.			
14.			
15.			
16.			
17.			
18.			
19.			
20.			

Exercise 9–9 COMPONENTS OF THE MEDICAL RECORD

Read the description of components found in a medical record and match the description with the name of the appropriate component. Choose the answer that best completes the description. Record the answer in the blank provided.

_____ 1. Contains information about the patient's past diseases and family members' past diseases.
 (a) Other specialized reports
 (b) Radiology reports
 (c) Immunizations
 (d) Medical history

_____ 2. A chronological record of a patient's visits to the physician.
 (a) Correspondence
 (b) Summary sheet
 (c) Progress notes
 (d) Discharge summary

_____ 3. Contains information about patient's insurance, employer, and possibly even a release of information for insurance purposes.
   (a) Summary sheet
   (b) Discharge summary
   (c) Consultation
   (d) Correspondence

_____ 4. Section that contains letters written about the patient and copies of medical records from other health care facilities.
   (a) Consultation
   (b) Correspondence
   (c) Progress notes
   (d) Discharge summary

_____ 5. Documents the results of a study on body tissue.
   (a) Radiology report
   (b) Pathology report
   (c) Consultation
   (d) Summary sheet

_____ 6. When a patient is referred to a specialist, the specialist will document the encounter with the patient in a report known as
   (a) Pathology report
   (b) Operative report
   (c) Correspondence
   (d) Consultation

_____ 7. A CBC and urinalysis are known as
   (a) Consultation
   (b) Progress notes
   (c) Laboratory reports
   (d) Other specialized reports

_____ 8. Report that documents a patient's condition on admission to a hospital.
   (a) Discharge summary
   (b) History and physical
   (c) Correspondence
   (d) Consultation

_____ 9. Report that documents a surgical procedure step by step.
   (a) Pathology report
   (b) Consultation
   (c) Operative report
   (d) Progress notes

_____ 10. An MRI or CT scan are examples of this type of report.
   (a) Pathology report
   (b) Discharge summary
   (c) Other specialized report
   (d) Radiology report

9
ACTIVITIES

ACTIVITY 9–1 Prepare a chart for each patient, using the patient list and chart numbers provided.

Materials needed

- 32 full-cut manila folders
- 1 permanent black marker

Prepare the folders for the patients' medical records as illustrated below.

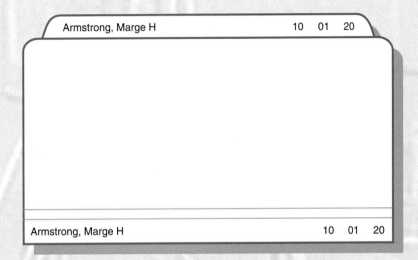

Last Name	First Name	MI	Chart Number
Armstrong	Marge	H	100120
Breckman	Jeanne	N	75600
Brenner	Inez	N	100121
Burlington	Allen	R	271911
French	Kirsten	M	641030
Garcia	Jose	N	120020
Garcia	Tamara	D	364602
Gordon	Amy	A	9520
MacLean	Tyler	C	649732
MacLean	Krista	A	348833
McLean	Mary	K	220164
McLean	Mark	B	28680
O'Henry	Gregory	A	320110
Olsen	Derek	R	10110
Olsen	Christian	B	401280
Olson	Christian	B	463278
Olson	Deanne	T	28632
Olson	Tara	D	647932
O'Malley	Timothy	E	209110
Pearsen	Michael	T	43220
Pearson	Steven	M	230184
Pearson	Susan	G	224764
Shepard	Alice	R	554148
Snow	Donna	M	210178
St. Michael	Adam	C	200123
Stein	Margaret	I	8330
Stevens	Evan	D	689723
Summerville	Paul	D	121087
Vasquez	Maria	T	621348
Walker	Ann	F	152634
Wang	Karen	J	230192
Webster	Peggy	A	171423

ACTIVITY 9–2   Using the charts prepared in Activity 9–1, place the charts in consecutive number order.

ACTIVITY 9–3   Using the charts prepared in Activity 9–1, place the charts in terminal digit order.

ACTIVITY 9–4   Using the charts prepared in Activity 9–1 and the color-coding chart in Table 9–1, color code the charts for alphabetical filing.

ACTIVITY 9–5   Using the charts prepared in Activity 9–1 and the color-coding chart in Table 9–1, color code the charts for consecutive number filing.

ACTIVITY 9–6   Using the charts prepared in Activity 9–1 and the color-coding chart in Table 9–1, color code the charts for terminal digit filing.

ACTIVITY 9–7   Using the progress notes page here, make a chart entry for today regarding an appointment made for Deanne Olson with Dr. Herbert next Monday at 4:00 PM. Locate Ms. Olson's chart number in the database in Lytec Medical 2001.

Horizons Healthcare Center – Progress Notes
Patient Name: Chart Number:

ACTIVITY 9–8   Research the medical records retention laws or recommendations for your state.

ACTIVITY 9–9   Research the AHIMA at www.ahima.org.

ACTIVITY 9–10 Prepare a release of information for Amy Gordon, a patient of Horizons Healthcare Center. Ms. Gordon would like her complete medical record from Noble Medical Center, 500 Elm Avenue, Farmington, to be sent to Horizons. Ms. Gordon's DOB and chart number can be located in the database in Lytec Medical 2001.

ACTIVITY 9–11 Obtain a tape of dictated medical reports from your instructor. Listen to the tapes as an example of how medical reports are dictated. If a transcriber is available, transcribe a complete medical report.

ACTIVITY 9–12 Consider the following situations. What is the appropriate response to the situation?

1. One of your coworkers at Horizons Healthcare is a personal acquaintance of a patient of the office. The patient has just undergone surgery for removal of a suspicious mass in the large intestine. Your coworker states she is hopeful that the mass was benign and then asks if the pathology report for the patient has been received yet. What do you say?

2. A celebrity is a surprise patient in the office one day. A coworker comments about asking the celebrity for an autograph. What do you say?

9
DISCUSSION

The following topics can be used for class discussion or for individual student essay.

DISCUSSION 9–1 Read the quotation at the beginning of the chapter. How does this quotation apply to the concepts presented in this chapter?

DISCUSSION 9–2 As it pertains to this chapter, discuss why special attention should be paid to what goes into the trash can in a medical office.

DISCUSSION 9–3 Discuss the application of the AHIMA Code of Ethics (available at www.ahima.org) to the position of a medical administrative assistant.

DISCUSSION 9–4 Discuss why quantitative analysis may be one of the most important health information management activities.

CHAPTER OUTLINE

THE BILLING PROCESS
  Registration
  Superbill
  The Billing Process from Beginning to End

BILLING BASICS
  What Does the Doctor Charge?
  Billing for Minors
  Missed Appointments — To Bill or Not To Bill
  Assignment of Benefits
  Fees for Medical Care

MEDICAL CODING
  Procedure Coding
  Diagnosis Coding
  The Coding Profession

BOOKKEEPING SYSTEMS
  Computerized Systems
  Pegboard

CREDIT
  Billing Patients
  Aging Accounts
  Collection

LEGAL AND ETHICAL ISSUES IN MEDICAL BILLING
  Confidentiality
  Billing Fraud
  Estate Claims
  Medical Records

SUMMARY

LEARNING OUTCOMES

On successful completion of this chapter, the student will be able to

1. Identify steps of the billing process.
2. Explain components of a superbill.
3. Identify proper manner for discussing physician's fees.
4. Explain assignment of benefits.
5. Identify how medical fees are determined.
6. Perform fundamental concepts of procedural coding.
7. Perform fundamental concepts of diagnosis coding.
8. Identify features of computerized and pegboard accounting systems.
9. Identify legal and ethical concepts and issues pertaining to billing and collection practices.
10. Describe cycle billing and accounts receivable aging.

CMA COMPETENCIES

1. Perform procedural coding.
2. Perform diagnostic coding.

3. Use a physician's fee schedule.
4. Post entries on a daysheet.
5. Perform accounts receivable procedures.
6. Perform billing and collection procedures.
7. Use computer software to maintain office systems.
8. Identify and respond to issues of confidentiality.
9. Perform within legal and ethical boundaries.

RMA COMPETENCIES

1. Know terminology associated with financial bookkeeping in the medical office.
2. Maintain and explain physicians' fee schedules.
3. Know coding systems used in insurance processing.
4. Code diagnoses and procedures.
5. Collect and post payments; manage patient ledgers.
6. Make financial arrangements with patients.
7. Prepare and mail itemized statements.
8. Know methods of billing.
9. Cycle billing procedures.
10. Identify delinquent accounts; take appropriate steps for collection.
11. Perform skip tracing.
12. Perform telephone collection procedures.
13. Know collection as related to bankruptcy and small claims cases.
14. Know accounts receivable procedures.
15. Use computer for billing and financial transactions.
16. Use procedures for ensuring the integrity and confidentiality of computer-stored information.

VOCABULARY

assignment of benefits
Certified Coding Specialist (CCS)
Certified Professional Coder (CPC)
conventions
CPT
cycle billing
diagnosis
dunning messages
Equal Credit Opportunity Act
Fair Debt Collection Practices Act
fee schedule
fraud
HCFA Common Procedure Coding System (HCPCS)
Health Care Financing Administration (HCFA)
ICD-9-CM
modifier
procedure
superbill

MEDICAL BILLING

When at last we are sure you've been properly pilled, then a few paper forms must be properly filled so that you and your heirs may be properly billed.

—*Dr. Seuss*, You're Only Old Once

A patient's office visit may be productive, but if the patient's charges are not billed correctly, that patient may decide to go elsewhere for medical care. Great care must be taken when processing charges and payments in the medical office. Patients' accounts must be kept up-to-date and must be accurate at all times.

Many components comprise the billing process, and an assistant must stay current on the constant changes that affect medical billing. An assistant who is thoroughly trained in billing processes is a tremendous asset to a medical office.

THE BILLING PROCESS

When someone hears the term *billing process,* all that may come to mind is a slip of paper on which charges are written. The billing process is far more than a slip of paper, however. The billing process begins at registration and ends after every charge has been paid and includes many steps in between. Depending on the size of the practice, a medical administrative assistant may be responsible for the entire billing process or may perform only specific parts, with other parts being performed in a separate billing department. Even if an assistant is not responsible for the entire process, a basic understanding will enable an assistant to help patients who have questions about their medical bills.

One of the most critical parts of the billing process takes place before the physician ever sees a patient. This critical part is the point at which a patient enters the medical office and registers for an appointment. At that point, vital information, such as patient's address, telephone number, and insurance company information, is gathered from the patient. This information is absolutely essential to provide enough information to bill the patient and file insurance claims as well as to reach the patient or the person responsible for the bill if there are problems with the bill or claim.

Registration

On entering a medical office, a patient stops at the front desk to check in for an appointment. If a patient is new to the office, registration is the time at which the following information is obtained from the patient (see Chapter 8):

- Patient's complete name and current address.
- Patient's date of birth.
- Patient's home phone number.
- Patient's employer's name, address, and telephone number.
- **Guarantor** information—complete name, address, and telephone number of party responsible for payment of account.
- Insurance company name, address, and policy number.

This information may be obtained via a verbal interview with the patient at the registration desk or by asking the patient to complete a registration form (see Fig. 8–2) containing the information needed for the registration process. The office

may even elect to mail a registration form to a new patient to allow the patient to complete the form ahead of time.

If a patient is an established (returning) patient to the practice, vital billing information, such as name, address, telephone number, and insurance company, is verified at the time of registration to be sure the office has correct information for billing.

Why is the registration process such an important part of the billing process? The information collected at this point is the information that will be used to generate the patient's monthly statement and any related insurance claims. Even one error at this point could mean that a statement does not reach the patient or that an insurance claim is filed incorrectly. Such billing delays can be frustrating to the patient and the physician, can create extra work for the office staff, and can cause delays in receiving payments for services rendered by the physicians in the medical office.

Superbill

After the registration information is obtained or verified, the assistant prepares a **superbill** (Fig. 10–1) to be included with the patient's chart during the office visit. A superbill is the document from which the patient's bill is generated. It contains the patient's diagnosis and a listing of the charges that are incurred during an office visit. Some facilities use different names for a superbill, such as *encounter form, charge slip, fee slip,* and *service record.* All of these terms denote an invoice for services rendered.

Superbills may be produced in either of two ways: they may be preprinted by a professional printing company or they may be generated via computer when the patient registers.

Preprinted superbills may be prepared with copies in duplicate, triplicate, or more. If necessary, a copy of the superbill can serve as a control copy. A control copy may be kept to make sure all bills are processed. When the physician's copy is sent to billing, it is matched with the control copy. Control copies that are not matched after a specific period of time will be researched to determine what happened to the original superbill and whether charges should be billed to the patient.

On rare occasions, a patient's superbill may be inadvertently misplaced or left between the pages of a patient's chart. If the charges for a patient are significantly delayed, a physician may choose to not bill that patient. For example, a superbill that has not been processed within 3 months after the visit may be considered too old, and the physician may not wish to bill the patient. Taking action in this situation is more or less a double-edged sword: if the physician bills the patient late or does not bill the patient at all, the physician's billing practices appear careless, and if the patient is concerned about the carelessness of the practice's billing processes, this may draw attention to the physician's practice in general. A patient might therefore infer that the physician operates a careless practice.

Computer-generated superbills are created after the patient's registration data have been verified and the assistant is

PATIENT NAME & ADDRESS	BIRTHDATE	EMPLOYER
	TELEPHONE #	INSURANCE CO. NAME
	EMERGENCY CONTACT #	GROUP #
RESPONSIBLE PARTY NAME	SOCIAL SECURITY #	POLICY #
RETURN APPOINTMENT		

COMMENTS:　　　　　　　**DIAGNOSIS:**

FORM 493206　COLWELL SYSTEMS 1-800.637.1140

OFFICE VISIT - NEW PATIENT

99201	Problem Focused H/E, SF
99202	Expanded Problem Focused H/E, SF
99203	Detailed H/E, LC
99204	Comprehensive H/E, MC

OFFICE VISIT - ESTABLISHED PATIENT

99212	Minimal
99213	Expanded Problem Focused H/E, LC
99214	Detailed H/E, MC

CONFIRMATORY CONSULTATIONS

| 99272 | Expanded Problem Focused H/E, SF |

ALLERGY

| 950__ | Allergy Testing |

X-RAYS

70120	Mastoids, <3 Views
70160	Nasal Bones, Complete, Min. 3 Views
70220	Sinuses, Complete, Min. 3 Views
70330	TMJ, Bilateral
70360	Neck, Soft Tissue

AUDIOLOGY

92541	Spont. Nystagmus Test w/Rec.
92542	Pos. Nystagmus Test w/Rec.
92543	Caloric Vestibular Test w/Rec.
92553	Pure Tone Audio., Air & Bone
92555	Speech Audio. Threshold
92557	Comp. Audio. Thresh/Speech Rec.
92567	Tympanometry
92585	Evoked Audiometry/CNS, Comp.

HEARING AIDS

	Hearing Aid Evaluation
	Hearing Aid Selection
	Hearing Aid Repair

IN-OFFICE SURGERY

30901	Nasal Caut., Ant., Simple
30903	Nasal Caut., Ant., Complex
30905	Nasal Caut., Post., Initial
30906	Nasal Caut., Post., Subseq.
31000	Maxillary Sinus Lavage
31231	Nasal Endos., Diag., Uni. or Bil.

IN-OFFICE SURGERY (CONT.)

31575	Fiberoptic Laryngoscopy, Diag.
69210	Removal Impacted Cerumen
69220	Debride Mastoid Cavity, Simple
69420*	Myringotomy w/Asp. or Infl.
69433	Tympanostomy Unilateral
-50	Tympanostomy Bilateral

MISCELLANEOUS

| 90782 | Therapeutic Inj. of Med., IM/SQ |
| | Specify: |

DIAGNOSIS

477.9	Allergic Rhinitis	784.0	Headache	380.10	Otitis Externa, Infective	465.9	URI
447.6	Arteritis	389.0	Hearing Loss - Conductive	381.4	Otitis Media, Nonsuppurative	478.4	Vocal Cord Polyps
493.9	Asthma	389.1	Hearing Loss - Sensorineural	527.2	Parotid Sialoadenitis	784.40	Voice Disturbance
350.2	Atypical Facial Pain	578.0	Hematemesis	475	Peritonsillar Abscess		
351.0	Bell's Palsy	786.3	Hemoptysis	472.1	Pharyngitis, Chronic		
491.9	Bronchitis, Chronic	784.49	Hoarseness	388.01	Presbyacusis		
682.1	Cervical Cellulitis & Abscess	474.1	Hypertrophy Tonsils & Adenoids	472.0	Rhinitis, Chronic		
784.2	Cervical Mass	380.4	Impacted Cerumen	527.2	Sialoadenitis Parotitis		
723.1	Cervical Pain	478.30	Laryngeal Paralysis	473.9	Sinusitis		
385.3	Cholesteatoma	464.0	Laryngitis, Acute	780.57	Sleep Apnea		
786.2	Cough	476.0	Laryngitis, Chronic	702.19	Sub. Keratosis		
470	Deviated Nasal Septum	528.6	Leukoplakia	527.5	Submaxillary Stones		
780.4	Dizziness	785.6	Lymph Node Enlargement	388.2	Sudden Hearing Loss		
787.2	Dysphagia	932	Nasal Foreign Body	246.9	Thyroid Disorder		
784.7	Epistaxis	802.0	Nasal Fracture, Closed	241.0	Thyroid Nodule		
381.81	Eustachian Tube Dysf.	471.9	Nasal Polyps	388.30	Tinnitus		
682.0	Facial Cellulitis & Abscess	478.1	Nasal Vestibulitis	463	Tonsillitis, Acute		
931	Foreign Body, Ear	460	Nasopharyngitis, Acute	474.0	Tonsillitis, Chronic		
529.6	Glossodynia	388.7	Otalgia	384.2	Tympanic Membrane Perf.		

Horizons Healthcare Center

123 Main Avenue
Farmington, ND 58000
Telephone (012) 555-4200

| PRIOR BALANCE | TODAY'S CHARGE | ADJUSTMENTS | TODAY'S PAYMENT | BALANCE DUE |
| | | | | |

Figure 10–1. A superbill lists common procedures performed and diagnoses of patients treated in the medical office and may contain complete patient information for billing purposes. (Form courtesy of Colwell Systems, St. Paul, Minn.)

ready to prepare the chart for the visit. This type of superbill may be customized to the physician's practice.

A computer can track the most common reasons for an office visit as well as track the illnesses and conditions the physician treats most often. This information will be printed on the computerized form. In an office in which physicians practice many different specialties, a computer could, essentially, customize a superbill for every physician in the practice. Having each physician's most-often-used information included on a customized superbill can save a significant amount of time when a physician identifies procedures to be billed, because the physician's most frequently used procedures and diagnoses are readily available for billing.

Computerized systems can also provide a control for superbills. The computer can assign a number to an office visit or superbill, and a report can be generated detailing the superbills that have not been entered into the system.

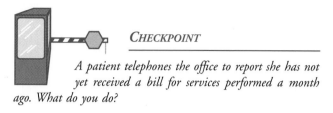

CHECKPOINT

A patient telephones the office to report she has not yet received a bill for services performed a month ago. What do you do?

Components

A superbill is divided into three parts: patient information, a list of procedures, and a list of diagnoses.

Patient Information. Depending on the needs of the practice, this section can vary greatly. Complete patient information (name, address, date of birth, and insurance information) may be included on the superbill. The information may be written on the form, or a computerized label may be generated to stick on the form.

Some superbills are very streamlined (Fig. 10–2) and may include only the bare essentials needed to produce a bill for the patient. Limited information necessary to identify the patient may be all that is included on the form. The rest of the data needed for billing can be retrieved at a later time during input into a computer billing system.

Procedures. A service provided for a patient in the course of medical treatment is known as a **procedure.** There are many types of procedures, such as office visits; surgical, laboratory, and x-ray tests; and immunizations. A patient may have more than one procedure for a single visit to the doctor.

Diagnoses. The cause of the patient's visit to the office is listed as the **diagnosis.** The diagnosis is the physician's determination of the patient's illness and is the reason for the office visit. A patient may have more than one or more reasons for seeing a physician. The diagnosis may be an illness, injury, or routine health treatment such as a physical examination or other checkup. All diagnoses pertinent to the visit should be listed on the superbill, with the diagnoses numbered in order of importance. The chief reason for the patient's visit is listed as diagnosis number 1, and any other diagnoses are listed subsequently.

The Billing Process from Beginning to End

Many parts of the billing process take place behind the scenes. In some instances, the patient rarely sees a copy of the superbill, receiving only a monthly statement of charges from the medical office.

Let's look at a typical superbill as it travels through the medical office (Fig. 10–3). As mentioned previously, the critical beginning step of the billing process is registration. A co-payment may be required when the patient registers.

After registration, the patient's superbill is attached to his or her medical record, and these documents are placed outside the examination room as the patient awaits the physician's visit. The physician brings the patient's chart and attached superbill into the examination room.

After the visit, the physician marks the procedures performed and the patient's diagnosis on the superbill. The physician may then collect the day's superbills in a stack and hand the superbills to the assistant at the end of the day for billing. In some situations, the physician may send the patient with the superbill to the front office. This may be bad practice, because patients may forget to return the superbill to the front desk. Sometimes, the physician may place the superbill in the chart so that the bill can be removed when the charts are reviewed for quantitative analysis in the records room. This practice also has drawbacks, because bills may become lost inside a patient's chart.

Perhaps the best practice for returning superbills to the front office for billing is to keep superbills in a specific location in the room in which the physician does paperwork. Such a location may be a shelf- or wall-mounted file or a manila folder. At the end of the day, the superbills can be collected and sent to the front office for billing.

However the superbills are collected, they are returned to the assistant for entering charges on the patient's account. After charges are made, information is collected to complete the patient's insurance claim, and the claim is sent to the insurance company. In some offices, claims for certain types of insurance may be done at a certain time of the month. The insurance claim process is reviewed in Chapter 11.

BILLING BASICS

What Does the Doctor Charge?

Occasionally, patients may inquire about the physician's fee for services. A common occurrence in the medical office is for patients to ask such questions as "How much does it cost for a strep test?" They sometimes do not realize that patients cannot come into the office and order whatever they want. An assistant might reply, "We are unable to perform only a strep test without the doctor's approval. You would need to see the doctor, and she would need to determine whether a strep test is necessary. If a strep test were ordered, there would be a charge for an office visit and for the test. Our office visits typically range from $X to $Y, and a strep test is $Z. If the doctor sees the need for any additional tests, those would be charged separately."

When giving an estimate of physician charges, an assistant should not give an absolute amount but should instead give a range of possible charges because each patient is unique and will have different needs for medical care. For example, a patient with a chronic medical condition such as diabetes may require additional time for an office visit and may need additional laboratory tests. A great deal of what is

Timothy Marks, M.D.
123 Main Avenue
Farmington, ND 58000
Telephone (012) 555-4200

NAME _____   DATE OF SERVICE _____

DESCRIPTION	CPT	FEE	DESCRIPTION	CPT	FEE	DESCRIPTION	CPT	FEE
NEW PATIENT			**PROCEDURES**			**LABORATORY**		
Problem Focused H/E, SF	99201		Anoscopy	46600		ANA	86038	
Expanded Problem Focused H/E, SF	99202		Audiometry, Pure Tone, Air	92552		Blood, Occult, Feces	82270	
Detailed H/E, LC	99203		Burn, 1st Degree, Local	16000		Automated Hemogram, CBC	85022	
Comprehensive H/E, MC	99204		Burn, Debridement, Small	16020*		Comp. Metabolic Panel	80053	
Comprehensive H/E, HC	99205		EKG w/Interp. & Report	93000		HCG Qualitative	84703	
ESTABLISHED PATIENT			EKG Tracing Only	93005		PSA, Total	84153	
Minimal	99211		F.B. Rem., Simple	10120*		Sed. Rate	85651	
Problem Focused H/E, SF	99212		F.B. Rem., Complex	10121		Strep Test	86403	
Expanded Problem Focused H/E, LC	99213		Hemorrhoid/External, Exc.	46320*		T.B. Tine Test	86585	
Detailed H/E, MC	99214		I&D Abscess, Simple	10060*		Thyroxine, Total	84436	
Comprehensive H/E, HC	99215		I&D Pilonidal Cyst, Simple	10080*		TSH	84443	
HOSPITAL CARE			I&D Sebaceous Cyst	10040*		Urinalysis, Stick w/Micro	81000	
Initial, New or Established			Impacted Cerumen Rem.	69210		Venipuncture, Routine	36415*	
Detailed H/E, SF or LC	99221		Injection, Ligament	20550*		Wet Mount	87210	
Subsequent, Established			Injection, Major Joint	20610*				
Problem Focused H/E, SF or LC	99231		Laceration Repair:					
Discharge, 30 Min. or Less	99238			120__		**IMMUNIZATIONS/INJECTIONS**		
EMERGENCY ROOM SERVICES			Lesion Removal:			DT, < 7 Yrs.	90702	
Problem Focused H/E, SF	99281		Curettement, Single	11055		Tetanus Toxoid	90703	
NURSING FACILITY			Destruction, Any, First Les.	17000*		Cholera	90725	
Detailed History/Comp.			Nail Removal, Simple, Single	11730*		Hepatitis B	9074_	
Exam, SF or LC, Initial	99301		Nail Removal, Perm.	11750		Influenza Virus Vaccine	906__	
Problem Focused Exam, SF or LC,			Removal Skin Tags up to 15	11200*		Measles	90705	
Subsequent	99311		Each Additional 10	11201		MMR	90707	
OTHER			Sigmoidoscopy, Flexible, Diagnostic	45330		Pneumonia Vaccine	90732	
After Hours	99050		Spirometry	94010		Injection IM/SQ	90782	
Sundays/Holidays	99054		Spirometry, Pre/Post Bronch.	94060				
Supplies:						**MISCELLANEOUS**		
	99070							

			DIAGNOSIS				
789.00	Abdominal Pain	722.6	Degenerative Disc Disease	242.90	Hyperthyroidism	V70.3	Physical Exam, Administrative
706.1	Acne	276.5	Dehydration	244.9	Hypothyroidism	486	Pneumonia, Organism Unspec.
477.9	Allergic Rhinitis	296.20	Depression	703.0	Ingrown Toenail	V22.2	Pregnancy
300.00	Anxiety	250.00	Diabetes	780.52	Insomnia	256.3	Premature Menopause
427.9	Arrhythmia	692.9	Eczema/Dermatitis	564.1	Irritable Bowel Syndrome	601.9	Prostatitis
493.90	Asthma	782.3	Edema	785.6	Lymphadenopathy	473.9	Sinusitis
427.31	Atrial Fibrillation	780.79	Fatigue	626.9	Menstrual Disorder	780.2	Syncope
490	Bronchitis	780.6	Fever	346.90	Migraine	465.9	URI
437.9	Cerebrovascular Disease	610.1	Fibrocystic Breast Disease	848.9	Muscle Strain	599.0	UTI, Site Unspec.
847.0	Cervical Strain	558.9	Gastroenteritis	728.85	Muscle Spasms	616.10	Vaginitis
786.50	Chest Pain	274.9	Gout	733.00	Osteoporosis	780.4	Vertigo
372.30	Conjunctivitis	784.0	Headache	382.9	Otitis Media	078.10	Warts
428.0	Congestive Heart Failure	785.3	Heart Murmur	V72.3	Pelvic Exam		
924.9	Contusion, Area Unspec.	272.0	Hypercholesterolemia	533.90	Peptic Ulcer Disease		
496	C.O.P.D.	272.4	Hyperlipidemia	462	Pharyngitis, Acute		
414.00	Coronary Artery Disease	401.9	Hypertension	V70.0	Physical Exam, General		

DIAGNOSIS (If not checked above)

PREVIOUS BALANCE	
TODAY'S TOTAL FEE	
TOTAL	
PAYMENT	
NEW BALANCE	

PHYSICIAN'S SIGNATURE _____

FORM 493202 COLWELL SYSTEMS 1.800.637.1140

Figure 10–2. Some superbills may contain only the information necessary to generate a computerized bill. (Form courtesy of Colwell Systems, St. Paul, Minn.)

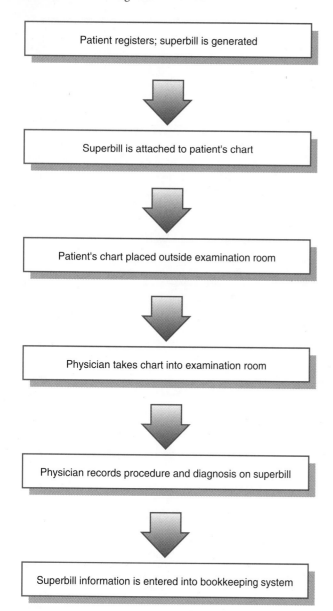

Patient registers; superbill is generated

Superbill is attached to patient's chart

Patient's chart placed outside examination room

Physician takes chart into examination room

Physician records procedure and diagnosis on superbill

Superbill information is entered into bookkeeping system

Figure 10–3. Many steps are included in the billing process.

required during a patient's encounter with the physician depends on the patient's condition and medical history.

When talking to a patient about charges for medical care, an assistant should state clearly that the charges given are merely an estimate. Depending on a patient's condition, a physician may decide to order additional tests or may spend extended time with the patient. Many variables exist within every patient visit.

When a patient inquires about the physician's charges, an assistant should encourage the patient to notify the office manager of any concerns the patient may have regarding charges for medical services. If a patient has financial hardship, a physician may have sample medications for the patient in lieu of a costlier prescription. If the patient has anxiety about the physician's charges, most offices are usually very willing to work with patients and to make arrangements for extended payment.

Charges for Minors

If a patient is a minor, the bill should always be addressed to an adult who is responsible for payment; the bill should not and cannot be addressed to the minor. Generally, a minor who is not emancipated cannot be held responsible for charges incurred. It is often very difficult, if not impossible, to hold a minor responsible for a bill.

In the case of divorce, a bill for services provided to a minor should be sent to a parent designated by the court to pay for medical expenses. In the absence of any court arrangements, the assistant should work with the minor's parents to establish a suitable billing arrangement of which both parents are aware. If there is no designation, a bill for services provided to a minor is usually sent to the parent presenting the child for treatment.

CHECKPOINT

A minor telephones the office and wishes to see a physician for information on birth control. The minor does not want her parents to know about the visit. Based on what you learned in Chapter 3 and in this chapter, what might your answer be?

Missed Appointments—To Bill or Not To Bill

What happens if a patient misses an appointment with a physician? Should the patient be charged for the appointment?

In most practices, physicians choose not to charge a patient for missing an appointment. Physicians realize that from time to time a patient may forget about an appointment. In a busy medical office, where a physician sees a few patients within the span of an hour, an occasional patient who forgets an appointment will probably not be noticed in the schedule.

In some practices, however, in which a physician sees only a few patients during the day (such as psychiatry, in which each patient is usually scheduled for an hour appointment), a physician may wish to charge the patient for the missed visit.

The American Medical Association's (AMA's) Council on Ethical and Judicial Affairs specifies that a patient can be charged for a missed appointment if the patient has been told in advance that there will be a charge for missed appointments. Providers who charge for missed appointments should make their policy clearly known to patients and may even wish to have patients sign a notice that they are aware that a charge will be made if an appointment is missed.

A medical office should be sure to make its policy on charging for missed appointments clear. Notices can be placed in monthly statements, or patients may be asked to sign a notification of such a policy.

Assignment of Benefits

Patients covered by insurance are usually encouraged to have their insurance claim payments sent directly to the physician's office. Such an arrangement is called **assignment of benefits.** The assignment of benefits authorization is located at the bottom of the patient registration form (see Fig. 8–2). A signature on such an authorization allows the insurance payments to be sent directly to the medical office.

Most medical offices prefer that patients assign their health benefits directly to the office, because the practice will receive any insurance benefits directly from the insurance company. The practice thus receives payment for at least a portion of its services. Patients who do not assign benefits to the clinic have the insurance benefits paid directly to themselves, and the practice may have to wait to receive payment from the patient. The medical office runs the risk of the patient keeping the payment and using the money for something else.

Fees for Medical Care

How does a dollar amount actually get on the patient's bill? Amounts for various procedures are determined long before the patient enters the clinic. Each medical practice establishes what is called a **fee schedule.** This schedule is a listing of every procedure done by the practice's physicians and a dollar amount to be charged for each procedure. Like any other commercial concern, medical offices must set prices. The fee schedule should be reviewed at least annually to determine whether any changes are warranted.

Charges for medical procedures vary throughout the country. Outside factors such as the local economy, cost of living, and competition all have an impact on what the physician charges for a medical procedure. Other items affecting the cost of medical services are such variables as the length of time the physician spends with the patient and the complexity of the patient's condition. A patient seen for congestive heart failure requires more complex decision-making on the physician's part and a longer office visit than does an otherwise healthy patient seen for an ear infection. The patient with heart failure would most likely incur a higher office charge because of the nature of his or her condition.

In addition, many insurance programs, such as government benefit programs (e.g., Medicare and Medicaid), have established maximum amounts that may be charged. If a medical office wishes to serve patients who receive these benefits, the office may be limited in the amount that may be charged. For more information on establishing fees, see Chapter 11.

▌ MEDICAL CODING

Coding refers to the practice of assigning a numerical or alphanumerical code to categorize a procedure that has been performed or a condition that has been treated. Use of an established system of procedure and diagnosis codes in the processes involved in medical billing enables health care providers, insurance companies, and government agencies to "speak the same language." Without a system of standardized codes, it would be difficult to establish uniformity in the description of medical conditions and disease and the procedures used to treat them.

Standardized systems (i.e., CPT and ICD coding systems; see next section) are used for a number of reasons. The use of codes means easier processing of insurance claims, which, in turn, means faster payment for the medical office. Codes are used to gather statistics, track the occurrence of disease, and aid in medical research. Codes may also be used by the medical office to tally the types of conditions most commonly treated by the physicians in the office as well as common procedures done by the physicians. Information from medical coding can help to plan for the health care needs of the population and can be used to further medical education and research.

When performing both procedure and diagnosis coding, you must be careful never to "overcode" or code something that did not occur. Knowingly and willingly performing such an act constitutes fraud and has legal penalties. Third-party payers occasionally review medical records to validate codes. Documentation from a patient's medical record must be able to support all codes used in billing for any patient's encounter.

There is so much to know about procedure and diagnosis coding that to perform each type of coding well would require an entire course of study. Expertise in coding can be developed only after in-depth study and actual work experience involving coding. The explanations of coding systems that follow are designed to help you become familiar with the structure and purpose of these coding systems.

Procedure Coding

The procedures for which the physician charges fees are identified by numerical codes called **CPT** codes. The CPT-4 manual is a listing of codes assigned to medical procedures performed by physicians. CPT-4 stands for *Current Procedural Terminology, 4th edition.* The AMA publishes CPT codes annually, and an AMA editorial panel reviews proposed changes to the CPT codes when the manual is updated each year.

CPT codes are used on a patient's insurance claim to identify procedures that the doctor performs. CPT provides a structured way to categorize medical procedures. By categorizing these procedures, statistics on procedures performed by physicians are gathered.

These codes are part of a larger coding system established by the Health Care Financing Administration (**HCFA,** pronounced "hik-fah"), an agency of the federal government now known as Centers for Medicare and Medicaid Services (CMS). This coding system is known as HCFA Common Procedure Coding System (**HCPCS,** pronounced "hik-piks"). The HCPCS system consists of the following three levels of codes:

- Level I codes are for physician procedures and services that are copyrighted by the AMA. If a patient is treated in a medical office or in a hospital, the physician's professional services are billed using a CPT code.
- Level II codes are for nonphysician services, supplies, and procedures not included in Level I.
- Level III codes are used at the local level for Medicare claims.

Sections of the CPT Manual

The CPT manual is divided into six sections of numerical codes, identified and arranged in the order listed in Table 10–1. In the beginning of each section, guidelines alert the user to special considerations when choosing a code in that section. Special instructions are also sometimes included at the beginning of certain groups of codes. The manual is arranged in numerical order with the exception of the Evaluation and Management (E&M) codes, which appear first in the manual.

Basics of Procedure Coding (CPT–HCPCS Level I)

In addition to the six sections of CPT codes, the manual contains an index that is located in the back of the book. When using the CPT manual, the index is always used first. The index introduction gives instructions for locating procedures within the index. Procedures are listed by

- condition (i.e., hematoma, cyst)
- anatomical site (i.e., carpal bone, hip)
- name of procedure (i.e., arthroscopy, cast)

This arrangement often makes it possible to arrive at the same procedure code by using different entries in the index. For example, the procedure code for a *tonsillectomy* could be located under *tonsils, excision; tonsillectomy;* or *excision, tonsils.*

When selecting CPT codes, it is very important for an assistant to have a general understanding of the procedure that has been done. Often in the listing of codes, there are slight variations listed for the procedures. If you are

PROCEDURE 10–1 Assign Procedure Codes for a Patient's Encounter

Materials Needed
- Medical records
- CPT-4 manual, current year's edition

1. Identify all procedures performed during a patient's encounter.
2. Locate the main term of each procedure code in the index by identifying the condition, anatomic site procedure, or service provided.
3. Look in the main term for any additional modifiers. Identify all codes that may fit the procedure.
4. Locate each of the codes from number 3 in the appropriate section of the CPT manual.
5. Read the description for each code and choose the code that best fits the procedure.*

Denotes a crucial step in the procedure. The student must complete this step satisfactorily in order to complete the procedure satisfactorily.

unfamiliar with the procedure, it is important to consult the physician as to the specifics of the procedure.

Procedure codes should never be chosen directly from the index. Always verify the codes by reading the description of the code listed in one of the six sections of the manual. Each procedure code description is almost always more detailed within each section than in the index. What may look like a good code in the index may not fit once the entire description is reviewed. Procedure Box 10–1 illustrates how to select a procedure code.

Modifiers

From time to time, procedures are performed under special circumstances. Perhaps a procedure was more complicated than usual, or maybe a physician wishes to reduce the costs of services for a patient. If special circumstances exist involving the patient's procedure, a **modifier** may be added after the CPT code to indicate the special circumstances. A modifier is used to communicate something different about the procedure or service that was provided. Modifiers that are applicable to each section are included in the section's introduction, and a complete listing of modifiers is located at the end of the manual.

A series of symbols is used throughout the manual to alert the user to special considerations about certain codes. The symbols are used to identify code revisions, new codes, codes that must be used with other codes, or surgical codes that include a procedure only.

Table 10–1. Organization of the CPT Manual

Section Name of CPT	Content of Codes
Evaluation and Management (E&M)	Physician visits, professional services
Anesthesia	Anesthetic administration
Surgery	Surgical procedures in all body systems
Radiology	X-ray, nuclear medicine, magnetic resonance imaging, computed tomographic scans
Pathology and Laboratory	Laboratory and pathology services
Medicine	Various procedures and services not listed elsewhere

Special Considerations

When performing coding for insurance claims, it is important to always use the current version of the CPT manual. Each year, several codes change or are dropped. If an out-of-date code is selected, it will cause the insurance company to deny a patient's claims and will cause unnecessary delay in receiving payment for health care services that are rendered.

Nonphysician Services (HCPCS Level II)

The second level of the HCFA Common Procedure Coding System contains codes that are assigned for many nonphysician services.

HCPCS level II codes are used to bill for such items as
- medical supplies (i.e., dressings and bandages, walkers, crutches, pacemakers)
- ambulance services
- medications
- medical equipment (i.e., wheelchairs)
- vision and hearing supplies and services
- nutrition counseling

Coding for HCPCS Level II supplies and services is done in much the same way as the coding for Level I. The assistant locates the supply or service in the index and verifies the code in the main section of the manual.

Diagnosis Coding

Diagnosis coding in the medical office is done using a system of numerical codes called the *International Classification of Diseases, 9th Revision, Clinical Modification* or **ICD-9-CM.** The ICD-9-CM is derived from the official version of the ICD-9, developed by the World Health Organization.

Divisions of the Manual

The ICD-9-CM consists of the following three parts:
- Volume 1, Tabular List of Diseases (in numerical order)
- Volume 2, Index of Diseases (in alphabetical order)
- Volume 3, Index and Tabular List of Procedures

The assistant will primarily use volumes 1 and 2 of the ICD-9-CM for coding the patient's diagnosis (Table 10–2). Volume 3 is used for coding services provided by a facility for inpatient hospital procedures. You will recall that a physician's professional services are coded with a CPT code. In the case of treatment provided for an inpatient, a CPT code will be used to identify the procedure or service provided by the physician, an ICD-9-CM procedure code will be used to identify the facility services provided for the procedure or service, and an ICD-9-CM diagnosis code will identify the patient's diagnosis.

As CPT assigns a numerical code to procedures, ICD-9-CM assigns a numerical code to a diagnosis. When coding a patient's superbill, the steps in Procedure Box 10–2 outline the basic process of selecting the correct diagnosis code for the patient's visit.

Table 10–2. Organization of ICD-9-CM, Volumes 1 and 2

Volume 1	
Chapter Name	**Codes**
Infectious and Parasitic Diseases	001-139
Neoplasms	140-239
Endocrinologic, Nutritional, and Metabolic Diseases and Immunity Disorders	240-279
Diseases of the Blood and Blood-Forming Organs	280-289
Mental Disorders	290-319
Diseases of the Nervous System and Sense Organs	320-389
Diseases of the Circulatory System	390-459
Diseases of the Respiratory System	460-519
Diseases of the Digestive System	520-579
Diseases of the Genitourinary System	580-629
Complications of Pregnancy, Childbirth, and the Puerperium	630-677
Diseases of the Skin and Subcutaneous Tissue	680-709
Diseases of the Musculoskeletal System and Connective Tissue	710-739
Congenital Anomalies	740-759
Certain Conditions Originating in the Perinatal Period	760-779
Symptoms, Signs and Ill-Defined Conditions	780-799
Injury and Poisoning	800-999

Supplementary Classification	
Classification of Factors Influencing Health Status and Contact with Health Service	V01-V82
Classification of External Causes of Injury and Poisoning	E800-E999

Appendices	
A	Morphology of Neoplasms
B	Glossary of Mental Disorders
C	Classification of Drugs by American Hospital Formulary Service List Number and Their ICD-9-CM Equivalents
D	Classification of Industrial Accidents According to Agency
E	List of Three-Digit Categories
F	Diagnoses Defined as Complications or Comorbidities

Volume 2
Index to Diseases and Injuries, alphabetic
Table of Drugs and Chemicals
Index to External Causes of Injuries and Poisonings

line the basic process of selecting the correct diagnosis code for the patient's visit.

Conventions Used in ICD-9-CM

Conventions are used throughout the ICD-9-CM manuals to point out special conditions related to codes. Depending on the type of ICD-9-CM manual used in the medical office, conventions used by ICD-9-CM may appear differently. The purpose of the conventions, however, is the same in all of the manuals—to alert the assistant to any special notations or conditions of selecting a particular code. A convention may be a symbol, such as a set of parentheses, or it may be an abbreviation, such as *NOS*.

A synopsis of some common conventions is shown in Figure 10–4. Each ICD-9-CM manual has detailed instructions to acquaint the assistant with the specific conventions used in the particular code book. Instructions are almost

PROCEDURE 10-2 *Assign Diagnosis Codes for a Patient's Encounter*

Materials Needed
- Medical records.
- ICD-9-CM manual, current year's edition.

1. Identify all diagnoses treated during a patient's encounter.
2. Determine the primary reason for the patient's office visit
3. Locate the main term of the diagnosis in the index (volume II).
4. Locate any modifiers beneath the main term.
5. Identify the numeric code referenced in volume II.
6. Locate the code from volume II in the tabular (numerical) listing (volume I) in the manual.
7. Read the description of the code. Determine whether the code fits the diagnosis given for the patient.*
8. Code any additional diagnoses listed in the patient's encounter by repeating steps 3–7.

*Denotes a crucial step in the procedure. The student must complete this step satisfactorily in order to complete the procedure satisfactorily.

always available in every coding manual, and anyone performing coding should become completely familiar with the instructions in the manual being used.

Updates for ICD-9-CM

The ICD-9-CM is updated annually on October 1. Changes are available in the *Federal Register, Coding Clinic,* and *American Health Information Management Association Journal.* It is important to use an updated version of the ICD-9-CM when coding to ensure proper processing of claims. Submitting old codes could mean a claim will be rejected by the insurance company.

The Coding Profession

Help is always available for anyone responsible for coding in the medical office. Many products are published that provide detailed examples, illustrations, and explanations of codes. As mentioned previously, there is much to know about coding. Educational programs in which coding is a key component may have several courses for procedure and diagnosis coding.

Examinations are available for individuals wishing to become a certified coder. Two coding certification designations are the Certified Professional Coder designation (**CPC**),

awarded by the American Academy of Professional Coders, and the Certified Coding Specialist (**CCS**), awarded by the American Health Information Management Association. Some coding certifications require specific training or work experience before a person is allowed to take a certification examination. Attainment of a coding certification demonstrates proficiency in coding and may be required by some employers who hire coders.

BOOKKEEPING SYSTEMS

Computerized Systems

Most medical offices today use some type of computerized billing system (Fig. 10–5). A computerized system has many advantages over the traditional pegboard system (discussed in the next section).

Not all computerized systems are alike. Features typically found in a computerized system are summarized in the following list:

ICD-9-CM Symbols and conventions with examples

NEC Not elsewhere classifiable. This category should be used only if the coder lacks the information to code to a more specific category.

Radiculitis (pressure) (vertebrogenic)
   729.2
   cervical NEC 723.4

NOS Not otherwise specified. The diagnosis cannot be found in another place.

723.4 Brachia neuritis or radiculitis NOS
    Cervical radiculitis
    Radicular syndrome of upper limbs

( ) Parentheses are used to include adjectives that may or may not be present in the diagnosis statement

Sprain, strain (joint) (ligament) (muscle)
    (tendon) 848.9
   abdominal wall (muscle) 848.8
   Achilles tendon 845.09
   acromioclavicular 840.0
   ankle 845.00
    and foot 845.00

[ ] Brackets are used to identify synonyms, substitute terms, or add information that clarifies the diagnosis statement.

524.60 Temporomandibular joint disorders, unspecified
    Temporomandibular joint-pain-dysfunction syndrome [TMJ]

Figure 10–4. ICD-9-CM symbols and conventions alert an assistant to special conditions concerning a diagnosis code.

- A database containing CPT codes and their associated costs can be maintained. When a code is entered, the current price of the procedure automatically appears on the patient's bill.
- A database containing ICD-9-CM codes can be maintained for identifying a patient's diagnosis on an insurance claim.
- Statistics needed for planning can be gathered.
- A patient's billing information, such as name, address, and insurance company, can be obtained from the program's database for easy billing.
- A patient's information can be accessed or updated from any computer location in the medical office if the office's computer system is networked.
- Past due accounts that may need attention for collection can be tracked.
- Reports for obtaining a clear picture of the business end of the practice can be run.
- Insurance claim information can be easily obtained and claims generated. Claims may even be filed electronically from the computer system.

For offices with computerized systems, a computer-input journal (Fig. 10–6) can be used to record cash, check, or credit card payments. This system uses a journal sheet, bank deposit slip, and cash receipt that are placed on top of a pegged control board. Receipts are aligned on top of the journal and bank deposit form, and entries are written once (Procedure Box 10–3).

When the journal sheet is complete, the bank deposit form is removed and accompanies the deposits to the bank. The journal is then used to post payments to the patient's account.

Pegboard

The pegboard system of billing (Fig. 10–7) is a record-keeping system that logs the business transactions of the medical office onto one sheet that is later tallied and posted to accounts. A pegboard is often referred to as a *one-write system* because transactions are recorded only once.

A journal sheet is placed on a control board containing a row of pegs. The control board and pegs help align the

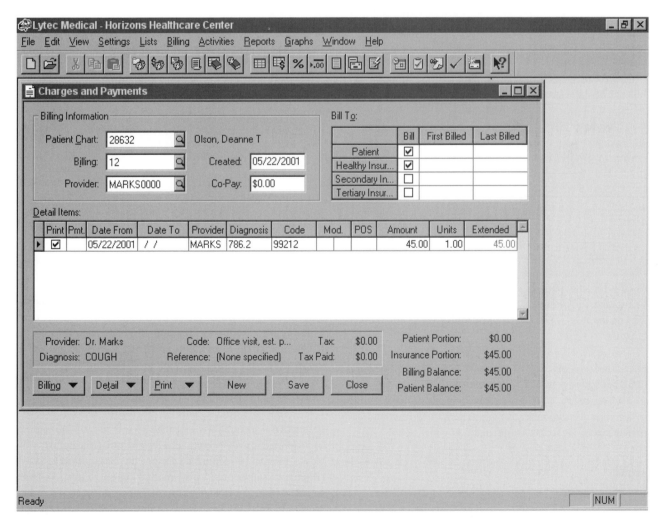

A

Figure 10–5. A computer system stores an assortment of information related to the billing process.

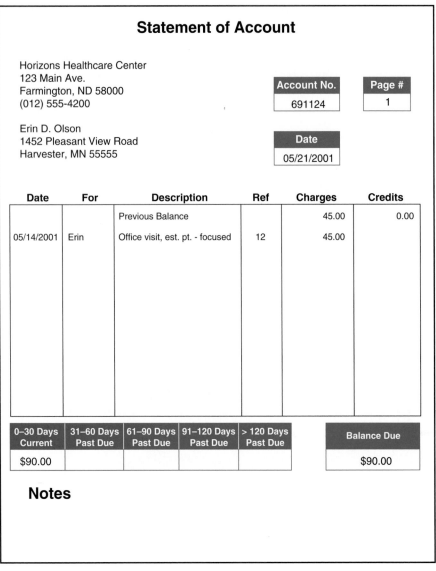

Statement of Account

Horizons Healthcare Center
123 Main Ave.
Farmington, ND 58000
(012) 555-4200

Account No.	Page #
691124	1

Erin D. Olson
1452 Pleasant View Road
Harvester, MN 55555

Date
05/21/2001

Date	For	Description	Ref	Charges	Credits
		Previous Balance		45.00	0.00
05/14/2001	Erin	Office visit, est. pt. - focused	12	45.00	

0–30 Days Current	31–60 Days Past Due	61–90 Days Past Due	91–120 Days Past Due	> 120 Days Past Due		Balance Due
$90.00						$90.00

Notes

B

Figure 10–5. *Continued.*

forms when amounts are entered. When a patient's charges and payments are received, these amounts are recorded on a receipt for the patient and on the journal sheet and patient's account ledger. Any possibility for errors is minimized, because sheets are totaled and cross-checked at the bottom.

This system is relatively low-cost, and errors are minimized because posting to accounts is reduced: the journal totals are entered into accounts rather than many single entries being made. This system can be more time-consuming to use, however, because all entries are handwritten and each patient's account ledger is updated manually.

CHECKPOINT

Your physician is contemplating switching from a pegboard system to a computerized system. What might be the advantages of a computerized system?

CREDIT

Usually, after a patient sees a physician in the medical office, he or she will receive a bill for services at a later date. This patient has received credit.

Credit may be as simple as incurring a charge and paying for it at another time. Many patients seen in most medical offices receive credit because they are not required to pay for office charges immediately after an office visit.

The federal **Equal Credit Opportunity Act** of 1975 requires that once credit is extended to one individual, it must be extended to all others. The law stipulates that an individual cannot be denied credit on the basis of race, color, religion, national origin, sex, marital status, or age. An individual cannot be denied credit if he or she receives public assistance. In other words, credit may be extended to people of any gender, race, or age—not only to men or to members of a particular race or to people 30 years of age and older. Such distinctions would be discrimination.

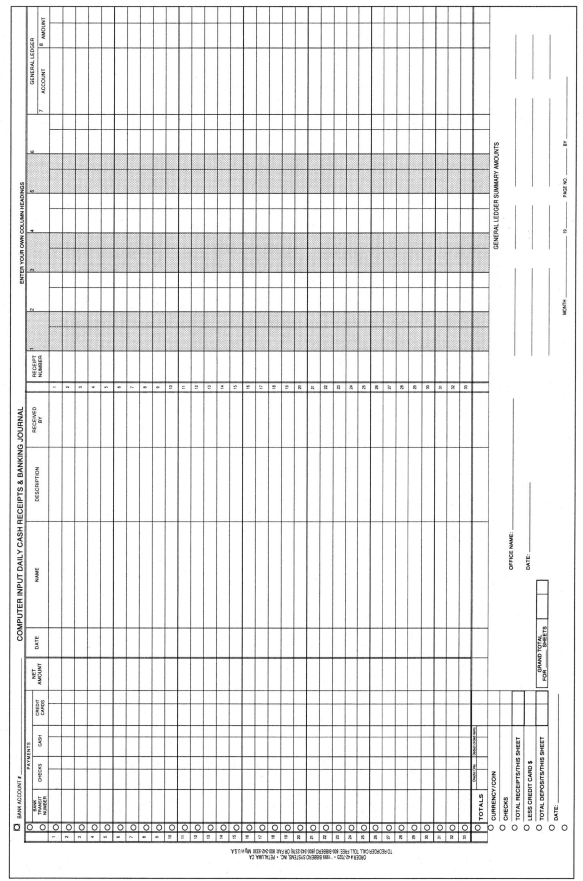

Figure 10–6. A computer input journal can be used to post transactions in a computer system. (Form courtesy of Bibbero Systems, Inc., Petaluma, Calif. Telephone, 800-242-2376. Fax, 800-242-9330. Available at www.bibbero.com.)

PROCEDURE 10–3 *Enter Patients' Charges into a Billing System*

Materials Needed
- Computer billing system or pegboard system
- Superbills from patient encounters

1. Gather the superbills to be recorded.
*2. Assign the correct procedure codes for each encounter.
*3. Assign the correct diagnosis codes for each encounter.
*4. Record the encounters in the billing system. If using a pegboard system, use the correct fee schedule for procedures. Enter the correct information in each billing category.

Denotes a crucial step in the procedure. The student must complete this step satisfactorily in order to complete the procedure satisfactorily.

PROCEDURE 10–4 *Produce Monthly Statements for Patient Accounts*

Materials Needed
- Patient account information (computer billing information or ledger cards)
- Outstanding charges and payments

1. Establish the statement due.
2. Determine which accounts should have a statement generated. If using a cycle billing system, only certain statements may need to be generated.
3. Post any outstanding charges to patient accounts.
4. Post any outstanding payments to patient accounts.
5. Print the statements.*

Denotes a crucial step in the procedure. The student must complete this step satisfactorily in order to complete the procedure satisfactorily.

Credit can be refused only because of inability to pay. Not everyone who asks for credit receives credit. When considering a patient for credit, the patient's income, expenses, debt, and credit history can be reviewed to determine whether the patient is credit-worthy. Assistants should remember and adhere to the following guidelines when determining a patient's request for credit:

- A patient's sex, race, national origin, or religion cannot be asked.
- A patent's marital status can be asked only if a spouse's income would be used to obtain credit. If asking about marital status, a creditor may ask whether the patient is married, single, or separated. Creditors are not allowed to ask whether a patient is divorced or widowed.
- You cannot ask for information about a patient's spouse unless the spouse will use the account or the patient needs to rely on the spouse's income.
- You cannot refuse to consider income because of its source (e.g., public assistance, pension funds, child support).

Billing Patients

Each month, a statement of a patient's account is generated. A statement contains a summary of charges and payments for the patient and any other family members on the account. Statements are printed and sent to the account's guarantor (Procedure Box 10–4). The guarantor is the individual responsible for payment of the account (see Chapter 8). A guarantor could be a patient, parent, spouse, or other individual.

Statements are usually sent to guarantors monthly; the size of the practice determines when the statements are generated.

Small practices may elect to mail out all statements at the end of the month. For large practices that send out hundreds or even thousands of statements each month, **cycle billing** can even out the medical office's workload. Cycle billing involves billing patients at intervals throughout the month. The practice's accounts are divided into equal groups, and each group is assigned a specific time of the month in which statements are done and mailed.

When using cycle billing, often the patient's last name is used to determine the day of the month the statement is to be billed (Table 10–3). Based on the information in Table 10–3, Harriet Anderson's bill would be sent out on the 1st of every month and Allen Williams's bill would be sent out on the 25th of every month. The payment due date for each statement will depend on the time of the month the statement was sent. Using cycle billing in a medical office enables the staff to carry on normal activities of the office and process statements and payments as a part of everyday activity.

Imagine that a practice has 1000 active accounts. If all accounts were billed on the last day of the month, an assistant would have to mail out statements in a sudden flurry of activity at the end of the month. Then, if all payments were due by the 20th of the month, the days surrounding

Table 10–3. Cycle Billing Schedule

Patient's Last Name	Date of Month
A–C	1st
D–G	5th
H–K	9th
L–N	13th
O–R	17th
S–U	21st
V–Z	25th

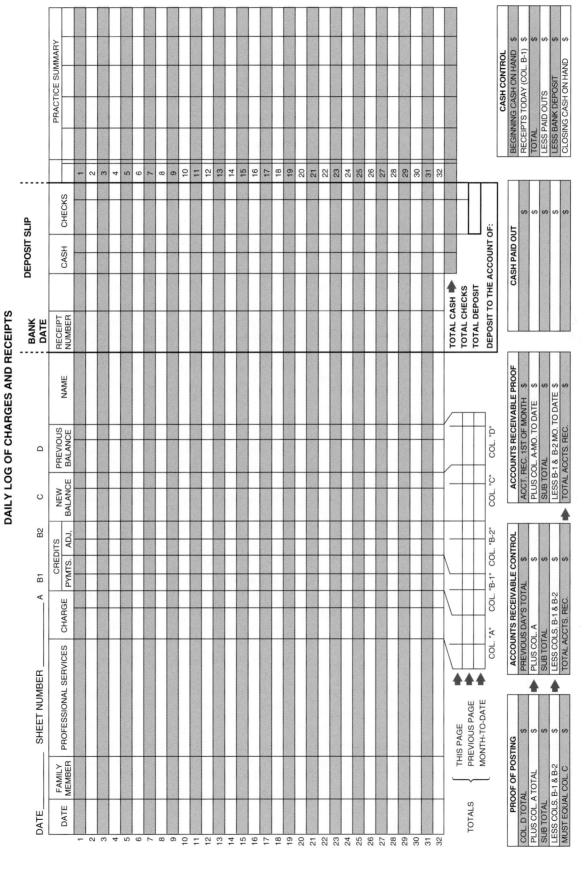

Figure 10–7. Transactions are recorded only once when using a pegboard system. (Courtesy of Colwell Systems, St. Paul, Minn.)

the 20th would be spent trying to get volumes of payments recorded in the patients' accounts.

Cycle billing spreads the work out over the course of the month. With this type of billing system, statements are constantly going out and payments are constantly coming in. Cycle billing also provides a steady flow of cash coming into the office.

Aging Accounts

Whatever bookkeeping system an office uses—computerized or traditional—an assistant should monitor account balances each month to determine whether an account has become seriously overdue. Accounts receivable aging categorizes the outstanding charges on a patient's bill and identifies how long the charge has been on the patient's account. Account balances are kept on 30-day intervals (e.g., fewer than 30 days or current, 31 to 60 days, 61 to 90 days, and more than 90 days). Tracking balances like this displays how old account charges are and enables an assistant to quickly see which balances may need attention for collection.

Let's take a look at the following two accounts:

Patient's Name	Susan Pearson	Matthew Stein
Account balance	$1000	$1000
Current balance (fewer than 30 days old)	$500	$0
Balance 31–60 days old	$300	$100
Balance 61–90 days old	$100	$50
Balance more than 90 days old	$100	$850

Although both account balances are the same, it is obvious that Mr. Stein's account needs some attention from the billing office. The distribution of the patients' balances is quite different. Aging accounts helps an assistant identify the accounts that may need some collection attention.

Collection

Occasionally in the course of business in the medical office, some patients do not pay their account. Most medical offices do pursue some type of collection action, but the degree to which a physician or practice pursues collection may vary widely.

Most physicians are used to providing some services for which they know they will never be reimbursed. Physicians provide some services on a charitable basis, but that does not mean that the physician will write off every account if the patient does not pay. Depending on the physician, overdue accounts may be targeted for collection.

Before pursuing any type of collection action on a patient's account, an assistant must consult the patient's physician to determine whether collection action is appropriate. The physician may not want to initiate any type of collection action if

a patient is suffering from a serious medical condition, is experiencing extreme financial hardship, or is going through an otherwise difficult situation. Many physicians feel that pursuing collection action when a patient is in such a situation would make them appear uncaring.

If a patient is currently undergoing chemotherapy for cancer, the physician is not likely to want the business office to call the patient about an overdue bill. Likewise, if a patient has other serious problems, such as an ill child or a recent job loss, the physician will likely not want to pursue collection. In addition to consulting a patient's physician, the assistant should check a patient's account to determine whether any outstanding insurance payments exist before initiating collection on the patient's account.

Collection Guidelines

Physicians in a practice should establish collection guidelines for an assistant to follow. Physicians may decide that accounts more than 60 days past due should be brought to their attention, or they may decide that only those accounts that have not had a payment for 3 months or more be brought to their attention. Physicians may also elect to have the assistant handle all collection.

Whatever the case may be, physicians in a practice should clearly communicate their personal philosophy of account collection and the collection activities of which they approve. Because the degree to which collection is pursued may affect the reputation of the practice, physicians should be chiefly responsible for establishing collection guidelines. Collection practices should also be in keeping with the Fair Debt Collection Practices Act as identified in the next section.

When collecting a patient's account, the assistant should remember that word will "get around" as to the physician's bill collecting practices. It is probably best for the reputation of the medical practice to use methods that are not aggressive. Today, patients may be unable to pay because of illness, but tomorrow, they may be able to pay and will remember the empathy shown by the practice in regard to the patient's medical charges. Aggressive collection practices could have a serious, detrimental effect on the image of the practice.

Fair Debt Collection Practices Act

The federal **Fair Debt Collection Practices Act** protects debtors against debt collectors who use unfair practices when collecting a debt. This law specifies the following:
- Collectors cannot use threats of violence.
- Collectors cannot use offensive language.
- Collectors cannot misrepresent themselves.

The law also sets the following requirements for debt collectors:
- When using a third party (i.e., a guarantor's relative or employer) to locate a debtor, the third party can be contacted only once.

- A debt collector cannot inform the third party that the individual is a debtor.
- A debt collector must use convenient hours—8 AM to 9 PM—to contact the debtor.
- A debt collector cannot contact the debtor at church or at special events.
- A debt collector cannot contact the debtor if the debtor states that he or she has an attorney.
- A debt collector cannot continue to contact a debtor if the debtor states in writing that he or she refuses to pay the debt or if the debtor says not to contact him or her again.

It is very important for any person conducting collection activity to follow these requirements. A debtor can sue a debt collector for violating the federal Fair Debt Collection Practices Act.

Initial Collection Methods

When collecting an overdue account, an assistant should remember to approach a guarantor sincerely and respectfully. The federal Fair Debt Collection Practices Act states that it is unlawful to threaten patients with action that the office does not intend to take. For instance, an assistant can't say "We will turn your account over to a collection agency if you don't pay the balance in one month," and then not do so.

When an account is past due, the first collection action is a gentle reminder that is printed on, stamped on, or enclosed with the patient's statement. Comments such as "Your account is past due" or "Your payment is overdue" are gentle reminders that the business office has noticed that payment has not arrived. These types of messages are known as **dunning messages.** A dunning message is any type of message that makes a request for payment of an account. If a physician decides not to pursue collection of a patient's account, the account should be marked "DO NOT DUN." Dun refers to repetitive action to collect.

Many computer systems can be set up to include dunning messages automatically on statements that are overdue. Messages can differ depending on the age of an account balance. If a physician has decided not to collect a patient's account, an assistant should be very careful to make sure that the patient's statement does not include a dunning message. Even if previous arrangements have been made with the billing department, a patient could become very upset if a message is included. The excuse that "the computer automatically puts it on" is not acceptable and is inappropriate. Although the statements may be computer generated, an assistant is still responsible for making sure the statements are done correctly.

Telephone Collection

Another action that can be used when collecting an account is to try and contact the guarantor by phone. Be-

cause a patient and a guarantor are not always the same person, an assistant should always ask to speak to the individual identified as the guarantor. An assistant must speak to the guarantor and to no one else about an overdue bill.

When collecting over the telephone, an assistant should remember a few basic principles, some of which have foundation in the law.
- Be respectful.
- Do not threaten action that you do not intend to take. That is unlawful.
- Call at a reasonable hour, between 8 AM and 9 PM. Calling outside a reasonable time could constitute harassment.
- Ask the patient to establish a payment schedule; get an agreement on a monthly payment.

Collection Letters

A collection letter (Fig. 10–8) is a formal notice to the patient that an account is overdue. Before a collection letter is sent, dunning messages should be used on a patient's statement, and an attempt should be made to contact the patient by telephone. The content of collection letters should be in keeping with legal and appropriate debt collection practices as mentioned previously. An assistant may want to keep a file of sample letters approved by the physician.

In-Person Collection

If a physician approves, an assistant may speak to a patient during a visit to the medical office. This type of collection practice can be difficult and uncomfortable for both the patient and the assistant and should be done only if privacy can be maintained during the conversation. If a physician does not want collection practices used in the office, the physician may suggest that the assistant simply ask whether a payment could be made on account.

Locating a Missing Guarantor

Occasionally, statements may be returned labeled *addressee unknown* or a guarantor's phone may no longer be in service. If one of these situations occurs, it may still be possible to locate a guarantor.

When searching for a missing guarantor, helpful information may be found in the medical record of any of the patients listed on the guarantor's account. If a patient completes a registration form such as the one pictured in Figure 8–2, information regarding the patient's nearest relative and employer may be given. Remember, you cannot reveal that the guarantor is a debtor and you can use the third party only once for this information; you could, however, ask whether the third party has a new address or telephone number for the guarantor. Also, do not forget to consult a telephone directory service. The guarantor may have a new listing in your local area.

Horizons Healthcare Center
123 Main Ave.
Farmington, ND 58000
(012) 555-4200

December 21, 200x

Mr. Jonathan Martin
1642 West 53rd Avenue
Harvester, MN 55555

Dear Mr. Martin:

I am writing today regarding the status of your account. Your account balance is currently $2,565.32, all of which is over 90 days past due. We have not received a payment on your account within the past 60 days.

Please contact our office immediately to work out a payment plan for your account.

Sincerely,

Taylor Hudson
Office Manager

TH/ma
enclosure

Figure 10–8. A collection letter may be used to collect on an account when other informal methods have not produced a response.

Private Agency Collection and Small Claims Court

On occasion, a physician may wish to use outside means to collect a debt. A patient's account may be sent to an outside collection agency that specializes in debt collection. A drawback to using an outside agency for collection of a patient's account is that the agency may use means to collect the account of which the physician does not approve and of which the physician may not even be aware. Outside collection agencies are often costly, keeping a hefty percentage of the total amount that is collected.

Small claims court collection is also an option for an office that may wish to pursue collection of an account. For a small fee, a claim can be filed with the court. There are limits on what can be collected in small claims court, and the use of this type of collection may not be suitable for a physician.

LEGAL AND ETHICAL ISSUES IN MEDICAL BILLING

Confidentiality

All medical billing information—whether it is a patient's superbill, monthly statement, or insurance claim—is as confidential as information in a patient's medical record. A patient's bill contains information pertaining to when a patient saw a physician as well as to what was done at the visit. A patient's superbill contains information on diagnosis and procedures related to an office visit as well as on the physician who provided treatment. A patient's insurance claim also contains procedure and diagnosis information.

Information from a patient's account should never be given to anyone without the patient's written permission.

An insurance company that calls the office must have the patient's authorization to release information from the patient's medical record that relates to specific charges. This release of information for billing purposes is usually obtained when a patient registers.

Billing Fraud

Fraudulent billing practices can cost consumers, insurance companies, and government agencies substantial amounts of money. **Fraud** in billing refers to knowingly and willfully billing for something that did not occur. Fraudulent billing practices are punishable by law. When billing a patient for services rendered, the medical administrative assistant should be careful and thorough in the completion of all the patient's charges.

Estate Claims

When a patient dies, it is important to determine whether any charges pertaining to the patient are owed. An assistant should review the obituaries in local area newspapers on a daily basis. Sometimes, a physician may notify an assistant of a patient's death; sometimes, a death certificate may arrive at the office for completion by the physician.

On hearing of a patient's death, an assistant should be mindful of the need for the patient's family to grieve but should also remember that the law often dictates how outstanding bills of the deceased are paid. Legal notices, such as the one shown in Figure 10–9, are printed in the newspaper in the county in which the decedent's will is probated. There may be a time limit in which any debtors of the decedent must file claims for payment against the estate. This claim is usually sent to the personal representative of the decedent's estate and is essentially a notice that the decedent owed money.

In the example shown in Figure 10–9, the state of North Dakota allows 4 months in which claims must be filed or they will not be allowed.

When should a bill be sent after a death? A reasonable period of time should elapse between a patient's death and the sending of a statement to the personal representative of the patient's estate. It would be uncaring to have a bill for medical care (especially if a patient died while under a physician's care) arrive within the first few weeks of a patient's death. If possible, an assistant should wait to send a bill until after this period.

A bill should be sent, however. Failing to send a bill after a patient's death may cause family members to question the motives of the physician. They may infer that the physician feels responsible in some way for the patient's death. Therefore, a deceased patient's statements should be sent for payment, but an assistant should avoid sending a statement within the initial period after the death. Laws for collecting from an estate vary from state to state, and it is important for an assistant to be aware of the local time limitations.

IN THE DISTRICT COURT OF WALKER COUNTY
STATE OF NORTH DAKOTA

In the Matter of the Estate of
Louis F. Knox, Deceased

NOTICE TO CREDITORS

NOTICE IS HEREBY GIVEN that the undersigned has been appointed personal representative of the above estate. All persons having claims against the said deceased are requested to present their claims within three months after the date of the first publication of this notice or said claims will be forever barred. Claims must either be presented to Paula Knox, personal representative of the estate, at 2468 Meadowview Road, Farmington, ND 58000, or filed with the Court.

Dated this 3rd day of September, 2001.

Paula A. Knox
Personal Representative
2468 Meadowview Road
Farmington, ND 58000

Lisa M. Howard
Attorney at law
P O Box 952B
Farmington, ND 58000
Attorney for Personal Representative
First publication on the 3rd day of September, 2001.
(September 3, 10, 17, 2001)

Figure 10–9. Legal notices inform creditors when claims for payment must be filed.

Medical Records

If a patient with a past due account requests that his medical records be sent to another physician, can the physician refuse to send the patient's record until the account is paid? The physician cannot refuse, according to the AMA's Council on Ethical and Judicial Affairs. The council states that it is unethical to withhold the release of a patient's medical record because a patient has an outstanding bill. Therefore, regardless of the patient's account balance, a patient's request for release of medical records should be accommodated.

SUMMARY

Many different activities are included in the billing process. Vital information regarding payment of a patient's charges is gathered at the point of registration. After registration, the superbill is generated and is used to document a patient's diagnosis and treatment for billing and insurance purposes. From the superbill, a patient's account is updated and insurance claims are generated. Medical coding uses a widely recognized system of numbers to categorize diagnoses and procedures provided for patients. These codes are used on insurance claim forms to describe diagnoses and procedures.

An assistant may be responsible for a portion of the billing process or may be responsible for the entire billing process in the medical office. Each month, statements are generated for each account. If an account becomes past due, it may be the assistant's responsibility to begin collecting on the account. Procedures used in the collection process should be approved by the physicians in the office and must stay within legal guidelines.

A medical administrative assistant should have a clear understanding of all of the activities involved in billing for medical services. A complete understanding of these components will enable an assistant to serve the patient in the best way possible.

You Are the Medical Administrative Assistant

A guarantor telephones you and begins asking questions regarding the monthly statement from the medical office in which you work. There is a charge of $100 for an office visit and a related laboratory test. The charge is for an office visit for the guarantor's spouse. The guarantor begins to ask questions, wanting to know what kind of test was done and what the diagnosis was for the visit. How do you respond?

Bibliography

American Medical Association: Code of Medical Ethics. Chicago, American Medical Association, 1997.

Buck CJ: Saunders' 2002 ICD-9-CM, volumes 1, 2, & 3 and HCPCS Level II. Philadelphia, WB Saunders, 2002.

Cheeseman HR: Contemporary Business Law. Upper Saddle River, NJ, Prentice Hall, 2000.

Fordney MT: Insurance Handbook for the Medical Office, 7th ed. Philadelphia, WB Saunders, 2001.

Newby C: From Patient to Payment: Insurance Procedures for the Medical Office, 2nd ed. Westerville, Ohio, Glencoe/McGraw-Hill, 1998.

Internet Resources

American Academy of Professional Coders.
Current Procedural Terminology.
Federal Trade Commission.
HCFA Common Procedure Coding System.
Health Insurance Association of America.
International Classification of Disease.

Exercise 10–1 TRUE OR FALSE

Read each statement and determine whether the statement is true or false. Record the answer in the blank provided. T = true; F = false.

_____ 1. A patient's registration information is verified at each office visit to ensure that the correct information is available for billing and insurance purposes.

_____ 2. Registration forms should not be mailed to new patients ahead of time.

_____ 3. Registration mistakes can be costly.

_____ 4. Control copies for superbills are used to ensure that all bills are accounted for.

_____ 5. Computer-generated superbills can be specialized for each physician.

_____ 6. When a patient inquires about the cost of a physician's services, the patient should be given an exact quote.

_____ 7. Delayed billing practices reflect poorly on a medical office as a whole.

_____ 8. If a medical administrative assistant is not responsible for generating patients' bills, it is not important for the assistant to know the components of the billing process.

_____ 9. A patient may be charged for only one procedure per office visit.

_____ 10. If a computer system is used for billing in the medical office, all information for the patient should be listed on the superbill.

_____ 11. An assistant should discourage any discussion of fees for medical services.

_____ 12. In the case of a child with divorced parents, the bill should always be sent to the patient's father.

_____ 13. If a patient has been notified in advance of charges for missed appointments, it is ethical to bill a patient for a missed appointment.

_____ 14. Most physicians will charge patients for a missed appointment.

_____ 15. It is generally preferred that patients assign their insurance benefits to a medical office.

_____ 16. If a patient does not assign insurance benefits to a medical office, payment to the office may be delayed.

_____ 17. A medical office establishes a fee for each service when the service is performed.

_____ 18. Some insurance programs have maximum amounts that are allowed to be charged for medical services.

_____ 19. Charges for medical services are the same across the country.

_____ 20. The CPT coding system assigns a numerical code to every procedure performed in the medical office.

_____ 21. A patient's medical record serves as documentation for procedures charged to the patient.

_____ 22. Coding is used for insurance billings in hospitals and physicians' offices.

_____ 23. The larger the practice, the more likely cycle billing should be used when billing patients.

_____ 24. A patient's physician should always be consulted before collection activity is taken on the patient's account.

_____ 25. Physicians should establish collection guidelines for the medical office.

_____ 26. Collection procedures used by an assistant will affect an office's reputation.

_____ 27. A superbill contains a summary of charges and payments on a patient's account.

_____ 28. Cycle billing means a patient's statement is sent out every other month.

Exercise 10–2 CHAPTER CONCEPTS

Read the statement or question and determine the answer that best fits the statement or question. Record the answer in the blank provided.

_____ 1. Which of the following is not necessary registration information when a patient visits a medical office for an appointment?

(a) Guarantor for the patient's account

(b) Patient's date of birth

(c) Patient's previous address

(d) Patient's employer

(e) Patient's insurance information

_____ 2. Which of the following is true about the billing process?
   (a) After completion, superbills should be placed in the patient's chart and the chart returned to the records room.
   (b) Patients should be asked to return their superbills to the front desk.
   (c) The nurse is responsible for recording a patient's procedure and diagnosis on the superbill.
   (d) Superbills should be collected in a specific location and returned to the front office at the end of each day.

_____ 3. Which of the following is true about billing for a missed appointment?
   (a) Patients should always be charged for missed appointments.
   (b) The AMA has notified physicians that it is illegal to charge for missed appointments.
   (c) A medical office should establish a policy for charges for missed appointments.
   (d) A physician who has only a few patients scheduled every day will probably not notice a missed appointment in the schedule.

_____ 4. When coding a patient's diagnosis, the first volume you should consult is
   (a) Volume I
   (b) Volume II
   (c) Volume III
   (d) Volume IV

_____ 5. "ICD" as in ICD-9-CM stands for
   (a) Information on Clinical Disorders
   (b) International Classification of Disease
   (c) Internal Coding of Diagnosis
   (d) International Coding of Disorders

_____ 6. The volume of the ICD-9-CM manual that is listed in numerical order is
   (a) Volume I
   (b) Volume II
   (c) Volume III
   (d) Volume IV

_____ 7. To obtain credit, a patient's marital status may be asked if
   (a) The patient is younger than 25 years of age.
   (b) The income of the patient's spouse will be used to obtain credit.
   (c) The patient is female.
   (d) The patient is covered by Medicare.

_____ 8. A patient can be refused credit if
   (a) Part of the patient's income is from public assistance.
   (b) The patient is younger than 21 years.
   (c) The patient is not a natural born citizen of the United States.
   (d) The patient is unable to pay because of insufficient income.

_____ 9. The first method used to attempt to collect a debt might be
   (a) Calling the guarantor at work.
   (b) Writing a letter to the guarantor.
   (c) Adding a dunning message to the guarantor's statement
   (d) Asking the patient in person for a payment.

_____ 10. Which of the following is true when billing a patient's estate?
   (a) The patient's bill should be sent immediately after the patient's death.
   (b) If the patient died while under the doctor's care, a bill should not be sent.
   (c) The bill should be sent to the patient's personal representative.
   (d) There is no time limit in which a patient's bill must be sent.

Exercise 10–3 PROCEDURE CODING

Using the correct edition of the CPT manual, identify the section of the CPT manual in which the following codes are located. Record the answer in the blank provided.

(a) Anesthesia   (c) Radiology   (e) Medicine
(b) Surgery   (d) Pathology and laboratory   (f) Evaluation and management

_____ 1. 80050   _____ 5. 71020   _____ 8. 73721

_____ 2. 29819   _____ 6. 01382   _____ 9. 80100

_____ 3. 99301   _____ 7. 99213   _____ 10. 90636

_____ 4. 93000

Identify the correct CPT code for the following professional services using the steps given in Procedure Box 10–1. Underline the main term found in the index and record the answer in the blank provided.

_____ 11. Emergency department visit, detailed history, and physical examination

_____ 12. Tubal ligation

_____ 13. Removal of 10 skin tags

_____ 14. Chest x-ray, complete, four views

_____ 15. I&D foot bursa

_____ 16. Excision of thyroid gland due to a malignant lesion

_____ 17. Repair of a strangulated umbilical hernia; patient is 3 years old.

_____ 18. Office visit, established patient, comprehensive history, and physical examination

_____ 19. Total bilirubin

_____ 20. Obstetric panel

_____ 21. Prothrombin time

_____ 22. Simple excision of nasal polyp

_____ 23. Routine obstetric care with antepartum and postpartum care with a vaginal delivery

_____ 24. Repair of three superficial lacerations (wounds) of the cheek—1 cm, 2 cm, 3 cm

_____ 25. Uncomplicated treatment of three rib fractures

Exercise 10–4 DIAGNOSIS CODING

Using a current edition of the ICD-9-CM manual, locate the diagnosis codes for the following diagnoses using the steps given in Procedure Box 10–2. Underline the main term found in the index and record the correct answers in the blanks provided.

_____ 1. Menometrorrhagia

_____ 2. Pharyngitis

_____ 3. Upper respiratory infection

_____ 4. Closed fracture of three ribs

_____ 5. Dupuytren's contracture

_____ 6. Carpal tunnel syndrome

_____ 7. Psoriasis

_____ 8. Physical examination for participation in sports competition

_____ 9. Localized atopic eczema

_____ 10. Varicose veins

_____ 11. Loose body in right knee

_____ 12. Benign hypertension

_____ 13. Partially torn medial meniscus

_____ 14. Morton's neuroma

_____ 15. Chronic cholecystitis with cholelithiasis

Exercise 10–5 COLLECTION PRACTICES

Read the following statements and determine whether the statement is good or bad practice when collecting a debt. Record your answers in the blanks provided. A = good practice; B = bad practice.

_____ 1. Consult with a physician regarding a patient's account status.

_____ 2. Contact a debtor at a public event.

_____ 3. Threaten a debtor.

_____ 4. Be polite.

_____ 5. Speak harshly.

_____ 6. Use foul language.

_____ 7. Call the debtor repeatedly in the middle of the night until a payment is received.

_____ 8. Call the debtor a "deadbeat."

_____ 9. Only speak to the guarantor about the debt.

_____ 10. Send the guarantor a letter explaining what charges are owed.

_____ 11. Talk about the debt to whomever answers the guarantor's phone.

_____ 12. If all else fails, turn the account over to a collection agency.

_____ 13. Ask the patient to commit to a monthly payment.

_____ 14. Refuse to release a patient's medical records until the patient's account is paid in full.

_____ 15. Call a guarantor's employer when the guarantor is not allowed to receive calls at work.

Exercise 10–6 MEDICAL BILLING—Pegboard

Using the patients listed in Activity 10–4, record the transactions for each encounter using a pegboard system. Use a fee schedule provided by your instructor.

10
ACTIVITIES

ACTIVITY 10–1 In your local newspaper, search for an example of a legal notice of estate claims similar to the one shown in Figure 10–9.

ACTIVITY 10–2 Draft a collection letter. Follow the guidelines for collection printed in this chapter as well as the guidelines for proper letter format given in Chapter 6.

ACTIVITY 10–3 Consider the following situations. What is the appropriate response to the situation given?

1. A patient telephones the office and asks how much a physical examination costs. What do you say?
2. A patient's account has a balance of $500 that is 120 days past due. No payment has ever been made toward the balance. Reminders and letters to the patient have produced no response. You must now phone the patient to attempt collection. What do you say?

ACTIVITY 10–4 *MEDICAL BILLING—computerized*

Using the Lytec Medical 2001 software provided with this text, process the charges for the patients listed.

To begin billing using Lytec Medical 2001

1. Open Lytec Medical 2001. At the main menu, click *Horizons Healthcare Center*. (Once the Horizons Healthcare Center practice is open, the practice name will appear on the title bar at the top of the window. You will also notice that the main menu selections have now expanded.)

2. On the main menu, click *billing;* then click *charges and payments.* The billing window will open.

3. View patients by clicking the *lookup* button (magnifying glass) on the right side of the chart box.

4. Find the patient to be billed on the patient list, highlight the patient's name, and click *OK.*

5. The charges and payments window for the selected patient will be displayed. Enter the following information for the patient's encounter in the identified boxes. (To move from field to field in this window, simply press the *Enter* key.)
   (a) *Billing number.* Accept the default number that appears in the box. (This box could also be used to record a superbill control number.)
   (b) *Provider number.* The provider recorded under the patient's registration information will appear in this box.
   (c) *Created.* Enter the visit date for the billing date.

(d) *Co-pay.* If the patient pays a co-payment with each office visit and the co-payment was entered in the patient's registration information, a co-payment will appear in this box. If a co-payment applies, a co-payment can also be entered manually. Accept the co-payment that appears for each patient.

(e) *Authorization.* If authorization from the patient's insurance company is required for the encounter with the physician, information will be entered in this box.

(f) Under the *bill to* portion of the window, a check mark should appear in the checkbox if the patient should receive a bill and the patient's insurance company should receive a claim form. If it does not appear, place a check in the *patient checkbox.* (If a check is not placed in the *patient checkbox,* the patient's charges will not appear on a monthly statement.) If an insurance company name appears on the primary insurance field, a check should be placed in the checkbox pertaining to that insurance. (To have the checkmark appear automatically in the charges and payments window, check the patient's registration data and be sure a checkmark appears in the *bill patient automatically* box.)

(g) Under *detail items,* enter the following information (pressing the *Enter* key after information is entered will advance the cursor to the next box):

I. *Print.* A check should appear in the *print checkbox.* This will print the transaction item on the patient's insurance claim.

II. *Payment.* When a payment is received on the patient's account, the payment may be applied to a specific item on the patient's account. If so, this field will be checked.

III. *Date from.* The current date appears in this box. Change the date to the patient's date of service.

IV. *Date to.* If a patient's charges apply to more than one day, the ending date should be entered in this box. Otherwise, leave the box blank.

V. *Provider.* The patient's assigned provider appears in this box. If the patient was seen by another provider, the provider can be selected by clicking the *lookup* button.

VI. *Diagnosis code.* Select a diagnosis code by clicking the *lookup* button. If the diagnosis code is not listed, it may be manually entered or it may be added to the master list when the *lookup* button is clicked.

VII. *Procedure code.* Select a procedure code by clicking the *lookup* button. If the procedure code is not listed, it may be manually entered or it may be added to the master list when the *lookup* button is clicked.

VIII. *Mod.* If a modifier applies to the procedure code listed, a two-digit modifier is entered in this box.

IX. *Amount.* If a fee schedule has been assigned to the patient, the cost of the procedure will automatically appear in the amount box. An amount can be entered to override any automatic charge.

X. *Units.* Enter the amount of times the procedure was done. The usual entry is 1.

XI. *Extended.* The number of units is multiplied by the amount to arrive at the extended amount. Once the *Enter* key is pressed after units, another line for billing will appear. If the patient has additional procedures to be entered, those procedures would be entered on the next line.

XII. After all of the information for a patient's bill has been entered, click the *Save* button at the bottom of the window. A new billing screen will be displayed, and information for another patient may be entered (start with number 3 listed earlier). When all bills have been entered, click *close* at the bottom of the window.

If a mistake is made after a line has been entered under detail items, click the line and choose *detail* at the bottom of the billing window. The *delete* option will delete the line currently in use. The *add* option will add a new blank line to the detail items portion of the billing window.

Process the following charges relating to the appointments entered in Chapter 7.

- Charges should be recorded under patient's regular provider.
- Locate the correct CPT and ICD-9 code(s) for each patient's encounter.

Date of Service	Patient	Diagnosis	Procedure(s)
10-7-02	Kirsten French	Sinusitis	Office visit, prob. focused
10-10-02	Timothy O'Malley	Benign lesion, arm	Excision of 1 benign lesion, 1.0 cm
10-8-02	Marge Armstrong	Internal hemorrhoids	Flexible sigmoidoscopy
10-7-02	Deanne Olson	Sinus infection	Office visit, prob. focused
10-9-02	Margaret Stein	DJD Physical examination	Preventative med px
10-8-02	Evan Stevens	Otitis media, acute	Office visit, prob. focused
10-7-02	Alice Shepard	UTI	Office visit, prob. focused Urinalysis (dip only)
10-7-02	Ann Walker	HA	Office visit, exp. prob. focused
10-7-02	Jose Garcia	FB eye Slit lamp examination to remove foreign body from the cornea	Office visit, prob. focused
10-11-02	Amy Gordon	Tinnitus	Office visit, prob. focused Screening test, hearing
10-9-02	Adam St. Michael	Ingrown toenail	Office visit, prob. focused I&D of paronychia
10-7-02	Tara Olson	Conjunctivitis	Office visit, prob. focused
10-9-02	Susan Pearson	Genital warts	Office visit, prob. focused
10-9-02	Christian Olsen	Hypertension Physical examination	Preventative med px
10-10-02	Tamara Garcia	Menometrorrhagia	Office visit, prob. focused
10-7-02	Inez Brenner	Pharyngitis	Office visit, prob. focused
10-8-02	Mark McLean	Urticaria	Office visit, prob. focused
10-7-02	Jeanne Breckman	Abdominal distention	Office visit, exp. prob. focused X-ray, abdomen, 1 view, AP

ACTIVITY 10–5 *STATEMENT MESSAGES—computerized*

Using the Lytec Medical 2001 software provided with this text, enter messages to be printed on each patient's statement.

To enter statement messages using Lytec Medical 2001

1. Open Lytec Medical 2001. At the main menu, click *Horizons Healthcare Center*. (Once the Horizons Healthcare Center practice is open, the practice name will appear on the title bar at the top of the window. You will also notice that the main menu selections have now expanded.)

2. On the main menu, click *settings*, then click *statement messages*. The statement messages window will open.

3. Enter messages to be printed on patients' statements by entering the following information on the appropriate lines:
Standard message: Thank you for your continued patronage.
Past Due 31–60 days: Please pay your account promptly.
Past Due 61–90 days: Your account is past due.
Past Due 91–120 days: Finance charges are assessed on balances over 90 days past due.
Past Due > 120 days: Please contact our credit office to arrange a payment schedule.
Patient Co–Pay: (Leave blank).
Not Covered by Insurance: We appreciate prompt payment of your account.

4. Click *OK* to add the changes to the statement messages.

ACTIVITY 10–6 *MEDICAL STATEMENTS—computerized*

Using the Lytec Medical 2001 software provided with this text, generate statements for October 2002.

To begin printing account statements using Lytec Medical 2001

1. Open Lytec Medical 2001. At the main menu, click *Horizons Healthcare Center*. (Once the Horizons Healthcare Center practice is open, the practice name will appear on the title bar at the top of the window. You will also notice that the main menu selections have expanded.)

2. On the main menu, click *billing;* then click *print statements.* The select custom form window will open. Choose *Standard statement with notes,* then click *open.* The print statements window will open.

3. Specify the following options for printing statements:
   Under the options tab
   Statement date: 10-31-02
   Statement messages: Standard and Dunning
   Sort Patients by: Name
   Place a check before *combine family members* and *balance forward format.*
   Minimum Patient Balance: $0.00
   Include Paid Billings: Current Month Only
   Under the range tab
   Providers: Print statements for all providers at Horizons Healthcare by clicking the *lookup* button and choosing the first provider (Dr. Marks) on the provider list and the last provider (Dr. Sanchez) on the provider list.

4. Click *Preview* to view the statements to be printed. Click the forward arrow to view each statement. Statements should appear for all patients entered in Exercise 10–6. (If they do not appear, check to make sure a checkmark is placed after patient in the *bill to* portion of the billing window.)

5. Print the statements by clicking the printer icon in the preview window.

10
DISCUSSION

The following topics can be used for class discussion or for individual student essay.

DISCUSSION 10–1 Read the quotation at the beginning of the chapter. What is the significance of this quotation?

DISCUSSION 10–2 Obtain a copy of a superbill from a medical office in your area. Discuss the following questions:

- What information is included on the superbill?
- Is the term *superbill* used by the medical office from which you obtained the form?
- How does this form compare with the superbills shown in Figures 10–1 and 10–2?

DISCUSSION 10–3 Is a patient's medical billing information as confidential as his or her medical record? Why?

DISCUSSION 10–4 Identify methods of tracking a guarantor who has moved and left no forwarding address.

CHAPTER OUTLINE

INSURANCE TERMINOLOGY

CENTERS FOR MEDICARE AND MEDICAID SERVICES
HCFA-1500 Claim Form
Preparing the HCFA-1500
Life Cycle of a Claim
Coordination of Benefits
Troubleshooting Claims
Timelines for Filing

TYPES OF INSURANCE PLANS
Fee-for-Service
Health Maintenance Organizations
Preferred Provider Organizations

GOVERNMENT PROGRAMS
Medicare
Medicaid
TRICARE
CHAMPVA
Workers' Compensation

PRIVATE HEALTH INSURANCE
Insurance Coverage
Blue Cross/Blue Shield
Disability Insurance
Long-Term Care Insurance

INSURANCE RESOURCES

CURRENT TOPICS IN HEALTH INSURANCE
Insurance Fraud and Abuse
Confidentiality
COBRA
Insurance Industry Statistics

SUMMARY

LEARNING OUTCOMES

On successful completion of this chapter, the student will be able to

1. Apply health insurance and benefits terminology.
2. Explain the components of an Explanation of Benefits (EOB) statement.
3. Complete an HCFA-1500 form.
4. Describe the life cycle of an insurance claim.
5. Identify reasons claims are denied.
6. Describe Blue Cross/Blue Shield coverage.
7. Describe group insurance coverage.
8. Describe Medicare eligibility and coverage.
9. Describe Medicaid eligibility and coverage.
10. Describe CHAMPUS/CHAMPVA eligibility and coverage.
11. Describe workers' compensation eligibility and coverage.
12. Describe short-term and long-term disability coverage.
13. Describe managed care policies.

CMA COMPETENCIES

1. Apply managed care policies and procedures.
2. Apply third-party guidelines.
3. Obtain managed care referrals and precertifications.
4. Complete insurance forms.
5. Identify and respond to issues of confidentiality.
6. Perform within legal and ethical boundaries.
7. Use computer software to maintain office systems.

RMA COMPETENCIES

1. Assist patients with insurance inquiries.
2. Know medical office terminology associated with health and accident insurance.
3. Know the major types of medical insurance programs encountered in the medical office, including government-sponsored, group, individual, and workers' compensation programs.
4. Complete and file forms for insurance claims.
5. Evaluate claims rejection.
6. Know billing requirements for insurance programs.
7. Use computer for billing and financial transactions.
8. Recognize legal responsibilities of the medical assistant.

VOCABULARY

assignment
beneficiary
birthday rule
capitation
claim
co-insurance
coordination of benefits (COB)
co-payment
deductible
explanation of benefits (EOB)
fee-for-service
fiscal intermediary
group insurance
group number
health maintenance organization
insurance contract
insured
insurer
managed care

HEALTH INSURANCE

We know that what happens in adolescence, in the teenage years, and in the young adult years often determines a person's quality of life later on.

—*David Satcher, MD, PhD, Surgeon General of the United States*

VOCABULARY (*Continued*)
participating provider (PAR)
policy
policyholder
precertifications
preferred provider organization (PPO)
premium
referral
subscriber
usual, customary, and reasonable (UCR) fee
workers' compensation

Note: Because health insurance regulations are continually updated and can change frequently, a medical administrative assistant should obtain insurance claim processing information directly from a specific insurance plan. This chapter is intended to be a guide to the types of issues that may arise when assisting patients with health insurance questions and claims processing. Information received directly from insurance plans is the definitive source of information about the insurance plan's benefits.

Today, many patients seeking health care have some type of coverage that will pay a portion or even all of their health care costs. For these patients, preparation of a statement summarizing charges is not sufficient: many individuals will need insurance claims filed to receive those benefits. Knowledge of medical insurance procedures is an integral part of the patient billing process. Medical office personnel spend many hours filing and collecting health benefits as a customer service for their patients. Claims for medical insurance benefits must be filed accurately and promptly to allow patients to collect their benefits in a timely manner.

INSURANCE TERMINOLOGY

When studying the various types of health insurance coverage and benefits, a medical administrative assistant must have a firm grasp of the specific language used in the health insurance industry.

An **insurance contract** or **policy** is an agreement between an insurance company, otherwise known as an **insurer,** and an individual or group of individuals. The insurance company agrees to provide payment for certain health care services in exchange for a monetary payment by the individual or group. A policy specifies what types of health care treatment are covered as well as the amounts that are payable.

The payment required for insurance coverage is known as a **premium.** A premium may be paid by an employer or an individual, or perhaps both may share the payment of the premium. Premiums may be paid on a monthly basis, or the parties may agree to another arrangement. In exchange for a paid premium, an insurance company agrees to provide insurance coverage pursuant to the terms of the contract or policy.

The terms **policyholder, insured,** and **subscriber** are synonymous and refer to the individual who holds the insurance policy. For instance, if one of the two working parents in a family of four has an insurance policy through an employer, that parent is known as the policyholder (or insured or subscriber). A **beneficiary** is an individual, such as the subscriber's spouse or dependent, who qualifies for benefits under that subscriber's policy.

In addition to paying any required premium, a policyholder may sometimes have to pay an additional cost, known as a **co-payment,** for health care services. A co-payment may need to be paid by a patient (or insured) each time the patient has a visit with a health care provider. A co-payment is a set amount (e.g., $10 or $15) that must be paid by a patient or policyholder for each encounter, regardless of the cost of the visit.

Consider the following examples: (1) Patient A's policy requires a $10 co-payment. The patient sees a physician for a sore throat and a "strep" screen for a total visit cost of $64. The patient must pay a $10 co-payment. (2) Patient B's policy also requires a $10 co-payment. The patient sees a physician for a complete physical examination, and diagnostic tests totaling more than $1500. Patient B also pays a $10 co-payment.

The co-payment does not change according to the amount of charges for a visit. Co-payments help hold down costs for the insurer, because a portion of every visit must be paid by a patient or insured, and the patient may think twice about seeing a physician for minor ailments.

Usually, when an insured patient receives services from a health care provider, a medical office files a **claim** to collect benefits from the patient's insurance company. A claim refers to any request to an insurance company or government insurance program for benefits on behalf of the insured. To collect insurance benefits, most medical offices file claims on behalf of their patients.

A **co-insurance** clause in an insurance contract greatly affects the amount the patient may need to pay for treatment. Co-insurance is a percentage of the claim required to be paid by the patient. In the previous example, if patients A and B both had a 20% co-insurance clause, patient B would pay far more for the visit than would patient A. This is because the total amount for patient B's visit is significantly higher than patient A's total amount. Policies may have co-payments, co-insurance, or both.

A **deductible** also affects the amount a patient must ultimately pay for medical services. A deductible is a specific amount that a patient must pay for health care services per year before insurance benefits will be paid. Deductibles are amounts that are larger than co-payments, for example, $100, $200, or $500. A policy may set a maximum deductible per patient as well as for an entire family.

For example, a policy's deductible may be $200 per family member or $500 for the entire family per year. If the policy covers a family of three, the first $200 of services for family member 1 and family member 2 will be applied toward the deductible. Only the first $100 of expenses for family member 3 will be applied toward the deductible because the maximum family deductible would be met. Likewise, if family member 1 incurred $50 more in expenses, those expenses would not be applied toward the deductible because the $200 limit would be met for the year.

Deductibles are usually applicable for charges from January 1 to December 31 of each year. Also, deductibles apply only to services that are covered under the terms of the insurance policy. Services not covered under an insurance policy are paid solely by the patient (or guarantor) and do not apply toward any deductible.

CENTERS FOR MEDICARE AND MEDICAID SERVICES

The Centers for Medicare and Medicaid Services (CMS), formerly known as the Health Care Financing Administration (HCFA), is an agency of the federal government. CMS manages the Medicare, Medicaid, and Children's Health Insurance Program and spends more than $360 billion per year on health care benefits. CMS's responsibilities include the following:

● Overseeing the operations of the state agencies and contractors that carry out the functions of CMS.
● Evaluating the quality of health care services.
● Studying the effectiveness of matters relating to health care services.
● Setting policy for payment for health care services.

HCFA-1500 Claim Form

Most medical office claims are filed on a standard claim form called the HCFA-1500 (Fig. 11–1). The HCFA-1500 was developed by HCFA for the purpose of standardizing the submission of claims sent in for payment of government benefits. It was gradually adopted for use by other insurance companies. The use of this standard form has helped to streamline claims submission for medical offices and claims processing for insurance companies. Table 11–1 lists HCFA guidelines for step-by-step completion of the HCFA-1500 for Medicare claims. Other insurance programs and private insurance companies such as Blue Cross/Blue Shield usually have their own specific requirements for completion of the HCFA-1500.

Table 11–1. Guidelines for Filing Insurance Claims*

Item Number	Patient Information
†1	Check the box that pertains to the insurance plan for the claim being filed.
	Blue Cross/Blue Shield—check the group health plan box.
	TRICARE—Enter name of military sponsor.
	Workers' Compensation—Use patient's social security number (SSN).
†1a	Enter the insured's policy identification (ID) number. This usually (but not always) is the insured's SSN.
	Workers' Compensation—enter the claim number.
†2	Enter the patient's last name, first name, and middle initial as shown on insurance card.
†3	Enter the patient's birth date using eight digits (MMDDYYYY) and identify patient's sex (M or F).
4	Enter the name of the insured. If the same as item 2, enter **SAME.**
	TRICARE—Enter name of military sponsor.
	Workers' Compensation—Enter name of patient's employer.
†5	Enter the patient's address and telephone number as identified on the form.
†6	Identify the relationship of the patient to the insured.
7	If #4 is completed, enter the insured's address and telephone number. If this information is the same as item 5, enter the word SAME.
8	Check the patient's marital status and employment and student status as they apply.
9	If the patient is covered by a secondary insurance policy, enter the policyholder's name of the secondary policy. If the information is the same, enter SAME.
9a	Enter policy number of secondary payer.
	Medicare—If Medicare is secondary, enter patient's ID number.
	Medigap—Enter **MEDIGAP, MGP,** or **MGAP** followed by the Medigap policy number.
9b	Enter the birth date (MM/DD/YYYY) and sex (M or F) of the secondary policyholder.
9c	If a secondary policy is from an employer, enter the employer's name. If the patient is a student but is also employed, enter patient's school name.
	Medicaid—Leave blank.
	Medicare—Leave blank.
	Medigap—Enter claims processing address from patient's Medigap card.
9d	Enter the name of the secondary insurance plan.
	Medigap—Enter the nine-digit payer ID of the Medigap insurer. If the payer ID is not available, enter the Medigap plan name.
†10a-c	Check the appropriate boxes "yes" or "no" as to whether this claim is a result of an employment, auto or other accident. Yes or no must be checked for each question.
10d	If the patient is covered by Medicaid, enter **MCD** followed by the patient's Medicaid number.
11	List the insured's group number in this box. If there is no group number, enter the insured's policy number.
	Medicare—If Medicare is the primary insurance, enter **NONE** and go to item 12.
	Workers' Compensation—Enter policy or group number of employer's workers' compensation plan.

(Continued)

Table 11–1. Guidelines for Filing Insurance Claims* *Continued*

Item Number

Patient Information

11a	Enter the insured's birth date (MM/DD/YYYY) and identify insured's sex (M or F) if insured is not the patient.
11b	Enter insured's employer's name, if policy was issued through the employer. *Medicare*—Leave blank. *Workers' Compensation*—Leave blank.
11c	Enter the plan name.
11d	Enter "yes" when a secondary insurance will be billed, then complete box 9 in its entirety. Enter "no" if no other plans. *Workers' Compensation*—Enter no.
12	The patient or authorized representative must sign and date this section of the form to authorize release of medical information to process the claim. This item also authorizes payment of Medicare benefits to the health care facility that accepts assignment. The notation "signature on file" (SOF) may be entered in this blank if the patient has signed a previous authorization and that authorization is kept on file at the facility.
13	The patient's signature or the notation of signature on file in this blank authorizes a health care facility to receive payments of insurance benefits from the patient's insurance company.

Provider Information

14	Enter an eight-digit date of current illness, injury or pregnancy. This field is required for treatment related to injury or pregnancy. Date of injury (DOI) must be entered if patient was injured.
15	Usually not required by most insurance plans.
16	*Workers' Compensation*—If patient is employed and unable to work due to a work-related injury, enter the dates patient is unable to work.
17	Enter the name of referring physician if applicable. *Managed care plans*—This field may be required if an authorization is required.
17a	*Managed care plans*—Use the payer ID number. *Medicare*—Enter the National Provider Identifier (NPI) of the provider listed in line 17.
18	Enter eight-digit date if medical services done pertain to a hospitalization.
19	Required only in special circumstances outlined in HCFA guidelines.
20	If outside laboratory tests were performed, the laboratory will bill the physician and the physician will bill insurance. If so, "yes" must be checked. *Medicare*—If yes is checked, enter purchase price under charges and complete information in item 32.
†21	Identify the ICD-9 codes related to the patient's diagnosis(es). Primary and secondary codes should be listed under item 1 and item 2, respectively. *Medicare*—If yes is checked in block 10 a, b, or c, an E code describing the injury is required.
22	*Medicaid*—Enter resubmission code and original reference number.
23	If applicable, enter a prior authorization number.
24	Up to six different items may be billed per claim. When a number of identical services are performed, enter on one line and enter number of days or units in 24g.
†24a	Enter eight-digit dates of service. When "from" and "to" dates are used, enter the number of days or units in 24g.
†24b	Enter the place of service code (see Box 11–1).
24c	May be required by some insurance plans, not required by Medicare. Use of a type of service code recognized by the insurance plan may provide further explanation of a procedure and may help prevent a claim denial.
†24d	Identify the procedure codes using the HCFA Common Procedure Coding System (HCPCS).
†24e	Reference the diagnosis code (1, 2, 3, or 4) in item 21 that applies to each procedure listed. Enter only one diagnosis code per line.
†24f	Enter the charge for each procedure.
†24g	Enter the number of times the procedure was performed or delivered. Some supplies list the quantity of supply delivered.
24h	*Medicaid*—This field is used if services are provided under EPSDT (Early Periodic Screening and Diagnostic Testing), a Medicaid program.
24i	Mark this field (usually an X is used) if service provided was an emergency.
24j-k	J-Check if coordination of benefits (COB) applies. K-Enter UPIN of physician (if group practice).
†25	Enter the Employer Identification number (EIN—federal tax ID) or SSN of the provider.
†26	Enter the patient's account number assigned by the provider.
27	*Medicare and TRICARE*—Check the appropriate box to identify whether the provider accepts assignment for Medicare benefits. If "yes" is entered, the provider agrees to accept payment from payer along with any co-payment and deductible as payment in full.
†28	Enter the total of charges listed in 24f, lines 1–6.
29	Enter the amount paid by the patient on charges related to this claim.
30	Subtract line 29 from line 28. *Medicare*—This field may be left blank.
†31	Enter the signature of the provider and date form was signed. Electronic signatures are acceptable.
32	If services were provided in a place other than the patient's home or the physician's office, identify the location where the services were performed.
†33	Enter the provider's billing name, address, and telephone number along with the NPI if the provider is not a member of a group practice.

*When completing the HCFA-1500 form, follow these basic instructions if no specific instructions are available from the insurance plan. Special instructions for certain insurance plans are included where applicable. A † denotes that the item number *must* be completed.

PLEASE
DO NOT
STAPLE
IN THIS
AREA

APPROVED OMB-0938-008

CARRIER

| | PICA | | **HEALTH INSURANCE CLAIM FORM** | PICA | | |

1. MEDICARE ☒ (Medicare #) MEDICAID ☐ (Medicaid #) CHAMPUS ☐ (Sponsor's SSN) CHAMPVA ☐ (VA File #) GROUP HEALTH PLAN ☐ (SSN or ID) FECA BLK LUNG ☐ (SSN) OTHER ☐ (ID)

1a. INSURED'S I.D. NUMBER 123XX6890B (FOR PROGRAM IN ITEM 1)

2. PATIENT'S NAME (Last Name, First Name, Middle Initial)
ARMSTRONG MARGE H

3. PATIENT'S BIRTH DATE MM 12 DD 20 YY 1922 SEX M ☐ F ☒

4. INSURED'S NAME (Last Name, First Name, Middle Initial)

5. PATIENT'S ADDRESS 732 SUNSET LANE

6. PATIENT RELATIONSHIP TO INSURED Self ☐ Spouse ☐ Child ☐ Other ☐

7. INSURED'S ADDRESS (No., Street)

CITY HARVESTER STATE MN

8. PATIENT STATUS Single ☐ Married ☐ Other ☐ Employed ☐ Full-Time Student ☐ Part-Time Student ☐

CITY STATE

ZIP CODE 55555 TELEPHONE (Include Area Code) (010) 555-2645

ZIP CODE TELEPHONE (Include Area Code) ( )

9. OTHER INSURED'S NAME (Last Name, First Name, Middle Initial)

10. IS PATIENT'S CONDITION RELATED TO:

11. INSURED'S POLICY GROUP OR FECA NUMBER NONE

a. OTHER INSURED'S POLICY OR GROUP NUMBER

a. EMPLOYMENT? (CURRENT OR PREVIOUS) YES ☐ NO ☐

a. INSURED'S DATE OF BIRTH MM DD YY SEX M ☐ F ☐

b. OTHER INSURED'S DATE OF BIRTH MM DD YY SEX M ☐ F ☐

b. AUTO ACCIDENT? PLACE (State) YES ☐ NO ☐

b. EMPLOYER'S NAME OR SCHOOL NAME

c. EMPLOYER'S NAME OR SCHOOL NAME

c. OTHER ACCIDENT? YES ☐ NO ☐

c. INSURANCE PLAN NAME OR PROGRAM NAME

d. INSURANCE PLAN NAME OR PROGRAM NAME

10d. RESERVED FOR LOCAL USE

d. IS THERE ANOTHER HEALTH BENEFIT PLAN? YES ☐ NO ☒ *If yes,* return to and complete item 9 a-d.

READ BACK OF FORM BEFORE COMPLETING & SIGNING THIS FORM.
12. PATIENT'S OR AUTHORIZED PERSON'S SIGNATURE I authorize the release of any medical or other information necessary to process this claim. I also request payment of government benefits either to myself or to the party who accepts assignment below.
SIGNED SOF DATE 12 22 2001

13. INSURED'S OR AUTHORIZED PERSON'S SIGNATURE I authorize payment of medical benefits to the undersigned physician or supplier for services described below.
SIGNED SOF

PATIENT AND INSURED INFORMATION

14. DATE OF CURRENT: ILLNESS (First symptom) OR INJURY (Accident) OR PREGNANCY (LMP) MM DD YY

15. IF PATIENT HAS HAD SAME OR SIMILAR ILLNESS. GIVE FIRST DATE MM DD YY

16. DATES PATIENT UNABLE TO WORK IN CURRENT OCCUPATION FROM MM DD YY TO MM DD YY

17. NAME OF REFERRING PHYSICIAN OR OTHER SOURCE

17a. I.D. NUMBER OF REFERRING PHYSICIAN

18. HOSPITALIZATION DATES RELATED TO CURRENT SERVICES FROM MM DD YY TO MM DD YY

19. RESERVED FOR LOCAL USE

20. OUTSIDE LAB? YES ☐ NO ☒ $ CHARGES

21. DIAGNOSIS OR NATURE OF ILLNESS OR INJURY. (RELATE ITEMS 1,2,3 OR 4 TO ITEM 24E BY LINE)
1. 715 04   3.
2.   4.

22. MEDICAID RESUBMISSION CODE ORIGINAL REF. NO.

23. PRIOR AUTHORIZATION NUMBER

24. A DATE(S) OF SERVICE From MM DD YY To MM DD YY	B Place of Service	C Type of Service	D PROCEDURES, SERVICES, OR SUPPLIES (Explain Unusual Circumstances) CPT/HCPCS MODIFIER	E DIAGNOSIS CODE	F $ CHARGES	G DAYS OR UNITS	H EPSDT Family Plan	I EMG	J COB	K RESERVED FOR LOCAL USE
1	12 22 2001	11		99213	1	60 00	1			
2	12 22 2001	11		73120	1	82 00	1			
3										
4										
5										
6										

25. FEDERAL TAX I.D. NUMBER ## 5623516 SSN ☐ EIN ☒

26. PATIENT'S ACCOUNT NO.

27. ACCEPT ASSIGNMENT? (For govt. claims, see back) YES ☒ NO ☐

28. TOTAL CHARGE $ 142 00

29. AMOUNT PAID $

30. BALANCE DUE $

31. SIGNATURE OF PHYSICIAN OR SUPPLIER INCLUDING DEGREES OR CREDENTIALS (I certify that the statements on the reverse apply to this bill and are made a part thereof.)
SIGNED MARY M SANCHEZ MD DATE 12-28-01

32. NAME AND ADDRESS OF FACILITY WHERE SERVICES WERE RENDERED (If other than home or office)

33. PHYSICIAN'S, SUPPLIER'S BILLING NAME, ADDRESS, ZIP CODE & PHONE #
HORIZONS HEALTHCARE CENTER
123 MAIN AVE.
FARMINGTON, ND 58000
PIN# 628###4 GRP# ##712

PHYSICIAN OR SUPPLIER INFORMATION

(APPROVED BY AMA COUNCIL ON MEDICAL SERVICE 8/88) **PLEASE PRINT OR TYPE** FORM HCFA-1500 (12-90) FORM OWCP-1500 FORM RRB-1500

Figure 11–1. The HCFA-1500 insurance claim form is used to file insurance claims for government and private insurance plans.

Preparing the HCFA-1500

Optical Character Recognition (OCR) equipment is often used to read a paper copy of an HCFA-1500. If the claims processor uses OCR equipment, providers must use HCFA-1500 claim forms that are printed in red ink. The ink is specialized and cannot be duplicated by a color PC printer. Scannable red HCFA-1500 forms must be ordered from the U.S. Government Printing Office, from a printing company, or from a local Medicare claims processor.

OCR scanning equipment requires that special procedures be followed to allow for the scanner to read the claim. When completing claim forms, a medical administrative assistant must

- Key the information on the claim using a computer printer or typewriter.
- Align the form properly. Information must appear in the correct position on the form.
- Print information on the form in black ink.
- Use all capital letters and no punctuation.
- Use a scannable font, such as Courier 12. Italics and script cannot be read.

Life Cycle of a Claim

Perhaps the most critical step of the insurance claim process takes place before a patient even sees the physician. Preparation for an insurance claim actually begins at the moment a patient registers for an appointment with a physician, when a medical administrative assistant obtains current insurance information from the patient and records the information for later use when processing the patient's insurance claim. This information can be obtained directly from the patient's insurance card (Fig. 11–2). The card

identifies the insurance company's name and address, policyholder, policy number, group number, information on how to contact the insurance company, and where to file claims.

A **group number** appears on many different insurance cards and is used to identify a group of people who all have the same policy and related benefits. An example of a group would be employees who all work for the same company. The policy number identifies individual policyholders within that group. Oftentimes, the policy number is the same number as the insured's social security number.

A medical administrative assistant records all information from the insurance card needed to submit the claim. That information is usually recorded in a computerized database used for patient billing but could also be written directly on the superbill. The information collected is the information that will be used to process a future insurance claim unless the patient reports an insurance change to the facility. At this point, the patient is ready to see the provider, and the superbill is generated according to the procedures given in Chapter 10.

After the superbill is completed and entered into the billing system, an HCFA-1500 claim form (Procedure Box 11–1) is created and sent to the patient's insurance company. Some claims are printed on paper and mailed to the insurance company. However, many facilities that process large numbers of insurance claims submit them electronically using computerized systems. These systems can spare the facility from using excessive stacks of paper and can also speed the actual processing and payment of the claims.

Once the insurance company receives the claim, the demographic or patient's information on the claim is checked. The patient's information on the claim is the information contained in boxes 1 through 13 shown in Figure 11–1. The patient's name is checked with the company's database to be sure that person is entitled to benefits from one of the

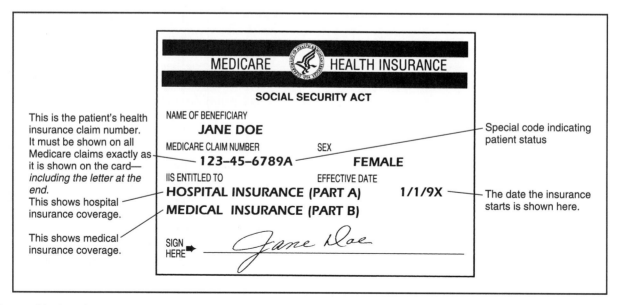

Figure 11–2. Information needed in processing insurance claims can be found on a patient's insurance card. (From Fordney MT: Insurance Handbook for the Medical Office, 7th ed. Philadelphia, WB Saunders, 2001, p. 354.)

PROCEDURE 11–1 *Complete an Insurance Claim Using the HCFA-1500*

Materials Needed

- Billing and insurance information for a patient
- Computer software or typewriter to complete form
- HCFA-1500 claim form

1. Obtain the billing information for the claim.
*2. Code the procedures and diagnoses for the claim.
*3. Obtain the patient's insurance information for the claim.
*4. Complete the HCFA-1500 claim form following the guidelines established by the insurance plan.

Denotes a crucial step in the procedure. The student must complete this step satisfactorily in order to complete the procedure satisfactorily.

Box 11–1   Place of Service Codes*

11	Provider's office
12	Home
21	Inpatient hospital
22	Outpatient hospital
23	Emergency room—hospital
24	Ambulatory surgical center
25	Birthing center
26	Military treatment center
31	Skilled nursing facility
32	Nursing facility
33	Custodial care facility
34	Hospice
41	Ambulance—land
42	Ambulance—air or water
50	Federally qualified health center
51	Inpatient psychiatric facility
52	Psychiatric facility partial hospitalization
53	Community mental health center
54	Intermediate care facility/mentally retarded
55	Residential substance abuse treatment facility
56	Psychiatric residential treatment center
60	Mass immunization center
61	Comprehensive rehabilitation facility
62	Comprehensive outpatient rehabilitation facility
65	End-stage renal disease treatment facility
71	State or local public health clinic
72	Rural health clinic
81	Independent laboratory
99	Other unlisted facility

*A complete description of the place of service codes is available at the Centers for Medicare and Medicaid Services Web site.

---

insurance company's plans. The policy number and group number are also verified to establish whether insurance coverage is available for that patient.

If "yes" is checked anywhere in box 10, the insurance plan may need to refer the claim back to the patient and ask for further information regarding a reported accident. Another entity may be responsible for payments pertaining to an accident. If a patient has been injured in an accident on someone else's property, property liability coverage may apply to the claim. If a patient has been injured in an auto accident, an auto policy—either the patient's or another responsible party's policy—will likely cover the claim. If a patient is injured at work, a workers' compensation claim will probably need to be filed.

Once all of the information in the top half of the HCFA-1500 is verified, the insurance company then proceeds to the bottom half of the claim form, boxes 14 through 33. Date of illness and date of service are checked to determine whether the patient was covered for benefits on those dates. The location of the health care service provided for the patient is noted with a place of service code in box 24b (Box 11–1). Procedure codes (box 24d) are verified to determine whether those procedures are covered under the policy benefits. Diagnosis codes (box 21) are also verified to determine whether the diagnosis is covered under the policy. The diagnosis and procedure codes are matched with each other to determine whether the procedure is related to or was appropriate treatment for the diagnosis. If the patient is covered under a managed care policy that may restrict the providers the patient is allowed to use, the provider name is checked against a list of authorized providers.

Once it has been determined that benefits should be provided for the health care services, the next step is for the insurer to determine the **usual, customary, and reasonable (UCR) fee** for the services provided. The UCR fee is the average amount charged by local physicians for the services performed. Insurers keep track of the UCR fee and may not pay any amounts greater than the UCR fee. If the provider charges more than the UCR fee, a UCR reduction will appear on the patient's explanation of benefits, which is defined later in this chapter.

Next, any co-payment due at the time of the visit is subtracted from the total bill, and any deductible that applies to the patient is applied. If the patient has a co-insurance clause in the policy, the co-insurance is then subtracted from the remaining amount of the bill. Co-insurance is usually a percentage of the total *approved* charges for which the insured is responsible. For further illustration of how co-payment, deductible, and co-insurance could be applied to a patient's charges, refer to Box 11–2.

With each claim submission, the insurance company then prepares an **explanation of benefits (EOB)** (Fig. 11–3) that explains what benefits will be paid and what (if any) subtractions have been made from the claim. Even if the claim is rejected, the reason for the rejection is listed on the EOB.

EXPLANATION OF BENEFITS

HEALTHY INSURANCE
1452 West Lake Road
Harvester, MN 55555
010-555-5555

THIS IS NOT AN INVOICE. This document explains the processing of charges submitted by your health care provider to this insurance plan. If you have questions regarding this claim, please contact 010-555-5551 from 8:00 to 5:00 Monday through Friday.

Claim Number	01 - 003 753 865
Date Received	9-11-2001
Date Processed	9-18-2001

Participating Provider	Horizons Healthcare Center
Date of Service	8-14-2001
Description of Service	Office visit, diagnostic laboratory
Provider Charges	$82.50
Usual, Customary, Reasonable Reduction	−12.50
Total Allowed Charges	$70.00
Co-payment	−10.00
Deductible	− 0.00
20% Co-insurance	−14.00
Charges Paid by Insurance Plan	$46.00
Amount You Owe to the Provider	$24.00

If you feel this explanation of benefits is in error, you may appeal this claim. Information on how to appeal is located in your insurance contract or at the number listed above.

Subscriber Information:

Policy number: 123xx6791

Christian B. Olson
1452 Pleasant View Road
Harvester, MN 55555

Figure 11–3. An Explanation of Benefits (EOB) lists the details on how an insurance claim was paid.

If the insurance plan will pay benefits on the claim, the plan writes a check for the benefit amount to either the patient or to the health care provider. The insurance benefits can be sent directly to the medical office if the patient has agreed to assign benefits to the facility. The assignment of benefits, which causes insurance payments to be sent directly to the health care provider, must be authorized by the patient (or guardian). A signed assignment of benefits is kept on file in the medical office. An authorization to release medical information and assignment of benefits can be found on the patient registration form as pictured in Figure 8–2.

Many government benefit programs provide by law a release of information and assignment of benefits (the patient does not need to sign a release and assignment), and paid benefits are sent directly to the health care facility. To identify a procedure and diagnosis on the claim form, a release of information for insurance purposes must be signed by the patient or guardian. This release also allows a copy of the patient's medical record pertaining to the visit to be sent to the insurance company if the insurance company requests more information to process the claim. Whenever an assistant releases information to an insurance company regarding a claim, great care must be taken to release only the information that pertains to the claim and nothing else.

Whether or not benefits are paid on a claim, a copy of the EOB is always sent to the medical office so that the office is aware of what has been paid and what has not been paid. A copy of the EOB is also sent to the insured to inform the insured of the processing of the claim.

When a health care facility receives a payment from the insurance carrier, the payment is applied to the charges that are being paid. This is an important step in the billing process, allowing the patient to be aware of how much money is left to pay for a visit.

Box 11-2 Insurance Charges

Jane Doe visits Dr. Sanchez for an office visit and routine laboratory tests. She incurs charges for health care of $200.00. Her private insurance company approves of the charges. She pays a $10 copayment for each visit, has a $100 deductible that has not yet been met this year, and has a 20% co-insurance clause in her insurance contract. The amount her insurance will pay for the visit is as follows:

Total approved charges*	$200.00
Co-payment	−10.00
	$190.00
Deductible	−100.00
	90.00
20% co-insurance	−40.00
Amount insurance company pays	$50.00

*If the charges for Jane's visit were not all approved by the insurer and a usual, customary, and reasonable fee reduction was taken, the patient may be charged for the reduction or the medical office may write off the reduction.

Box 11-3 Determining the Primary Insurance Carrier

If an individual is covered by two or more policies, the policies will likely pay in the following order:
1. Workers' compensation.
2. Any applicable liability insurance (e.g., property insurance, auto insurance, usually for claims related to accident).
3. Employer-sponsored insurance.
4. Medicare.
5. TRICARE and CHAMPVA.
6. Medigap supplemental insurance.
7. Medicaid.

Coordination of Benefits

If the patient has a secondary insurance policy listed in box 9 of the HCFA-1500, the insurance plan receiving the claim will need to verify whether it is the primary insurance for the patient. The primary insurance is the insurance plan that is first responsible for payment of any benefits.

If an individual has two or more insurance policies providing coverage for a service, **coordination of benefits (COB)** will take place. Coordination of benefits occurs so that a health expense is not paid for more than once.

Following is how COB works: If a patient's encounter costing $400 is covered by two insurance plans and the first plan pays $320 of the charges, the second plan will pay only a maximum of $80. Both plans' combined benefits will not exceed the total charges.

Many insurance plans have COB provisions in the plan. If there were no coordination of benefits, people might actually "make" money by seeing a health care provider. To determine what type of plan should be listed as primary when coverage exists from two or more companies, refer to Box 11-3 for a listing of the priority of insurance coverages.

Coordination of benefits will take place if a patient is covered by two different types of insurance plans or if a patient is covered by two group or individual policies. Here is another COB example: Suppose a family of four (father, mother, two children) has two policies providing health care coverage obtained through their employers. The father has a policy through his employer and the mother through her employer. In this case, the father's policy is always the father's primary policy; the mother's policy is his secondary policy. The opposite is true for the mother. Her policy is her primary policy, and the father's policy is her secondary policy.

How is it determined which policy covers their dependents first? Dependents are covered by the policy of the parent that has a birthday closest to the beginning of the year. This is known as the **birthday rule.** When implementing this rule, the year of the policyholder's birth is disregarded. For instance, if, in the family previously mentioned, the father's birthday is 5-4-59 and the mother's is 4-4-61, the mother's policy would cover the dependents first even though she is younger. For further explanation of this concept, see the scenario in Box 11-4.

Troubleshooting Claims

It is extremely important for every step of the claims preparation process to be done carefully and without

Box 11-4 Birthday Rule

John and Jane Doe have 2 children, ages 14 and 12. John has an insurance policy (A) through his employer providing family coverage. Jane has a policy (B) through her employer also providing family coverage. John's birthday is 10-19-63, and Jane's birthday is 4-4-64. The primary and secondary policies for the family are as follows:

	Primary Policy	Secondary Policy
John	A	B
Jane	B	A
Dependents	B	A

Using the birthday rule to determine which policy covers the dependents first, B would cover the dependents first because Jane's birthday (4-4) occurs before John's birthday (10-19) during the year. Even though John is older than Jane, the year is disregarded when determining the policy for primary coverage.

mistakes. When a mistake occurs anywhere during the process, the claim will likely be rejected by the insurance company. Mistakes on insurance claims consist of any information that is missing, incorrect, or incomplete and are very costly. Delays in claim processing cost additional time on the part of the office staff to correct and refile the claim. This also slows payments coming in to the office, thus reducing the cash flow. Delays and mistakes can also frustrate a patient, possibly even causing the patient to seek health care elsewhere.

When a medical office receives notice of a claim rejection, a medical administrative assistant must review the accuracy of the information on the HCFA-1500.

The claim rejection will list the reason for the rejection. An error on the upper portion of the claim can be remedied by verifying the information with the data in the patient's file. This information can usually be found in the patient's medical record or financial record. The patient's address, insurance company, policy number, and group number should be verified by an assistant at each appointment to ensure accuracy of the information when the insurance claim is generated. A misspelling or incorrect information entered on the form (i.e., a group number listed as a policy number) is enough to cause the claim to be rejected. If the data in the patient's medical record do not agree with the information on the claim form, a medical administrative assistant may need to contact the patient to check the accuracy of the information. Once the correct information has been obtained, a corrected claim form should be generated and sent to the insurance company for processing.

If the claim has been rejected for reasons related to the information on the lower half of the HCFA form, that information may also need to be verified with the information in the patient's medical record. Dates of service, as well as procedures and diagnoses, can be confirmed with the medical record of the patient's visit. A rejection can also occur because information such as an employer identification number or facility billing information has been entered incorrectly.

Timelines for Filing

Insurance claims should be filed as quickly as possible after the patient's visit. Many offices process all of their insurance claims on a regular (generally monthly) schedule. Also, most insurance plans have specific deadlines for filing claims (e.g., all claims must be filed by the end of the next calendar year). For instance, a claim for services provided on 7-9-01 could be filed no later than 12-31-02.

TYPES OF INSURANCE PLANS

Insurance plans are set up in a variety of ways. Some of the types of plans are fee-for-service, Health Maintenance Organization (HMO), and Preferred Provider Organization

(PPO). Each of these insurance plans has its own unique characteristics, but many plans use some of the more desirable characteristics of each type of insurance in order to attract customers.

A common practice in health care today is controlling health care costs through **managed care.** Many of the insurance plans or programs highlighted in this chapter have adopted some type of managed care controls to help curtail health care costs.

The general concept of managed care is that accessibility to health care is managed by the insurance company or the health care provider, or both (thus, *managed* care). Managed care often restricts the patient's ability to choose a health care provider. In the past, patients were essentially free to go to almost any health care provider they wished.

Under managed care, a network of primary care physicians and specialists is established. When seeking medical care, the patient first consults a primary care provider. That provider may treat the patient or, if necessary, may refer the patient to a specialist. Sometimes, a patient is required to select a specific primary care provider to help coordinate health care services. A patient may be required to see a physician within the network in order to receive maximum benefits from the insurance plan and may be required to receive a referral from a primary care physician in order to see a specialist.

Before a surgical procedure can be done for a managed care patient, a **precertification** from an insurance plan may be necessary. Precertification is an insurance plan's approval for a health care provider to provide a health care service to a patient. Treatment for emergencies is allowed to be given as needed, and, when the danger has passed, a patient may be required to notify an insurance plan of the emergency treatment.

Fee-for-Service

A **fee-for-service** insurance plan pays fees for the services obtained by its insured. When a patient sees a physician for a visit, the insurance company reimburses the physician for the service provided. If a patient does not see a physician in a particular month, the insurance company pays the physician nothing.

Fee-for-service plans very often allow patients to choose their own provider for health care services. Patients may go back and forth among various providers. Patients can go to any facility they want, whenever they want. No pre-approval may be required when seeking health care services; as mentioned previously, however, some fee-for-service plans have instituted some restrictions as found in other types of plans. These restrictions might include limiting patients to a specific network of physicians or requiring approval before seeing a specialist.

Costs for a fee-for-service plan include payment of a monthly premium for the coverage, and, typically, a deductible per individual or family and a co-insurance. Most fee-for-service plans do have a maximum deductible and maximum out-of-pocket expense that the individual or family may have to pay in a single year for health care.

Health Maintenance Organizations

A **health maintenance organization** (**HMO**) is a prepaid plan that provides all the care a patient may need in exchange for a flat monthly fee or premium. This concept is known as *capitation*. No matter how often a patient uses an HMO's health care services, the monthly fee remains the same. With capitation, the physician collects a monthly fee for every patient in the HMO in exchange for providing all of the patient's health care. In this type of arrangement, physicians count on some patients not using any of their services to compensate for those patients who do use their services.

Unlike a fee-for-service plan, subscribers are not free to see whomever they choose for health care. They must see someone who is a provider listed under the HMO. The only exception to this rule is in the case of an emergency or if the HMO cannot provide the care (e.g., the HMO does not have a specialist in a certain area). In an emergency, a patient is almost always allowed to seek care outside the HMO. If a patient is admitted to a hospital that is not in the HMO, the patient will likely be moved to a hospital within the HMO as soon as the patient's condition permits.

The fundamental idea behind HMOs is health maintenance. An HMO typically includes in its policies coverage for preventive care, such as physical examinations, routine eye examinations, pap smears, mammograms, immunizations, and other medical services. The reasoning is that patients will schedule themselves for regular checkups, thereby catching a potential problem before it becomes a big problem. For example, if a patient, during a physical examination, discovers he has high blood pressure, it can be treated before it becomes dangerously high and the patient has a stroke. Because the HMO is providing a patient's total health care, it is to the HMO's benefit to treat health problems before they become costly.

To control costs related to health care, HMOs customarily require a patient to choose a physician as their primary care physician. This means that the patient must see the specified primary care physician for all care (barring emergencies) and the primary care physician provides the basic health care needs of the patient. If the patient requires the services of a specialist, a **referral** must be approved by the primary care physician. A referral is the approval from the primary care physician for the patient to receive the services of a specialist. This control measure helps the HMO control costs by eliminating unnecessary visits to specialists.

Providers in HMOs may be located all in the same building, or independent groups of providers in various locations may join in an HMO contract to provide coverage for patients. The independent group of providers is referred to as an *independent practice association* (IPA). If a patient chooses to see a provider not included in the HMO or IPA,

coverage for that visit may be greatly reduced or may even be nonexistent.

HMOs typically require a co-payment with each visit to the provider. Co-payments for office visits are usually about $10; co-payments for emergency room visits are frequently somewhat higher ($30 to $40).

Preferred Provider Organizations

A **preferred provider organization** (**PPO**) provides a network of providers or preferred providers who contract with the PPO to provide services at a discount for members of the PPO.

A PPO may require patients to choose a primary care physician or primary care clinic. A primary care clinic choice allows the patient to choose from a group of providers in one clinic location. Patients choosing to see providers outside of a designated primary care clinic will likely receive reduced coverage for health care services.

By requiring patients to select a primary care physician or clinic, the PPO, like the HMO, can control costs related to a patient's health care. Patients are usually required to pay a co-payment with each office visit. Unlike the HMO, however, which receives only a flat monthly fee for each patient, the PPO operates like a fee-for-service plan. With each patient visit, in conjunction with the co-payment given by the patient, the health care provider bills the PPO for each service that is provided.

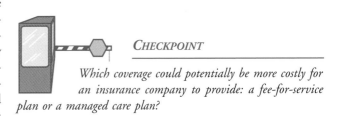

CHECKPOINT

Which coverage could potentially be more costly for an insurance company to provide: a fee-for-service plan or a managed care plan?

GOVERNMENT PROGRAMS

Medicare

The Medicare program, the largest health insurance program in the United States, is managed by CMS and provides coverage to more than 38 million people at an annual cost of almost $200 billion. Medicare is a federal program that provides health care benefits for individuals 65 years and older, certain individuals who are disabled, and patients with kidney transplants or those undergoing dialysis. Individuals who are eligible for social security or railroad retirement benefits are eligible for Medicare.

Medicare was established in 1965 as part of the Social Security Act. Medicare was designed to provide health care services for the elderly. CMS (formerly HCFA) was established in 1977 to oversee both Medicare and Medicaid, which are discussed later in this chapter.

Medicare Coverage and Enrollment

The Medicare program is composed of two parts: Part A, hospital insurance, and Part B, supplementary medical insurance. In 1997, a new, third part of Medicare, Part C, known as Medicare+Choice, was established to provide managed care services to persons enrolled in Parts A and B. In the past few years, Medicare HMOs have become available in some parts of the country, but Medicare is generally managed on a fee-for-service basis.

Persons aged 65 and older who are entitled to social security or railroad retirement benefits are automatically enrolled in Medicare. If an individual has not reached age 65 but is receiving social security benefits or railroad retirement benefits, that person is automatically enrolled in Parts A and B of Medicare. Likewise, if an individual is disabled, he or she will automatically be enrolled in Medicare in their 25th month of disability.

Not everyone is automatically enrolled in Medicare. Individuals who do not fit the examples mentioned need to apply for Medicare. This includes individuals who do not currently receive social security or railroad retirement benefits and patients with kidney disease. Persons may go to their local social security office to apply for Medicare.

Part A Premiums

For people who qualify, there is no charge for Part A Medicare coverage. To qualify, a person (1) must have worked at least 10 years in Medicare-covered employment, (2) must be 65 years old or older, (3) must be disabled and receiving social security or railroad retirement disability benefits for 24 months, or (4) must have kidney failure treated with dialysis or transplantation.

For those people who cannot meet the requirements for premium-free Part A, the coverage may still be available if they pay a premium. A premium is charged only if the patient meets one of the following conditions:

- The patient has less than 30 quarters of Medicare-covered employment. In 2002, this premium was $319 per month.
- The patient has 30 to 39 quarters of Medicare-covered employment. In 2002, this premium was $175 per month.

Part A Coverage and Deductibles

Part A coverage for Medicare provides payment assistance for the following: inpatient hospital charges, skilled nursing facility (nursing home) services, home health services, and hospice care. Medicare Part A also provides coverage for medically necessary hospital services such as semiprivate room charges, meals, regular nursing services, rehabilitation services, drugs, medical supplies, laboratory tests, x-ray, operating and recovery room charges, and intensive care and coronary care services. Medically unnecessary services such as telephone, television, or private-duty nurses in the hospital room are not covered by Medicare.

For Medicare to pay for hospitalization charges, the following criteria must be met:

1. A doctor prescribes inpatient hospital care for an illness or injury.
2. The patient's illness or injury requires care that can be provided only in a hospital.
3. The hospital is approved by Medicare.
4. The hospital's Utilization Review Committee or Peer Review Organization (PRO) did not disapprove the patient's stay.

Medicare also pays for home health care services and necessary medical equipment. There is no deductible for home health services. Home health services are covered if the following conditions are met:

1. The patient requires intermittent skilled nursing care, physical therapy, or speech-language pathology services.
2. The patient is confined to home.
3. The patient's doctor determines that the patient needs home health care and devises a plan for care in the patient's home.
4. The home health agency participates in Medicare.

Hospice care is also provided to Medicare beneficiaries. Hospice care, for the terminally ill, is focused on relieving the patient's pain and providing comfort to the patient and family members. Medicare pays most of the charges related to hospice care when the patient meets the following conditions:

1. The patient's doctor or doctors certify that the patient is terminally ill.
2. The patient chooses to receive hospice benefits instead of standard Medicare benefits.
3. The hospice care provider participates in Medicare.

Part A Deductible

In 2002, the deductible for Part A coverage was $812 per benefit period. A benefit period begins when a patient is admitted to a hospital and ends when the patient has been out of the hospital for 60 consecutive days. The deductible applies to the first 60 days of hospitalization. If the patient is hospitalized for longer than 60 days a co-insurance of $203 applies for each day the patient is hospitalized from the 61st to the 90th day of each benefit period. If the patient is hospitalized for 91 to 150 days, a $406 per day co-insurance applies for each day of the period between the 91st and 150th day. If the patient is placed in a skilled nursing facility, a co-insurance of $101.50 per day from the 21st to the 100th day of the benefit period applies. Once a benefit period ends, a new benefit period can begin. A summary of important Medicare deductibles, premiums, and co-insurance amounts for Part A and B is shown in Table 11–2.

Part B Coverage

Medicare Part B provides coverage for a variety of medical expenses, including physician services (both inpatient and

Table 11–2. Summary of Medicare Deductibles, Co-insurance, and Premiums for the Year 2002

	Medicare Part A	Medicare Part B
Deductible	$812 per benefit period	$100 per year
Co-insurance	$203 per day for the 61st to 90th day of benefit period	20% of Medicare-approved charges (less deductible)
	$406 per day for the 91st to 150th day for each lifetime reserve day (total of 60 lifetime reserve days—nonrenewable)	
Premium	None unless individual has fewer than 10 years of Medicare-covered employment	$54 per month

outpatient physician services), outpatient hospital services, clinical laboratory tests, medical equipment, ambulance services, influenza vaccines, home health services, and other specified health services and supplies. Of course, to be covered, services must be medically necessary or a prescribed preventative.

Part B Premiums, Deductible, and Co-insurance

In 2002, the monthly premium for Medicare Part B was $54. If an eligible individual fails to enroll in Medicare Part B within the initial enrollment period in which the individual is eligible, a penalty will be assessed if the individual decides to enroll at a later date. A 10% surcharge is added to the Part B premium for every year in which an eligible individual fails to enroll. If a patient waited to enroll for two years, a penalty of 20% would be added to the cost of the yearly premium.

The deductible for Medicare Part B in 2002 was $100 per person. A co-insurance also applies to Medicare Part B claims. The co-insurance is 20% of the Medicare-approved amount (less deductible) for the claim.

Processing of Medicare Claims

To facilitate the processing of Medicare claims, the federal government has elected to contract for claims processing services. A **fiscal intermediary** (or carrier or agent depending on what type of claim is processed) is an insurance company that has contracted to process claims for a government benefit program.

After the claim is processed, the intermediary sends the patient a Medicare Summary Notice (MSN), Medicare's version of an EOB, detailing what Medicare will pay and what the patient must pay related to the claim. The intermediary handles all questions regarding the benefits listed on the claim.

Intermediaries are responsible for determining costs and reimbursement amounts, maintaining records, establishing controls, safeguarding against fraud and abuse or excess use, making payments to providers for services, and assisting providers and beneficiaries when needed.

Medicare Assignment

Physicians and other health care providers who accept Medicare **assignment** agree to accept the amount that

Medicare approves for services as payment in full. These providers who accept assignment are known as **participating providers (PAR)**. If a patient sees a PAR, the patient will not need to pay more than the deductible and 20% co-insurance. Accepting Medicare assignment means the patient will pay less. For an example of how assignment affects the amount a patient owes for health care, see Table 11–3.

Medigap

Because Medicare does not completely cover all costs related to medical care, private companies offer insurance policies referred to as *Medigap policies* that will cover the costs that Medicare does not cover. Medigap policies may cover Medicare deductibles and co-insurance or services not covered by Medicare, or both. Thus, a Medigap policy "bridges the gap," more or less, between what Medicare allows and what Medicare pays.

Ten basic Medigap plans offer a variety of benefits. If an eligible enrollee purchases a policy during an open-enrollment period, the enrollee cannot be charged higher premiums because of poor health. A 6-month open-enrollment period usually begins when a Medicare B recipient reaches age 65.

Table 11–3. Comparison of Medicare Assignment

	Physician 1 (accepts assignment) Patient A (has met deductible for year)	Physician 2 (does not accept assignment) Patient B (has met deductible for year)
A. Doctor charges	$250	$250
B. Medicare allows	$200	$200
C. Minus deductible	0	0
D. Subtotal	$200	$200
E. Co-insurance (20% of D)	$40	$40
F. Amount Medicare pays (D − E)	$160	$160
G. Patient pays (C + E)	$40	$40 + (*) = $70

*This amount equals 15% × B, or 15% × (A − B), whichever is lower. If a provider does not accept assignment, the provider is permitted to charge the Medicare-approved amount plus 15%. A provider who does not accept assignment may charge the patient more for services. Federal law prohibits a provider from charging more than 15% over Medicare's approved amount.

Medicaid

The Medicaid program became law in 1965 with the passage of Title XIX of the Social Security Act. Medicaid, or medical assistance, was created to ensure adequate medical coverage for needy individuals.

An insurance program funded by both federal and state dollars, Medicaid covers nearly 36 million people. The federal government establishes minimal coverages for Medicaid but allows each state to set income guidelines, determine additional coverages, establish reimbursement rates, and administer its own program. Because of the wide latitude given to the state governments, Medicaid coverage can vary greatly among states.

Medicaid Eligibility

Medicaid provides coverage for many individuals who would otherwise likely go without medical care. To receive federal funds for a Medicaid program, a state must provide coverage to specific groups of individuals, some of whom are low-income families with children, supplemental security income (SSI) recipients, infants born to Medicaid-eligible pregnant women, children younger than age 6, and pregnant women whose income is below 133% of the federal poverty level.

States also have the option of adding coverage for specific groups. Many states provide Medicaid benefits for individuals who are medically needy. A medically needy individual may have an income that is greater than the Medicaid limits but may have sizable or catastrophic medical expenses. Persons who wish to obtain information about eligibility for Medicaid and to apply for Medicaid benefits in their state should contact their local Medicaid agency. Information on the location of local Medicaid offices is available at the CMS Web site.

Medicaid Coverage

As mentioned previously, to receive federal funds for Medicaid, all states must provide the following basic health care services:

- Inpatient and outpatient hospital services.
- Physician services.
- Nursing facility services for individuals aged 21 and older.
- Medical and surgical dental services.
- Home health care for persons eligible for nursing facility services.
- Family planning services and supplies.
- Rural health clinic services.
- Laboratory and x-ray services.
- Pediatric and family nurse practitioner services.
- Federally qualified health center services.
- Nurse midwife services.
- Early and periodic screening, diagnosis, and treatment (EPSDT) services for individuals younger than age 21.

- Prenatal care.
- Vaccinations for children.

Each state may then decide what other types of coverage the state will provide for each Medicaid beneficiary. Some of the additional services provided may include the following:

- Vision services, including eyeglasses.
- Nursing facility services for persons younger than age 21.
- Intermediate care/nursing facility services.
- Prescribed medications.
- Tuberculosis-related services for persons with tuberculosis.
- Prosthetic devices.
- Dental services.

In some instances, a state may determine that a beneficiary is overusing Medicaid services. In this situation, the state may restrict the patient to a certain number of physician visits, or it may require that the patient see a certain physician or benefits will not be paid. Some states use the term *lock-in* to describe this restriction. A patient is essentially locked in because the patient has overused or abused Medicaid services. Lock-in patients may see a physician other than their designated physician only in cases of emergency.

Medicaid Payments

Medicaid benefits are paid directly to the health care provider. Any provider accepting Medicaid patients and requesting reimbursement for Medicaid services is required to accept payment for Medicaid-approved amounts as payments in full. This includes the portion Medicaid pays as well as any co-payment or deductible paid by the patient. Some states may have small co-payments or deductibles for which the patient is responsible. These amounts cannot be charged for family planning or emergency services. Also, certain Medicaid beneficiaries, pregnant women, children, and some hospital or nursing home patients, are exempt from these co-payment or deductible amounts.

Many elderly patients are covered by both Medicare and Medicaid. In the case of benefits for health services received for these patients as well as for patients with other coverages, Medicaid is always the secondary payer or "payer of last resort." All other health insurance benefits must be exhausted before Medicaid will pay benefits.

When serving a Medicaid patient, a medical administrative assistant should be sure to not use the term "welfare" when referring to Medicaid. This term conjures up such a negative image in the mind of most individuals that it is best never to use the term in the medical office.

TRICARE

Formerly known as CHAMPUS (Civilian Health and Medical Program of the Uniformed Services), TRICARE is a health care benefit program for active-duty and retired military personnel and their families. Three plans are available under TRICARE: TRICARE Prime, TRICARE Extra, and TRICARE Standard.

TRICARE Prime provides health care coverage for active-duty and retired military personnel and their families who wish to enroll. TRICARE Prime operates much like an HMO operates. Preventive care such as physical examinations, pap smears, mammograms, and prostate screening are provided for enrollees. Care provided to TRICARE Prime enrollees is usually given at military hospitals and clinics.

TRICARE Extra operates much like a PPO operates. Individuals are able to seek health care from a civilian provider in a network of providers. No enrollment is required with TRICARE Extra. Eligible individuals can choose a network provider and need to pay a share of the costs of health care.

TRICARE Standard is close to what used to be known as CHAMPUS and provides care for family members who wish to use civilian health care providers. Like TRICARE Extra, there is no enrollment in TRICARE Standard; of the TRICARE options, this option is often the most expensive, however. This is because an eligible individual may choose any health care provider; they are not limited to a specific network of providers. Individuals who choose TRICARE Standard have an annual deductible and also pay a percentage of charges over allowed rates. Health care providers who do not accept assignment of TRICARE benefits may charge patients any extra amounts over allowed rates.

CHAMPVA

In 1973, the Veterans Health Care Expansion Act created a health insurance benefits program that provided health care coverage for dependents of veterans who have a total, permanent service-connected disability, survivors of veterans who died because of a service-connected disability or who at the time of death were totally disabled from a service-connected condition, and survivors of persons who died in the line of duty. This program is known as the Civilian Health and Medical Program of the Veterans Administration, or CHAMPVA. The program is separate from TRICARE. Individuals are eligible for CHAMPVA provided they are not eligible for TRICARE. The military member on which TRICARE or CHAMPVA eligibility is based is known as a *sponsor,* and the individuals receiving insurance benefits are known as *beneficiaries.* CHAMPVA covers health care services and supplies that are medically or psychologically necessary.

Workers' Compensation

Workers' compensation (workers' comp) programs cover employees who suffer from work-related injuries, diseases, illnesses, or even death. Each state is responsible for structuring the workers' compensation system within the state. Depending on that structure, employers may be able to provide workers' comp insurance in one or more of the following ways: (1) state-funded program, (2) self-insured program, (3) private insurance coverage, or (4) a combination of any of the three.

Workers' compensation insurance provides medical treatment benefits for workers with job-related conditions and pays a portion of wages lost to an employee who is unable to work because of a work-related condition. Death and burial benefits are also available to help cover some of the expenses incurred and income lost as a result of a work-related death. If a worker is permanently injured, vocational rehabilitation may be available to retrain the injured worker for work in another type of employment. Restrictions on workers' compensation coverage may exist if a worker was negligent.

Examples of occurrences that may be covered under workers' compensation include the following:

- An employee setting up a display falls off a ladder and breaks an arm.
- A nurse assistant lifts a patient and herniates a disk.
- A health care worker experiences a needle stick and needs testing for the human immunodeficiency virus.
- A medical transcriptionist suffers from pain due to carpal tunnel syndrome.
- A fast-food employee sustains third-degree burns from a hot grease spill.
- A sales manager is killed in a car accident while en route to a work-related meeting.
- A factory worker has permanent hearing loss due to excessive noise.

When a worker is injured, it is important for the worker to complete a first report of injury to document the circumstances of the injury. Time limitations usually exist as to when the report must be completed and when the employer must be notified of a work-related injury. Limitations can range from a few days to almost a month. Requirements for filing an injury report vary from state to state. Information should be obtained from the state for current reporting guidelines.

Premiums for workers' compensation insurance are paid by the employer and are determined by the number of employees and by the type of work performed by the business. The more risky the work, the more costly the premium.

Some states have consultive services available to employers who wish to reduce their workers' compensation claims. These services counsel employers and employees on accident prevention and workplace safety and may also include inspection services.

PRIVATE HEALTH INSURANCE

There are many private insurance companies throughout the United States that offer health insurance coverage in exchange for a premium. Many people get health insurance through their jobs. This type of health insurance is called **group insurance.** Group insurance is usually the cheapest method for an individual to obtain insurance because, in many instances, the employer helps to pay all or a portion of the cost of the insurance. Although individuals can purchase a health insurance policy on their own, a large number of policies are sold through group insurance plans provided by employers.

Insurance Coverage

The types of benefits provided by most insurance companies are divided into two main categories: basic and major medical. Basic coverage generally pays for charges related to hospitalization, such as hospital room, treatment, procedures, medications, diagnostic tests, and supplies necessary to the hospitalization. Major medical coverage typically covers those types of services provided outside the hospital, such as office visits and prescription medications.

Blue Cross/Blue Shield

The Blue Cross/Blue Shield Association (BCBSA) is a national association composed of independently owned and operated Blue Cross/Blue Shield Plans. The BCBSA provides business support and sets quality standards that the individual Plans must meet. These Plans, in order to use the BCBS name, must apply for a license to offer health insurance within a predefined geographic area. For large employers that span a several-state area or the entire country, the Association helps coordinate the insurance coverage available to those groups.

The BCBS group originated from two separate insurance plans: Blue Cross, which provided hospital coverage, and Blue Shield, which provided coverage for physician services. Most corporations today operate as a combined BCBS organization.

Every individual BCBS plan is managed by a board of directors whose membership consists of a majority of public members (people not employed in a health care organization). Approximately one of every four Americans is insured by a BCBS plan.

When a group of physicians agrees to join a BCBS organization and provide services for the organization, it is known as a participating provider (PAR). Similar to Medicare, this means that the physician agrees to a payment amount established by the plan. The amount paid will likely be determined by the usual, customary, and reasonable (UCR) fee, which is an amount usually charged for a particular service.

Just as in the Medicare example given earlier, the designation of PAR means a cost savings to the patient. If a provider is a PAR, the provider agrees to accept the payment made by the insurance company (plus any deductible, co-insurance and co-payment) as payment in full for the services rendered. In other words, if a physician charges $100 for a service and the UCR is $75, the difference of $25 is discounted off the patient's bill.

Disability Insurance

Disability insurance provides partial income replacement for individuals if they become unable to work. Disability insurance does not cover the cost of medical care but instead provides benefit payments to policyholders who lose income because of an incapacity to work.

Coverage may be paid for or purchased from an individual's employer. Disability insurance policies are also available from private insurance companies on an individual basis. Disability coverage can be purchased for loss of income on a short-term or long-term basis.

Long-Term Care Insurance

Nursing home costs can easily exceed $100 per day. Nursing home insurance helps cover costs of nursing home care. Coverage for nursing home care is usually not covered by health insurance, and Medicare provides few coverages. Nursing home insurance helps fill in the gap left by other insurance programs.

Nursing home care can quickly exhaust an elderly couple's lifetime of saving. In 1988, Congress enacted legislation designed to protect a nursing home resident's spouse from losing needed financial resources.

When an individual is placed in a nursing home and is expected to stay for at least 30 days, the couple may apply for Medicaid. An assessment of the couple's assets is conducted, and exemptions for home, household goods, automobile, and burial funds are established. The amount remaining after the exemptions and any state maximums is considered to be available for care of the resident. This legislation helps protect a healthy spouse from having to spend all the couple's resources on nursing home care with little or nothing left to pay the spouse's own living expenses.

INSURANCE RESOURCES

The study of health insurance is quite vast, and many excellent references are available for the medical administrative assistant who requires a more extensive review of the subject. The *Insurance Handbook for the Medical Office,* by Marilyn T. Fordney, provides a more detailed look at the complexities of the health insurance industry. In addition to federal and state regulations, every health insurance program provides information on its specific guidelines for processing of insurance claims.

Many excellent Internet sources are available to provide access to up-to-date information about industry requirements. The Federal Government's CMS Web site contains a wealth of information related to Medicaid, Medicare, and government regulations pertaining to health care insurance (Table 11–4). Within the Medicaid portion of the site,

Table 11–4. CMS Regional Offices

Region	Address and Telephone Number	States Covered
I. Boston Regional Office	John F. Kennedy Federal Building Room 2325 Boston, MA 02203-0003 617-565-1232	Connecticut Maine Massachusetts New Hampshire Rhode Island Vermont
II. New York Regional Office	26 Federal Plaza Room 3811 New York, New York 10278-0063 212-264-3657	New Jersey New York Puerto Rico Virgin Islands
III. Philadelphia Regional Office	The Public Ledger Building 150 South Independence Mall West Suite 216 Philadelphia, Pennsylvania 19106 215-861-4140	Delaware District of Columbia Maryland Pennsylvania Virginia West Virginia
IV. Atlanta Regional Office	Atlanta Federal Center 61 Forsyth Street, S. W., Suite 4T20 Atlanta, Georgia 30303-8909 404-562-7500	Alabama North Carolina South Carolina Florida Georgia Kentucky Mississippi Tennessee
V. Chicago Regional Office	233 North Michigan Avenue Suite 600 Chicago, Illinois 60601 312-886-6432	Illinois Indiana Michigan Minnesota Ohio Wisconsin
VI. Dallas Regional Office	1301 Young Street, 8th Floor Dallas, Texas 75202 214-767-6423	Arkansas Louisiana New Mexico Oklahoma Texas
VII. Kansas City Regional Office	Richard Bolling Federal Building 601 East 12 Street, Room 235 Kansas City, Missouri 64106-2808 816-426-2866	Iowa Kansas Missouri Nebraska
VIII. Denver Regional Office	Federal Office Building, Room 522 1961 Stout Street Denver, Colorado 80294-3538 303-844-4024	Colorado Montana North Dakota South Dakota Utah Wyoming
IX. San Francisco Regional Office	75 Hawthorne Street 4th and 5th Floors San Francisco, California 94105-3903 415-744-3501	American Samoa Arizona California Commonwealth of Northern Marianas Islands Guam Hawaii Nevada
X. Seattle Regional Office	2201 Sixth Avenue, MS/RX-40 Seattle, Washington 98121-2500 206-615-2354	Alaska Idaho Oregon Washington

information on state Medicaid agencies and programs is available. Additional Internet resources are found in the bibliography section of this chapter.

CURRENT TOPICS IN HEALTH INSURANCE

Insurance Fraud and Abuse

Health care insurance programs face a tremendous problem in trying to combat fraud and abuse in obtaining health insurance benefits. Fraud can be defined as an intentional act committed by an individual who knows the act to be false or deceptive in order to receive a benefit for himself or someone else. Insurance fraud and abuse are estimated to cost American taxpayers billions of dollars each year. HCFA has recently stepped up efforts to reduce fraud and abuse and in turn to reduce the huge amounts of money that are lost each year. Federal and state agencies often work together in a cooperative effort to expose and combat this problem.

Committing insurance fraud and abuse is a willful and conscious act. Following are some examples of the acts that perpetrators intentionally carry out to take advantage of insurance programs:

- Billing for office visits that never occurred.
- Billing for procedures never done.
- Billing used items as new.
- Billing for unnecessary tests.
- Paying kickbacks for referrals.
- Inflating charges for procedures.
- Falsifying credentials.
- Misrepresenting a patient's diagnosis for greater payment of benefits.

CMS issues fraud alerts that identify schemes used to defraud Medicare. Information is available on the CMS Web site. Providers who suspect fraudulent billing practices should report the suspected perpetrator to the state insurance commissioner's office or other appropriate agency.

Confidentiality

As is with many activities in the medical office, insurance claims processing involves dealing with sensitive medical information. Information about dates of treatment, diagnoses, procedures, and providers is confidential and should not be given or sent to any party unless the patient has authorized release of the information. Telephone inquiries from insurance companies must be carefully scrutinized. In general, it is best to handle these inquiries by asking the insurance company for the patient's name, the insured's name, and the reason for the inquiry and by taking a message regarding the inquiry. The patient's record can then be checked for a release of information, and the information can be mailed directly to the insurance company if the release has been done.

COBRA

Federal law established in 1985 known as COBRA (Consolidated Omnibus Budget Reconciliation Act of 1985) requires that an employee be allowed to continue health insurance coverage if the employee is laid off or if the employee leaves the job. The continuation of health insurance is for a specific period of time. A drawback is that the employee will probably have to pay the entire premium. COBRA also applies if an individual divorces but a former spouse was covered.

Insurance Industry Statistics

Not all Americans are covered by health insurance. In 2000, 14% of the U.S. population (38.6 million people) did not have health insurance coverage. Of all people who had health insurance in 2000, 24.2% were covered by a government program. Of these individuals, 13.4% were covered by Medicare, 10.3% by Medicaid, and 3.0% by military health care.

Although some individuals are not covered by an insurance plan, most individuals are covered by some type of plan. To ensure prompt and informed customer service in the medical office, the medical administrative assistant should be knowledgeable about health insurance regulations and procedures.

SUMMARY

The insurance claims process is an important customer service function that is provided by a medical administrative assistant for the patients of the medical office. In smaller offices, an assistant may be responsible for the entire claims process. In larger offices, a separate billing and insurance department may be responsible for filing insurance claims. Whatever the setup of the medical office, assistants must know the claims process so that they can assist patients with insurance claim filing and related questions.

Federal and state governments establish regulations that the insurance industry is required to follow. An assistant should consult CMS or the insurance plan for current information on insurance requirements and claims processing.

> ### YOU ARE THE MEDICAL ADMINISTRATIVE ASSISTANT
>
> *You have received an EOB that states that an incorrect policy number was listed on a claim form. What do you do?*

Bibliography

Brown J: Medical Insurance Made Easy. Philadelphia, WB Saunders, 2000.

Fordney MT, Follis JJ: Administrative Medical Assisting, 4th ed. Albany, NY, Delmar, 1998.

Fordney MT: Insurance Handbook for the Medical Office, 7th ed. Philadelphia, WB Saunders, 2001.

Newby C: From Patient to Payment: Insurance Procedures for the Medical Office. Westerville, Ohio, Glencoe McGraw-Hill, 1998.

Internet Resources

Agency for Health Care Research and Quality and the National Council on Patient Information and Education: Checkup on Health Insurance Choices.

Blue Cross/Blue Shield.

Centers for Medicare and Medicaid Services.

CHAMPVA.

MEDICARE.

Ohio Bureau of Workers' Compensation Resources.

Texas Workers' Compensation Commission.

TRICARE.

TRIWEST Healthcare Alliance (TRICARE Program overview).

REVIEW EXERCISES

Exercise 11–1 TRUE OR FALSE

Read each statement and determine whether the statement is true or false. Record the answer in the blank provided. T = true; F = false.

_____ 1. When an individual is employed, insurance premiums are always paid by the employer.

_____ 2. Co-payments help hold down insurance costs for an insurance plan.

_____ 3. Health insurance policies identify what types of treatments are covered by the policy.

_____ 4. The greater the charges for an office visit, the greater the patient's co-payment.

_____ 5. A patient's deductible usually must be met for the year before any insurance benefits will be paid.

_____ 6. Health insurance policies may have a maximum deductible amount that a family will have to pay in a year.

_____ 7. To draw special attention to new information on an HCFA-1500 claim form, the information should be printed in italics.

_____ 8. Assignment of benefits means that the health care provider must accept what the insurance company allows as payment in full for services provided.

_____ 9. A release of information for insurance purposes is necessary to send information to a patient's insurance company.

_____ 10. An MSN is essentially the same type of form as an EOB.

_____ 11. With a fee-for-service insurance plan, an insurance company pays a health provider only if services are performed.

_____ 12. With an HMO, a health care provider is paid a fee to provide all health care for a patient.

_____ 13. Medicare provides health care coverage for some individuals who are younger than 65 years.

_____ 14. Medicare+Choice offers managed care plans for individuals who have Medicare Part A and Part B.

_____ 15. Medicare is administered by each state, so benefits vary from state to state.

_____ 16. Premiums may be charged for both Parts A and B of Medicare.

_____ 17. Medicare Part A covers hospital charges.

_____ 18. Hospice care and home health care are provided by Medicare as long as certain conditions are met.

_____ 19. It is the responsibility of the fiscal intermediary to monitor Medicare claims for fraud and abuse.

_____ 20. Persons with a large income may be eligible to receive Medicaid benefits if they are medically needy.

_____ 21. Because each state determines Medicaid eligibility and additional benefits, Medicaid coverage can vary widely from state to state.

_____ 22. Each state is free to decide what coverage will be provided under Medicaid.

_____ 23. If Medicaid does not cover all of a physician's charges, a physician may bill the patient for the remainder of the charges.

_____ 24. Workers' compensation covers a worker's injuries that occur on the job.

_____ 25. A first report of injury for a workers' compensation claim must be done within 1 year of the injury.

_____ 26. Employees are responsible for paying their own workers' compensation premiums.

_____ 27. Major medical covers catastrophic medical expenses resulting from hospitalization.

_____ 28. Patient registration is a critical part of the insurance claim process.

_____ 29. Physicians must personally sign every HCFA-1500 claim form before it is sent to the insurance company.

_____ 30. Vocational rehabilitation is sometimes provided by workers' compensation for an injured worker.

Exercise 11–2 INSURANCE TERMINOLOGY

Match the terms in the list with the correct definition. Record the answer in the blank provided. Each answer is used only once.

(a) Assignment
(b) Beneficiary
(c) Birthday rule
(d) Claim
(e) Co-insurance
(f) Coordination of benefits
(g) Co-payment

(h) Deductible
(i) Explanation of benefits
(j) Fiscal intermediary
(k) Insured, policyholder, subscriber
(l) Insurance contract, policy
(m) Managed care

(n) Participating provider
(o) Precertification
(p) Premium
(q) Referral
(r) Usual, customary, reasonable fee
(s) Workers' compensation

_____ 1. Agreement between an insurance company and an individual (or group of individuals) in which the insurance company agrees to provide insurance coverage in exchange for a premium.

_____ 2. A type of insurance that provides benefits for employees who are injured on the job.

_____ 3. Request to an insurance company to receive insurance benefits.

_____ 4. An individual who holds an insurance policy.

_____ 5. An insurance plan's approval for a patient to receive a health care procedure from a health care provider.

_____ 6. An individual who qualifies for benefits under a subscriber's policy.

_____ 7. An insurance company that has contracted to process claims for a government health benefits program.

_____ 8. Dependents are covered by the policy of the parent who has a birthday closest to the beginning of the year.

_____ 9. A set amount that must be paid by a patient for each encounter with a physician.

_____ 10. Accessibility to health care is controlled by the insurance company or health care provider.

_____ 11. A percentage of a claim is paid by a patient.

_____ 12. Monetary payment paid for insurance coverage.

_____ 13. A specific amount a patient must pay for health care services per year before insurance benefits are paid.

_____ 14. An agreement to accept the amount that Medicare approves for services as payment in full.

_____ 15. An insurance clause that ensured health expenses are not paid for more than once.

_____ 16. Providers who accept assignment.

_____ 17. Approval from a primary care physician for a patient to receive services from a specialist.

_____ 18. Describes what insurance benefits will be paid and what subtractions have been made from an insurance claim.

_____ 19. The average amount charged by local physicians for health care services.

Exercise 11–3 CHAPTER CONCEPTS

Read each statement or question and choose the answer that best completes the statement or question. Record the answer in the blank provided. Each answer is used only once.

_____ 1. Which of the following does not belong?
   (a) Insured   (c) Beneficiary
   (b) Policyholder   (d) Subscriber

_____ 2. Which of the following is not true about preparing an HCFA-1500 for processing by OCR equipment?
   (a) Forms must be printed in a special type of red ink.
   (b) Information should be entered by a computer or typewriter and should be entirely in capital letters.
   (c) A scannable font such as Courier 12 should be used.
   (d) Punctuation should be used where needed when entering information on the form.

_____ 3. A family of six (father, mother, four children) has two insurance policies covering all family members. Each parent has full family coverage through his or her employer. Which policy will cover the children?
   (a) The policy that was in effect first.
   (b) The father's policy.
   (c) The mother's policy.
   (d) The policy of the parent whose birthday occurs first in the year.
   (e) The policy of the parent who was born first.

_____ 4. An insurance claim has been rejected by the insurance company. All of the following might be done to resubmit the claim except:
   (a) Check the patient's medical record to determine whether the procedure and diagnosis were correct.
   (b) Verify the insurance information by calling the patient.
   (c) Confirm the insurance information by checking the office's computer database.
   (d) Notify the patient that he will have to resubmit the claim.

_____ 5. All of the following are true about Medicare except:
   (a) Patients must be 65 years old to receive Medicare.
   (b) Medicare Part B covers physician services provided in a clinic setting.
   (c) CMS oversees Medicare.
   (d) Patients with kidney transplants are eligible for Medicare.

_____ 6. The deductible for Medicare Part B is
   (a) $54 per year.   (c) $812 per year.
   (b) $100 per year.   (d) There is no deductible.

_____ 7. If a patient is covered under Medicare and Medicaid for an office visit, which insurance is primary?
   (a) Medicare.
   (b) Medicaid.

_____ 8. Medicaid is a health benefits program that is administered by the
   (a) Federal government.   (c) City government.
   (b) State government.   (d) Centers for Medicare and Medicaid Services.

_____ 9. Which group is covered under Medicare?
   (a) People who have retired from their jobs.
   (b) People who cannot afford health insurance and have children.
   (c) People 65 and older who are retired and receive social security or railroad retirement benefits.
   (d) People who are partially disabled.

_____ 10. The proper format for entering a date on an HCFA-1500 is
   (a) 03 08 1983.   (c) March 8, 1983.
   (b) 03-08-83.   (d) 83 03 08.

_____ 11. A patient's encounter with a physician has 10 different procedures that need to be billed for the visit. How many claim forms are required to be completed for the encounter?
   (a) 1   (c) 5
   (b) 2   (d) 10

_____ 12. The proper format for entering a patient's name on an HCFA-1500 is
  (a) Shepard, Alice R.   (d) ALICE R SHEPARD.
  (b) SHEPARD, ALICE R.   (e) SHEPARD ALICE R.
  (c) Alice R. Shepard.

_____ 13. A child is covered under both parents' group insurance policies. The father's birth date is 5-12-62, and the mother's birth date is 3-14-61. Which policy is primary for the child?
  (a) Father
  (b) Mother
  (c) Neither

_____ 14. A patient is injured while at work. Identify the policy that likely provides primary coverage.
  (a) Liability policy
  (b) Long-term care policy
  (c) Group insurance policy
  (d) Workers' compensation
  (e) Medicaid

_____ 15. If a patient has Medicare and Medigap, which plan will provide the primary insurance coverage for the patient?
  (a) Medicare
  (b) Medigap
  (c) Whichever plan provides the most benefits

_____ 16. The portion of each bill that a Medicare B patient must pay is
  (a) $0.   (c) 20%.
  (b) $20.   (d) $100.

_____ 17. All of the following are true about Medicaid except:
  (a) State and federal funds are used to fund Medicaid.
  (b) Each state must provide certain minimum coverage for all Medicaid recipients.
  (c) If Medicaid cannot pay a patient's entire bill, a physician can bill the patient for the remainder of the bill.
  (d) Co-payments may be required for some Medicaid services.

_____ 18. If a patient is injured and unable to work, which box on the HCFA-1500 should be completed?
  (a) Box 18   (d) B and C only
  (b) Box 14   (e) All of the above
  (c) Box 16

_____ 19. The procedure code for services provided to a patient is located in which box on the HCFA-1500?
  (a) Box 21   (c) Box 24D
  (b) Box 23   (d) Box 24C

_____ 20. Which box on the HCFA-1500 identifies how many times a procedure was performed for a patient?
  (a) Box 24C   (c) Box 24J
  (b) Box 24G   (d) Box 24F

Exercise 11–4 LIFE CYCLE OF AN INSURANCE CLAIM

Read the following steps in the insurance claim process and number the steps in the order in which they occur. Record the number in the blank provided.

_____ The superbill is generated.

_____ The HCFA form is completed and sent to the insurance plan.

_____ The insurance plan determines the UCR fees.

_____ The superbill is completed.

_____ Any insurance payment received by a health care provider is applied to the appropriate charges on the patient's account.

_____ The patient's information on HCFA-1500 is verified by the insurance company.

_____ The EOB is prepared, subtracting any co-payment, deductible, or co-insurance.

_____ The provider's information on HCFA-1500 is verified by the insurance company.

_____ The patient's insurance information is obtained at registration.

_____ If the insurance plan owes benefits, a check is prepared for either the patient or the health care provider.

_____ A copy of the EOB is sent to the patient and the provider. Any check for payment of benefits is also sent.

Exercise 11–5 MEDICARE COMPUTATIONS

Read the following scenarios and determine the amounts requested in each scenario. Horizons Healthcare Center accepts assignment for all Medicare patients. Record your answers in the blanks provided. Use rates for year 2002 when calculating amounts.

1. Linda Larson has Medicare Part B coverage. She sees Dr. Sanchez for an office visit and laboratory tests pertaining to diabetes. Ms. Larson has already met her deductible this year. The charges for the visit and tests are $325, of which Medicare allows only $300.
   Identify the following amounts:
   (a) Amount discounted from Ms. Larson's charges _____
   (b) Amount Medicare pays _____
   (c) Amount Ms. Larson pays _____

2. Abner Wright has Medicare Part B coverage. He sees Dr. Marks for an office visit and diagnostic tests pertaining to arthritis. He has already met his deductible for the year. The charges for the visit and tests are $800, of which Medicare allows only $684.
   Identify the following amounts:
   (a) Amount discounted from Mr. Wright's charges _____
   (b) Amount Medicare pays _____
   (c) Amount Mr. Wright pays _____

3. Martha Maye has Medicare Part B coverage. She sees Dr. O'Brian for an office visit and diagnostic tests pertaining to influenza. She has not met her deductible for the year. The charges for the visit and tests are $250, of which Medicare allows only $225.
   Identify the following amounts:
   (a) Amount discounted from Ms. Maye's charges _____
   (b) Amount Medicare pays _____
   (c) Amount Ms. Maye pays _____

4. Martha Maye has Medicare Part B coverage. She sees Dr. O'Brian again for an additional office visit and tests pertaining to influenza. She has now met her deductible for the year. The charges for the visit and tests are $330, of which Medicare allows only $286.
   Identify the following amounts:
   (a) Amount discounted from Ms. Maye's charges _____
   (b) Amount Medicare pays _____
   (c) Amount Ms. Maye pays _____

5. Marge Armstrong has a urinary tract infection and sees Dr. Sanchez for an office visit and diagnostic tests. She has already met her Medicare Part B deductible for the year. The charges for the visit and tests are $126, of which Medicare allows only $84.
   Identify the following amounts:
   (a) Amount discounted from Ms. Armstrong's charges _____
   (b) Amount Medicare pays _____
   (c) Amount Ms. Armstrong pays _____

6. Amy Gordon has been having blackouts and sees Dr. O'Brian for an office visit and numerous tests. Her Medicare Part B deductible has not been met for the year. The charges for the visit and tests are $1232, of which Medicare allows $998.
   Identify the following amounts:
   (a) Amount discounted from Ms. Gordon's charges _____
   (b) Amount Medicare pays _____
   (c) Amount Ms. Gordon pays _____

7. Arthur Hunter sees Dr. Marks for an office visit and diagnostic tests pertaining to cellulitis. He has paid $50 toward his Medicare Part B deductible for the year. The charges for the visit and tests are $400, of which Medicare allows only $350.
   Identify the following amounts:
   (a) Amount discounted from Mr. Hunter's charges _____
   (b) Amount Medicare pays _____
   (c) Amount Mr. Hunter pays _____

8. Charles Webster sees Dr. Marks for an office visit and diagnostic tests pertaining to bladder problems. He has Medicare Part A and has not paid any deductible this year. The charges for the visit and tests are $200.
   Identify the following amounts:
   (a) Amount discounted from Mr. Webster's charges _____
   (b) Amount Medicare pays _____
   (c) Amount Mr. Webster pays _____

9. Mr. Webster (as mentioned in question 8) is found to have a kidney infection and is hospitalized at Horizons Healthcare Center for 5 days. The charges for his hospital stay total $5317, of which Medicare allows $4645. Mr. Webster has not been hospitalized at all for the past year.
   Identify the following amounts:
   (a) Amount discounted from Mr. Webster's charges _____
   (b) Amount Medicare pays _____
   (c) Amount Mr. Webster pays _____

Exercise 11–6 OTHER INSURANCE COMPUTATIONS

Read the following scenarios and determine the amounts requested in each scenario. Horizons Healthcare Center accepts assignment for all BCBS patients. Record your answers in the blanks provided.

1. Susan Miller has BCBS coverage and sees Dr. Sanchez for an ankle fracture. The total charges for the initial treatment of the fracture are $863, of which BCBS has a UCR reduction of $92. Ms. Miller has not yet paid her $200 deductible for the year. She has no co-payment required for the visit and has a 20% co-insurance in her contract.
   Identify the following amounts:
   (a) Amount discounted from Ms. Miller's charges _____
   (b) Amount BCBS pays _____
   (c) Amount Ms. Miller pays _____

2. Rayanne Roberts has BCBS coverage and sees Dr. O'Brian for a foreign body in her eye. Total charges for the office visit and slit lamp examination are $162. BCBS allows all charges, and Ms. Roberts has met her deductible for the year. She has a $10 co-payment for each visit and a 20% co-insurance clause in her contract.
   Identify the following amounts:
   (a) Amount discounted from Ms. Roberts' charges _____
   (b) Amount BCBS pays _____
   (c) Amount Ms. Roberts pays _____

3. Nan Johnson has Medicaid coverage. She sees Dr. O'Brian for an office visit regarding otalgia. Ms. Johnson has no deductible requirement but has a $3 co-payment for each office visit. The charges for the visit are $48, of which Medicaid allows only $36.
   Identify the following amounts:
   (a) Amount discounted from Ms. Johnson's charges _____
   (b) Amount Medicaid pays _____
   (c) Amount Ms. Johnson pays _____

4. Henry Sherman has Priced Right insurance coverage. He sees Dr. Marks for an office visit and laboratory tests pertaining to gout. Horizons Healthcare does not accept assignment for Priced Right insurance and will bill the patient for any UCR reduction taken by the insurance company. Mr. Sherman has already met his deductible this year. The charges for the visit and tests are $164, of which Priced Right insurance allows only $124. A $10 co-payment and 20% co-insurance also pertains to Mr. Sherman's charges. Identify the following amounts:

   (a) Amount discounted from Mr. Sherman's charges   _____

   (b) Amount Priced Right pays   _____

   (c) Amount Mr. Sherman pays   _____

5. Kaye Evenson has Medicaid coverage and is a lock-in patient at another clinic. She sees Dr. O'Brian for an office visit that is not urgent. Medicaid does not provide coverage. Ms. Evenson has no deductible requirement but has a $3 co-payment for each office visit. The charges for the visit are $48. Identify the following amounts:

   (a) Amount discounted from Ms. Evenson's charges   _____

   (b) Amount Medicaid pays   _____

   (c) Amount Ms. Evenson pays   _____

Exercise 11–7 HCFA-1500 CLAIM FORM

Look at the HCFA-1500 as pictured in Figure 11–1 and identify the following:

Patient's name   _____

Insured's name   _____

Primary insurance name   _____

Secondary insurance name   _____

Primary insurance policy number   _____

Date patient was seen by physician   _____

Name of patient's diagnosis(es)   _____

Name of procedure(s) done for patient   _____

Physician who provided services   _____

Location where services were provided   _____

11

ACTIVITIES

ACTIVITY 11–1 Using Lytec Medical 2001 software provided with this text, prepare insurance claims for the following patients. (To complete this exercise, billing exercise 10–6 must have been completed.)

To begin preparing insurance claims using Lytec Medical 2001:

1. Open Lytec Medical 2001. At the main menu, click *Horizons Healthcare Center*. (Once the Horizons Healthcare Center practice is open, the practice name will appear on the title bar at the top of the window. You will also notice that the main menu selections have now expanded.)

2. On the main menu, click *billing*, then click *print insurance claims*. The select custom form window will open.

3. Highlight standard form and click *open*. The print insurance claims window will open.

4. Make the following selections:
   (a) Print claim types: primary.
   (b) Diagnoses per page: 4 (By leaving all other options blank, all outstanding claims will be generated.)

5. Click *preview.* The claims for the charges made in billing exercise 10–6 should appear. If the claims are correct, click the *printer* button in the preview window.

If claims do not appear, go back to the charges and payments window under the billing option. Look up all billings from exercise 10–6. In the *bill to* portion of the window, a check must appear next to the primary insurance company. If a check does not appear, insert a check and redo this exercise.

If you wish to reprint claims after you complete this exercise, you must choose the reprint insurance claims option under the billing menu.

ACTIVITY 11–2 Obtain a policy handbook for an insurance policy that provides coverage for people in your local area. Identify the following:
   (a) Deductible
   (b) Co-payment
   (c) Co-insurance
   (d) What the policy covers
   (e) What the policy excludes
   (f) Does the policy require selection of a primary care physician or clinic?

ACTIVITY 11–3 Obtain guidelines for submitting claims from your local BCBS office, another commercial health insurance company, or your local Medicaid office, or all three.

ACTIVITY 11–4 Explain the purpose of the release of information statement on Figure 8–2 to a patient.

ACTIVITY 11–5 Compare one of the HCFA-1500 claim forms prepared in Activity 11–1 with the instructions provided in Table 11–1. Are the computerized forms consistent with the instructions in the table? If not, are any differences significant enough to affect the processing of a claim?

11
DISCUSSION

The following topics can be used for class discussion or for individual student essay.

DISCUSSION 11–1 Read the quotation at the beginning of the chapter. What type of insurance plan follows the philosophy of this quotation?

DISCUSSION 11–2 A health care provider agrees to accept Medicare assignment. Is this beneficial for patients? Why or why not?

Directing the Activities of the Medical Office

CHAPTER OUTLINE

ORGANIZATIONAL STRUCTURE OF THE MEDICAL OFFICE
Types of Ownership
Organizational Hierarchy

HEALTH CARE ORGANIZATIONS
Joint Commission on Accreditation of Healthcare Organizations
Facility Safety
Occupational Safety and Health Administration
Clinical Laboratory Improvement Amendments Program

OTHER OFFICE SUPPORT RESPONSIBILITIES
Office Supplies
Office Meetings and Communications
Travel Planning

SUMMARY

LEARNING OUTCOMES

On successful completion of this chapter, the student will be able to

1. Identify types of ownership of medical facilities.
2. Explain the function of the Joint Commission on Accreditation of Healthcare Organizations and the purpose of accreditation.
3. Examine facility safety, the Occupational Safety and Health Administration (OSHA), and OSHA requirements.
4. Explain ergonomics and recognize its importance.
5. Define the function of the Clinical Laboratory Improvement Amendments.
6. Explain the stocking of office supplies.
7. Explain effective methods of interoffice communication.
8. Demonstrate planning considerations for meetings.
9. Explain coordination of travel arrangements.

CMA COMPETENCIES

1. Perform an inventory of supplies and equipment.

RMA COMPETENCIES

1. Maintain inventory of medical and office supplies and equipment.
2. Arrange for equipment maintenance and report and maintain warranty/services files.
3. Know Occupational Safety and Health Administration (OSHA) guidelines and comply with regulations.

VOCABULARY

corporation
ergonomics
Material Safety Data Sheet (MSDS)
minutes
musculoskeletal disorders (MSDs)
partnership
sole proprietorship
standard precautions

BUSINESS OPERATIONS OF THE MEDICAL OFFICE

There is a time in the life of every problem when it is big enough to see, yet small enough to solve.

—Mike Leavitt

Medical practices vary widely in size and scope of practice, and a manager is responsible for various activities in the office. The assistant's role in office management is determined by the arrangement and needs of the organization. This chapter examines the fundamental considerations of organizing and operating a medical practice. An understanding of the organizational makeup of the medical office and functions that support the operation of the medical office is necessary to help a medical administrative assistant develop a "big picture" of the organization—how it works and what supportive functions are necessary to keep the office running smoothly.

ORGANIZATIONAL STRUCTURE OF THE MEDICAL OFFICE

Types of Ownership

Medical practices can be structured in various ways to accommodate the physicians practicing within the organization. Medical practices may be incorporated, with the physicians as shareholders of the corporation. A **corporation** is a recognized separate entity and operates independently of its employees and stockholders. Health care systems that organize as a medical practice and hospital may choose to operate as a for-profit or as a nonprofit corporation. Organizing as a corporation is advantageous because the organizational structure stays intact and does not need to be reorganized as physicians come and go from the organization. Also, individual physicians may be protected from actions attributed to the corporation.

Some independent physicians choose not to incorporate and instead operate a practice as a **sole proprietorship.** A sole proprietor assumes all liabilities for the practice and receives all of the income for the practice. With this type of business arrangement, a physician makes all business decisions and could be on call 24 hours a day. This business arrangement means that a physician assumes personal liability for the actions of the practice. A sole proprietor physician may risk losing personal assets in a suit against the practice. Sole proprietorships were much more common in the earlier part of this century and have been declining with the advent of group practices operating as corporations.

Two or more physicians who do not wish to incorporate may choose to form a **partnership.** Partner physicians share all income and expenses of a practice. A disadvantage of a partnership is that one partner may be found liable for the actions of another partner. An advantage of working in a partnership or working for a corporation is that the partnership or corporation can purchase equipment that might otherwise be too expensive for a sole proprietor to purchase.

Financial Interests of Physicians

In today's medical community, it is common for physicians to have part or full ownership of health-related businesses such as pharmacies, home health agencies, laboratories, nurs-ing homes, or other medically related services. Although such ownership is legal, the ethical standards of the American Medical Association state that a physician's financial interest in a company should not influence the physician's decision-making and that a physician should never place personal financial interest above a patient's best interest. It is a patient's prerogative to choose where prescriptions and other medical products and services will be purchased.

This ethical standard is evident in the everyday practice of physicians. Consider the following example: When a physician decides that a prescription is necessary to treat a patient, the physician either writes the prescription or telephones a pharmacy to fill the prescription. When a written prescription is given, the patient may fill the prescription wherever he or she chooses. If a physician telephones a pharmacy, the physician asks the patient which pharmacy should be called. A physician does not automatically telephone a pharmacy of the physician's choice; the physician lets the patient decide where the prescription will be purchased.

Many practices make it a point of notifying patients of a physician's financial interest in a health-related business that may be connected to the medical office. A notice may be legally required to be posted in the office to inform patients of a physician's ownership in the equipment or business.

Organizational Hierarchy

Depending on the nature of the medical office, the size of the office staff can vary from just a few people to hundreds and, in the case of large facilities, even thousands.

When the hierarchy of a medical organization is established, employees are usually divided into groups related to the nature of their work. That is, the clinical staff, consisting of registered nurses, licensed practical nurses, certified nurse assistants, and clinical medical assistants, usually report to the same superior because their job duties are somewhat similar. Supervisors have work experience related to the group that they supervise. A registered nurse, not an accountant, is a logical choice to manage the nursing staff. An accountant would be a logical choice to manage the business office, however.

Of course, if the organization consists of only 5 to 10 employees, it may not be necessary, or even possible, to hire a professional to manage each group in the office. In this case, key personnel may be assigned duties within the office. Professional services can then be contracted on an as-needed or regular basis.

Following is an example of how the contracting of certain professional services might work: A key person of the office staff (e.g., a medical administrative assistant) may collect financial information, such as charges and payments to patients' accounts and payroll information. Monthly totals are tabulated by the assistant and given to an outside accounting firm for maintaining the accounts of the office and for filing necessary government reports such as those required for payroll.

Large corporate practices are typically managed by a board of directors. The board may be elected by the shareholders of the corporation and may consist of staff physicians, retired physicians, community leaders, and key people of the organization. The board then elects a chairperson from the group to conduct board meetings. These meetings consist of reports from key personnel within the organization and any matters that require the attention of the board. Examples of key personnel of an organization are a chief of medical staff, chief financial officer, human resources director, and facilities manager.

It is important for everyone to know the hierarchy of the medical organization in which they are employed and to understand the importance of the organizational hierarchy. An organizational hierarchy is developed to establish a chain of command for accountability and decision-making. If there is a question or concern about the procedures of the medical office, an assistant should communicate with the individual most directly responsible for the procedure in question.

Consider the following situation: An assistant has a question regarding a physician's wishes for scheduling patients for physical examinations. Depending on the hierarchy of the organization, the situation could be handled in one of two ways. (1) If the assistant is a supervisor in charge of the registration and appointment services for a larger medical practice, the assistant probably talks directly with the physician to determine the appropriate method for scheduling patients. The assistant then communicates the decision of the physician to the rest of the registration and appointment staff. (2) If the assistant is a member of the registration and appointment services staff and has another assistant as an immediate supervisor, the staff assistant speaks with the supervisor, and the supervisor, in turn, speaks with the physician, if necessary. The supervisor then returns to the assistant and the rest of the staff and reports the physician's decision.

An assistant should never go above an immediate supervisor unless the situation is urgent and following the chain of command would cause a delay in handling the situation or injury or harm could come to someone. Another reason for not following the chain of command is when the problem is with the supervisor. In such cases, the assistant may need to use personal judgment as to what action is appropriate. If possible, a supervisor should be given an opportunity to correct any situations for which the supervisor may be responsible. Circumventing an immediate supervisor may provoke some unnecessarily tense situations in the medical office. Always try to resolve a problem directly with the supervisor first.

HEALTH CARE ORGANIZATIONS

Joint Commission on Accreditation of Healthcare Organizations

A key component in operating a medical facility is accreditation by a recognized accreditation agency. Health care organizations all across the country participate in various types of accreditation processes. Some health care organizations are reviewed by outside accreditation agencies and some by respective state government organizations. States have licensing authority over health care organizations but may accept other accreditation in lieu of inspection by a state agency.

The Joint Commission on Accreditation of Healthcare Organizations (JCAHO) is an independent national organization that reviews the practices of many types of health care organizations, such as hospitals, home health agencies, mental health providers, ambulatory care facilities, laboratories, and nursing homes. The accreditation process involves reviewing a health care facility's operations and determining whether the services the facility provides meet predetermined quality standards of JCAHO. Accreditation is often tied to the ability to conduct business as a health care organization.

Accreditation may or may not be voluntary. Many states require that health care organizations be accredited by a recognized organization in order to obtain and maintain a license to do business in the state. Accreditation by JCAHO may also satisfy Medicare certification requirements.

The accreditation process consists of a health care facility conducting a careful study of its organizational practices and documenting the practices in a written response. This study process, called a self-study, requires the organization to conduct an in-depth review of all procedures and policies used in the everyday operation of the health care facility. Procedures and policies are reviewed in the self-study, along with the documented evidence of how those procedures and processes are carried out within the organization.

The self-study process is often an eye-opening experience for the organization because it examines what is and is not working within the organization. After the self-study is completed, an investigative team consisting of industry experts conducts an on-site visit to verify that the organization is indeed meeting the standards as established by JCAHO. At the end of the on-site visit, the team reports their recommendation on accreditation to the organization and files a report with the Joint Commission. The JCAHO then determines whether to grant the accreditation recommendations of the on-site team. If the health care facility wishes to appeal an unfavorable decision of the Joint Commission, it is allowed to do so. More information on JCAHO is available at the Joint Commission's Web site.

Facility Safety

In addition to accreditation from a nationally recognized agency, safe work practices and a safe work environment are essential to the success of a medical practice. The management team of the medical practice must effectively and continually communicate to all employees the importance of safety in the workplace. A single incident because of an unsafe environment or unsafe practices can ruin an otherwise successful practice. The management team as well as all employees of the organization should stress workplace safety and expect everyone to ensure a safe workplace.

Occupational Safety and Health Administration

Setting standards to ensure safe workplaces is the chief responsibility of the Occupational Safety and Health Administration (OSHA, pronounced "o-sha"). OSHA was created by the Occupational Safety and Health Act of 1970 and applies to all employers and employees, with the exception of self-employed persons, farms in which only family members are employed, work sites (i.e., mining, nuclear energy) that are covered by other federal statutes, and employees of certain identified state and local governments.

OSHA carries out its responsibility by setting workplace standards and conducting workplace inspections to ensure that standards are being met. Employers are responsible for knowing the standards that apply to their workplace, eliminating any hazardous conditions, and making sure employees comply with applicable standards.

OSHA establishes standards that impose basic requirements for ensuring a safe workplace. The Personal Protective Equipment Standard requires that employers provide employees with personal protective equipment necessary to do their job. This equipment must be provided at no cost to the employee. Examples of protective equipment in a medical office include latex gloves, splashguards for eyes, and other protective coverings that may be necessary for performing a task in the office.

Employee Injury

If an employee injury occurs, OSHA form 101 (Fig. 12–1) is used to report the incident and describe in detail the injury or illness that has occurred. An insurance or workers' compensation form may be substituted for form 101 if it provides the same type of information. Form 101 contains information about the name and location of the employer; the name, address, age, sex, and occupation of the injured or ill employee; information about the incident that caused the employee's injury or illness; information about the injury or illness itself; and information regarding the treating physician and hospital (if the employee was hospitalized). OSHA forms must be kept a minimum of 5 years after the end of the calendar year in which the incident occurred. For instance, a report for an incident occurring on July 9, 2000, would need to be kept until December 31, 2005.

If a work-related death occurs or three or more employees require hospitalization because of a work-related accident, the employer is required to contact the nearest OSHA office within 8 hours of the accident. This time requirement is necessary in case an investigation of an accident is needed to ensure that workplace standards were being met at the time of the accident.

Employers found in violation of OSHA standards are subject to a fine for each offense, and if an employer knows of a serious violation and does not attempt to correct it, the violation may be punishable by a fine and incarceration.

Ergonomics

A very common type of work-related injury occurs when work done by an employee is done incorrectly or is done in improper conditions. If a job task is not suited to an employee, that employee may sustain a work injury because of job conditions.

If a task does not match the physical capacity of an employee, a musculoskeletal injury is likely to result. A musculoskeletal disorder (MSD) is an injury or disorder of the muscles, nerves, tendons, ligaments, and joints and does not include injury resulting from trips or falls. MSDs are likely to appear in employees who use repetitive motions throughout the day, lift heavy objects, or perform a task in an awkward position. An example of a common MSD is carpal tunnel syndrome. Office personnel who perform repetitive motions as part of their job are especially susceptible to MSDs.

The largest work-related type of injury, MSDs make up one third of all work-related injuries as reported to the Bureau of Labor Statistics every year. In 1997, MSDs accounted for 626,000 lost workdays and $1 of every $3 that was spent on workers' compensation claims. Some employees may become permanently disabled because of an MSD and may not even be able to perform simple tasks like combing hair or picking up a child.

An improperly designed workstation (e.g., a chair that is nonadjustable or a desk that is too high) that results in a worker performing a task in an unnatural position may lead to injury. Often, something as simple as an adjustable chair can prevent a work-related injury. The concept of **ergonomics** involves fitting the work to the worker. Results of OSHA studies reveal that ergonomics programs for injury prevention help reduce injuries in the workplace. Studies by the National Research Council/National Academy of Sciences have demonstrated a direct, positive correlation between ergonomics education and a reduction in work-related musculoskeletal disorders (Fig. 12–2).

Because of the large number of work-related disorders, all employees of the medical office should be educated about the hazards that may cause a work-related injury. To reduce the chance of injury, an employer can monitor the following situations

- Proper lifting techniques should be used to avoid back injury.
- Computer workstations should be at an appropriate ergonomic height for the employee. Computer keyboards should be at a comfortable height to relieve pressure on shoulders and upper back, and monitors should be at eye level and should have a nonglare screen.
- Employees working at computer stations or at other tasks for long periods should take frequent breaks to relax muscles in use.
- Appropriate lighting should be available for the task at hand.
- Proper ventilation should be ensured throughout the building. Air cleaning services should be regularly employed to clean ductwork and remove dust and other foreign particles that accumulate in air systems. Improper or dirty ventilation systems can cause employee illness.

Occupational Safety and Health Administration
Supplementary Record of
Occupational Injuries and Illnesses

U.S. Department of Labor

This form is required by Public Law 91-596 and must be kept in the establishment for 5 years.

Failure to maintain can result in the issuance of citations and assessment of penalties.

Case or File No.

Form Approved
O.M.B. No. 1218-0176

See OMB Disclosure
Statement on reverse.

Employer

1. Name

2. Mail address (No. and street, city or town, State, and zip code)

3. Location, if different from mail address

Injured or Ill Employee

4 Name (First, middle, and last)

Social Security No.

5. Home address (No. and street, city or town, State, and zip code)

6. Age

7. Sex (Check one)   Male ☐   Female ☐

8. Occupation (Enter regular job title, not the specific activity he was performing at the time of injury.)

9. Department (Enter name of department or division in which the injured person is regularly employed, even though he may have been temporarily

working in another department at the time of injury.)

The Accident or Exposure to Occupational Illness

If accident or exposure occurred on employer's premises, give address of plant or establishment in which it occurred. Do not indicated department or division within the plant or establishment.

If accident occurred outside employer's premises at an identifiable address, give that address. If it occurred on a public highway or at any other place which cannot be identified by number

and street, please provide place references locating the place of injury as accurately as possible.

10. Place of accident or exposure (No. and street, city or town, State, and zip code)

11. Was place of accident or exposure on employer's premises?   Yes ☐   No ☐

12. What was the employee doing when injured? (Be specific. If he was using tools or equipment or handling material, name them and tell what he was doing with them.)

13. How did the accident occur? (Describe fully the events which resulted in the injury or occupational illness. Tell what happened and how it happened. Name any objects or substances

involved and tell how they were involved. Give full details on all factors which led or contributed to the accident. Use separate sheet for additional space.)

Occupational Injury or Occupational Illness

14. Describe the injury or illness in detail and indicate the part of body affected. (E.g., amputation of right index finger at second joint; fracture of ribs; lead poisoning; dermatitis of left hand, etc.)

15. Name the object or substance which directly injured the employee. (For example, the machine or thing he struck against or which struck him; the vapor or poison he inhaled or swallowed;

the chemical or radiation which irriatated his skin; or in cases of strains, hernias, etc., the thing he was lifting, pulling, etc.)

16. Date of injury or initial diagnosis of occupational illness

17. Did employee die? (Check one)   Yes ☐   No ☐

Other

18. Name and address of physician

19. If hospitalized, name and address of hospital

Date of report	Prepared by	Official position

OSHA No. 101 (Feb. 1981)

(See Next Page/Reverse)

Figure 12–1. Occupational Safety and Health Administration form 101 documents the circumstances of an employee injury. (From U.S. Department of Labor. U.S. Government Printing Office, 1981.)

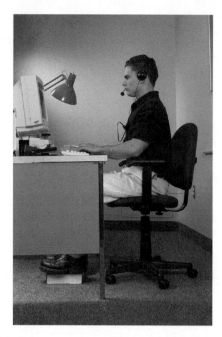

Figure 12–2. Proper attention to ergonomics reduces the chances of a work-related injury.

Employee Rights under the Occupational Safety and Health Act

The Occupational Safety and Health Act also protects employee rights on the job. Employees have the right to complain to OSHA about safety and health conditions in their workplace and to have their identities kept confidential. Employees are allowed to participate in workplace inspections and may challenge the time OSHA allows for the employer to comply with any violations. Also, if an employee feels he or she has been discriminated against, the employee must notify OSHA within 30 days of the time the employee became aware of the discrimination.

CHECKPOINT

A medical office employee trips and falls over some boxes in the medical records room. One of the staff physicians examines the employee, obtains x-rays of the employee's wrist, and determines that the x-rays are negative and that the employee has sustained only a wrist sprain. Because the worker is already employed by the clinic, the services are performed at no charge. Should anything else be done by the employee?

Material Safety Data Sheet

All products that are potentially hazardous to a person's health must be appropriately labeled, and the facility must keep information on file documenting the contents of the products and actions that should be taken if an employee has improper exposure to the products. Employees must also be educated about what should be done if they come into contact with a hazardous substance.

Product information is recorded on a Material Safety Data Sheet (MSDS) (Fig. 12–3). An MSDS details the ingredients of the product as well as first aid measures to take in case of wrongful exposure to the product (e.g., a product splashes the eye). All facilities with hazardous substances are required to have an MSDS on file for every hazardous substance. MSDS are usually included with shipments of substances.

OSHA Information

Information on OSHA standards is published in the *Federal Register,* which is available in many public libraries. Additional information about OSHA standards and regulations is also available at the federal government Web site.

Blood-Borne Pathogens and Standard Precautions

In 1991, OSHA established the Occupational Exposure to Blood-Borne Pathogens Standard. This standard is designed to protect health care workers from pathogens that may be distributed by means of blood and other bodily fluids and applies to all employees who have occupational exposure to these potentially infectious materials.

All employees who handle a specimen of blood or other bodily fluids should exercise **standard precautions.** The term *standard precautions* refers to the treatment of all human blood and certain bodily fluids as potentially infectious for pathogens such as the human immunodeficiency virus or hepatitis. Whether an office employee knows the patient is not important. Every medical office employee—or anyone—coming into contact with any bodily fluids at any time should treat those fluids as potentially infectious. Examples of bodily fluids included in this standard are human blood; semen; vaginal secretions; cerebrospinal, synovial, pleural, pericardial, peritoneal, and amniotic fluid; any body fluid contaminated with blood or saliva in dental procedures; and unfixed human tissues or organs (other than intact skin).

When a medical administrative assistant comes in contact with any type of potentially infectious bodily fluid, precautions should be taken. For instance, if a patient drips blood from a laceration on the registration desk, the assistant should consult the physician's written instructions for cleaning and disinfecting the area. These instructions should be on hand at all times and will likely include using an approved disinfectant and the use of appropriate equipment, such as wearing gloves during the decontamination of the area (Fig. 12–4).

Any employee who is potentially contaminated with a blood-borne pathogen should complete an incident report (OSHA or workers' compensation, or both) immediately after the incident. If an employee requires testing because of a possible exposure, the expenses for that testing are usually covered under workers' compensation plans.

MATERIAL SAFETY DATA SHEET

MSDS NO. 396
PAGE 1

SECTION 1   IDENTIFICATION

MANUFACTURER'S NAME: Corelis Corporation
ADDRESS: P.O. Box 93
Camden, NJ 08106

IDENTITY: 2% Aqueous Glutaraldehyde Solution

PRODUCT CODE: 3345

TRADE NAME: Aldecyde

SYNONYMS: None

CHEMICAL FAMILY: Aldehydes

RTECS #: MA 2450000 (Active)

HAZARD RATING – HEALTH: 3 (Serious Hazard)

EMERGENCY TELEPHONE NUMBER: 1 (800) 733-8690

TELEPHONE NUMBER FOR INFORMATION: 1 (800) 331-0766

ISSUED: 10/99

PREPARED BY: Regulatory Affairs

MOLECULAR FORMULA: $OHCC_3H_6CHO$ (Active)

MOLECULAR WEIGHT: 100

FLAMMABILITY: 0   REACTIVITY:0   SPECIFIC: NONE

SECTION 2   HAZARDOUS INGREDIENTS/IDENTITY INFORMATION

COMPONENTS (SPECIFIC CHEMICAL IDENTITY)	CAS #	%	OSHA PEL	ACGIH TLV	OSHA 1910.1200
Glutaraldehyde (active)	111-30-8	2	0.2ppm, C	0.2ppm, C	n/a
Inert buffer salts	n/a		None	None	Nonhazardous
Water	7732-18-5	98	None	None	Nonhazardous

SECTION 3   PHYSICAL/CHEMICAL CHARACTERISTICS

APPEARANCE AND ODOR: 2 components: colorless fluid and liquid salts; turns green when activated. Sharp odor masked with peppermint fragrance.

BOILING POINT: 212°F

VAPOR PRESSURE (mm Hg): same as water

VAPOR DENSITY (AIR=1): same as water

SOLUBILITY IN WATER: complete

FREEZING POINT: same as water

SPECIFIC GRAVITY (H_2O=1): 1.003 g/cc

MELTING POINT: n/a

EVAPORATION RATE (H_2O=1): 0.98

pH: 8

ODOR THRESHOLD: .04 ppm, detectable. (ACGIH)

SECTION 4   FIRE AND EXPLOSION HAZARD DATA

FLASH POINT (METHOD USED): None   FLAMMABLE LIMITS – LEL: nd   UEL: nd

EXTINGUISHING MEDIA: If water is evaporated, material can burn. Use carbon dioxide or dry chemical for small fires. Use foam (alcohol, polymer or ordinary) or water fog for large fires.

SPECIAL FIRE FIGHTING PROCEDURES: Self-contained breathing apparatus and protective clothing should be available to fireman.

UNUSUAL FIRE AND EXPLOSION HAZARDS: None

TOXIC GASES PRODUCED: None

SECTION 5   REACTIVITY DATA

STABILITY: 212°F

INCOMPATIBILITY (MATERIALS TO AVOID): None

HAZARDOUS DECOMPOSITION OR BYPRODUCTS: None

HAZARDOUS POLYMERIZATION: Will not occur

CONDITIONS TO AVOID: None

Figure 12–3. A Material Safety Data Sheet identifies the chemical makeup of a hazardous substance and identifies remedies to use in case of exposure. (From Bonewit-West K: Clinical Procedures for Medical Assistants, 5th ed. Philadelphia, WB Saunders, 2000, pp 161–163.)

MATERIAL SAFETY DATA SHEET	MSDS NO. 396
	PAGE 2

SECTION 6   HEALTH HAZARD DATA

ROUTE(S) OF ENTRY – INHALATION: yes   SKIN: yes   INGESTION: yes   EYE: yes

SIGNS AND SYMPTOMS OF EXPOSURE:

EYES: Contact with eyes causes damage.

SKIN: Can cause skin sensitization. Avoid skin contact.

INHALATION: Vapors may be irritating and cause headache, chest discomfort, symptoms of bronchitis.

INGESTION: May cause nausea, vomiting and general systemic illness.

EMERGENCY AND FIRST AID PROCEDURE:

EYES: Flush thoroughly with water. Get medical attention.

SKIN: Flush thoroughly with water. If irritation persists, get medical attention.

INHALATION: Remove to fresh air. If symptoms persist, get medical attention.

INGESTION: Do not induce vomiting. Drink copious amount of milk. Get medical attention.

HEALTH HAZARDS (ACUTE AND CHRONIC):
  Acute: As listed above under Signs and Symptoms of Exposure
  Chronic: None known from currently available information.

MEDICAL CONDITIONS GENERALLY AGGRAVATED BY EXPOSURE: None known from currently available information.

LISTED AS CARCINOGEN BY –   NTP: yes   IARC MONOGRAPHS: no   OSHA: no

TOXICITY:	ORAL LD50 (Rat)	Toxicity Rating 1: 500-5000 mg/kg.
	OCULAR (Rabbit)	Toxicity Rating 2: Irritating or moderately persisting more than seven days with.
	DERMAL LD50 (Rabbit)	None by dermal route.
	INHALATION LC50 (Rabbit)	Irritating but non-toxic at highest concentration achieved (2.89 ppm).

SECTION 7   PRECAUTIONS FOR SAFE HANDLING AND USE

STEPS TO BE TAKE IN CASE MATERIAL IS RELEASED OR SPILLED: For LARGE spills, use ammonium carbonate to "neutralize" glutaraldehyde odor. Collect liquid and discard it. For SMALL spills, wipe with sponge or mop down area with an equal mixture of household ammonia and water. Flush with large quantities of water.

WASTE DISPOSAL METHOD: Triple rinse empty container with water and dispose in an incinerator or landfill approved for pesticide containers. Discard solution with large quantities of water.

EPA HAZARDOUS WASTE NUMBER: n/a

PRECAUTIONS TO BE TAKEN IN HANDLING AND STORING: Use normal storage and handling requirements.

SECTION 8   TRANSPORTATION DATA AND ADDITIONAL INFORMATION

DOMESTIC (D.O.T.): Aldehydes, N.O.S.	INTERNATIONAL (I.M.O.): Aldehydes, N.O.S.
PROPER SHIPPING NAME: Glutaraldehyde	PROPER SHIPPING NAME: Glutaraldehyde
HAZARD CLASS: None	HAZARD CLASS: None
LABELS: None Needed	LABELS: None Needed
REPORTABLE QUANTITY: None	UN/NA: 1989

Figure 12–3. *Continued*

Clinical Laboratory Improvement Amendments Program

Health care laboratory facilities must undergo inspection in order to conduct laboratory tests. All laboratory testing (with the exception of research testing) is regulated by the Clinical Laboratory Improvement Amendments (CLIA) as passed by Congress in 1988. CLIA was enacted to ensure that quality standards are followed in clinical laboratory testing. All health care facilities conducting laboratory testing on specimens from human beings for the purposes of providing diagnosis or treatment require CLIA certification. Laboratories may be exempt from CLIA certification if the laboratory has been inspected and accredited by an approved agency or if it is located in a CLIA-exempt state (in which case the state inspects the laboratory).

MATERIAL SAFETY DATA SHEET	MSDS NO. 396
	PAGE 3

SECTION 9   CONTROL MEASURES

VENTILATION:
   ROUTINE: Product should be used in a covered container. Use with standard room ventilation (air conditioning); natural draft.
   EMERGENCY: Enhanced ventilation

RESPIRATORY PROTECTION:
   ROUTINE: None required
   EMERGENCY: Organic vapor cartridge, canister mask

EYE PROTECTION:
   ROUTINE: Safety glasses recommended
   EMERGENCY: Safety glasses

SKIN PROTECTION:
   ROUTINE: Impervious gloves
   EMERGENCY: Impervious gloves; Protective clothing; Rubber boots

WORK/HYGIENIC PRACTICES: Avoid contamination of food

SECTION 10   SPECIAL REQUIREMENTS

None

KEY:	n/a	= Not Applicable
	nd	= Not Determined
	C	= Ceiling
	PEL	= Permissible Exposure Level
	RTECS	= Registry of Toxic Effects of Chemical Substances
	*	= Trademark

Figure 12–3. *Continued*

OTHER OFFICE SUPPORT RESPONSIBILITIES

It may be the assistant's duty to perform some supportive functions that are necessary to keep the office running smoothly. Depending on the nature of the practice, an assistant may need to perform a variety of supportive functions to avoid interruption of services.

Office Supplies

It is often an assistant's responsibility to maintain a stock of office supplies necessary to complete the tasks of the front office. A well-equipped medical office should have a 6-month stock of office supplies on hand. Items such as pens, pencils, note pads, chart supplies, appointment reminders, and office forms are used daily, and an adequate supply must be available.

A quick inventory of supplies should be done once a month to monitor the supply stock and to order any items that may be needed within the 6 months. A log of inventory and supply orders can be kept to monitor the frequency of ordering. To determine the average monthly usage of a supply, the log can be reviewed when supplies are ordered. Maintaining a 6-month supply of materials should minimize the amount of ordering that is necessary but will not overstock the supply

cabinet. Of course, the amount of office supplies that can be stocked will depend on the amount of storage space available. A larger supply generally saves money because larger quantities are usually able to be purchased at a discount.

Ordering insufficient quantities of supplies (i.e., a 1-month supply of telephone message pads) to save money will actually cost the practice money in the long run because the item will need to be constantly reordered. Frequent reordering requires a great deal of time that might be better spent elsewhere in the office. The stock of office supplies should be replenished

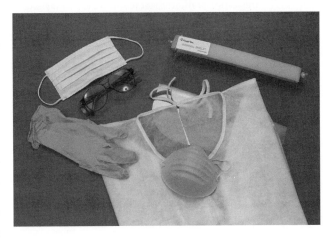

Figure 12–4. All employees are provided with the protective equipment necessary to perform their jobs within the medical office.

to minimize the frequency of reordering, with the shelf life of the supply kept in mind. Supply orders that may last years should be avoided because some items may become unusable or may become outdated.

Supply Scams

The office supply business has had some unscrupulous business practices associated with the industry. An assistant should be aware of office supply scams. One of the practices that is sometimes used is to send the office a document that looks like an invoice but is really an offer to order some merchandise. An assistant, on looking at the document, may believe that it is an invoice and may authorize a check to be written for the supplies. Because many people work in an office, an assistant may believe that someone else ordered the merchandise. To avoid this situation, all invoices should be reviewed carefully, and it should be determined whether the material was legitimately ordered. Whenever supplies are received, they should be counted and checked with the packing slip. The packing slip can then be attached to the invoice, verifying that all merchandise was received.

Another scam is a solicitation over the telephone in which an office receives a call to verify the make of the office copier and the number of copies that are tallied on the machine. The caller then says that the office's address will need to be verified and requests an authorization to ship copier supplies. An assistant may inadvertently say yes (thinking someone else originally ordered the supplies), and soon a large order of supplies—along with an invoice—arrives.

To avoid falling victim to such a scam when purchasing office supplies, an assistant should conduct business only with reputable local businesses or with nationally recognized office supply companies. Keeping the practice's business with well-known suppliers may save a few surprises down the road.

Office Meetings and Communications

Communication between the physicians of the practice and the office staff is critical to the success of the organization. The larger the office staff, the more difficult it may be to communicate information to everyone in the office. Depending on the type of information that is necessary to disseminate, interoffice memos or meetings are effective ways of keeping communication open in the office.

A meeting should be called (1) when input from the office staff may be necessary to solve a situation, (2) when a matter is crucial to the practice and office staff may need an opportunity to ask questions, or (3) when the supervisor needs to be sure information is clearly understood. If information merely needs to be circulated, an interoffice memo or e-mail should suffice to communicate that information.

Interoffice Memo

Many times it is necessary to inform the office staff of simple changes in policy and procedure. Whenever possible, information should be disseminated in an interoffice memo (see Fig. 6–13) instead of at an employee meeting.

Memos are advantageous because everyone gets a written copy of the information, and a memo serves as documentation of the information that was communicated. Memos can be sent expediently via e-mail, by leaving the memo in an employee mailbox, or by posting the information in a prominent place in the office. Distribution of routine information can be done quickly, the assistant does not need to find a convenient time to schedule a meeting, and employees are not required to sit through a meeting. An interoffice memo can be cost-effective, because many medical offices often pay employees to attend office meetings.

Memos do have some disadvantages, however. The author of the memo must be sure everyone who needs the memo sees a copy of it. If the subject is complicated, the memo may be misunderstood. Complicated subjects are usually better communicated in person to give employees a chance to ask questions for clarification.

Office Meetings

Meetings are an effective way to communicate practice information (Fig. 12–5). Office meetings should be held on a regular basis to give employees a chance to get together to discuss concerns relevant to the practice. A meeting should be productive and time well spent. Meetings are not effective if they simply become an "oral memo." The office management must decide if information needs to be disseminated via memo or meeting.

Meetings offer several advantages. Important information can be given, and the office management can ask for feedback or check for understanding of the information during the meeting time. At meetings, employees usually have a chance to work together to solve a problem or, sometimes, to get to know one another better.

Meetings also have disadvantages. It is often difficult to find a convenient time for a meeting. If all employees are not present at the meeting, the information will not be

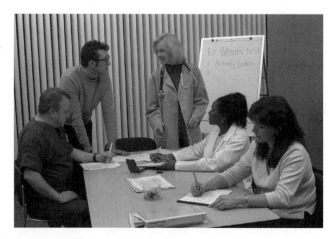

Figure 12–5. A staff meeting provides an excellent opportunity to communicate important information about the practice.

HORIZONS MEDICAL CENTER
Monthly Staff Meeting
Agenda for July 11, 2001 8:00 a.m.
Room C12

1. Office cleaning services
2. Training for new phone system
3. Annual Family Practice Conference,
   October 24–25, 2001, Minneapolis, MN
4. Expansion planned for 2002–2003
5. Other

Figure 12–6. An agenda identifies the topics to be covered in a meeting.

received by everyone. If the practice pays employees to attend meetings, a meeting may be costly.

When planning a meeting, an agenda (Fig. 12–6) is prepared to inform the participants about the subject matter of the meeting and to serve as a plan for the person conducting the meeting. As mentioned previously, a meeting should be productive, and any information that can be communicated by means of a memo should not be included in a meeting. The participants must feel as though a meeting has been worthwhile and has accomplished something. Otherwise, participants may be tempted to skip future meetings.

PROCEDURE 12–1 *Prepare a Meeting Agenda*

Materials Needed
- Information about the meeting
- Computer

1. Identify the meeting date, time, and place.
2. Identify the agenda items to be discussed and the order of discussion.
3. List the agenda items in order of discussion.
4. Proofread the agenda for typos and grammatical errors.
*5. Print a copy of the agenda.
6. Make the required number of copies of the agenda and distribute them to designated individuals.

Denotes crucial step in procedure. Student must complete this step satisfactorily in order to complete the procedure satisfactorily.

Depending on the size of the medical practice, an office meeting may include all staff or may be conducted for specific employees of the practice (i.e., nursing or office staff). It is sometimes very helpful if all departments can attend because more often than not, the items discussed may have some significance to others in the office staff. All meetings should be conducted in a well-organized manner, with sufficient time allotted for discussion of important agenda items. The individual conducting the meeting should allow attendees to ask questions and to offer feedback if necessary (Procedure Box 12–1).

A recorder should be appointed to write down the **minutes** (Fig. 12–7) of the meeting. Minutes are a summary of the information and discussion that occurred during the meeting. After the meeting, minutes should be produced in written form and distributed to all persons attending the meeting or to those with an interest in the minutes. The minutes serve as a written archive of the information given in the meeting and should be kept in a specific location in the office for future reference (Procedure Box 12–2).

Other Meetings

Occasionally, an assistant may need to host meetings for outside groups. The practice may host patient education seminars or profession-related workshops for employees or outside groups or may conduct meetings for other business purposes.

Whatever the reason for a meeting, an assistant is usually responsible for any arrangements. Several items must be considered when meetings are scheduled. These include the following:

PROCEDURE 12–2 *Prepare Minutes of a Meeting*

Materials Needed
- Meeting agenda
- Attendance at the meeting
- Laptop computer or paper and pencil

1. Identify the meeting date, time, and place.
2. Obtain a copy of the agenda.
3. Attend the meeting and list those present at the meeting.
4. During the meeting, take notes regarding meeting discussion. Record the minutes in chronological order.
5. Prepare the minutes using the format provided in Chapter 12.
*6. Proofread the minutes for typos and grammatical errors.
7. Print a copy of the minutes.
8. Make the required number of copies of the minutes and distribute them to designated individuals.

Denotes crucial step in procedure. Student must complete this step satisfactorily in order to complete the procedure satisfactorily.

HORIZONS MEDICAL CENTER
Minutes of Monthly Staff Meeting
July 11, 2001 8:00 a.m.
Room C12

Staff members present: Patrick Scott, Rae Smith, Margaret Gordon, Robert Dorland, Jackie Sears, Amy Dixon, Connie Michaels, Taylor Hudson, Dr. O'Brian, Dr. Marks, Dr. Sanchez

Office cleaning services–So Bright Cleaning Services has been contracted to provide cleaning services for the office starting on August 1, 2001. Office staff is asked to communicate any services that are not satisfactory to Taylor, the office manager, and she will speak with the supervisor of the cleaning crew.

Training for new phone system–A new telephone system was recently purchased and will be installed the last week in September. The system has several new features and the company is providing free training immediately after installation. It is important that all employees attend. Anyone requesting vacation days is asked to reconsider as this training cannot be repeated.

Annual Family Practice Conference, October 26–27, 2001, Minneapolis, MN–The conference will be held on the date noted above. The office would like to pay for at least 4 staff members to attend and bring back information to share with the rest of the staff. Conference brochures were distributed and Patrick, Amy, and Connie will attend. There is room for one more, so if anyone is interested, contact Taylor immediately.

Expansion planned for 2002–2003–The clinic physicians have just finished meeting with architects regarding the addition of office space. HMC is expecting to add a physician in each of the following areas: OB-GYN, orthopedics, and dermatology. The architects will be distributing surveys to all employees regarding uses and needs for space within the office. When the survey is received, please complete it and return to Taylor ASAP.

No other business was discussed.

CM
Prepared by Connie Michaels

Figure 12–7. Minutes of a meeting provide a written record of what transpired during the meeting.

Size of Room. Obviously, the number of people expected to attend the meeting will influence where the meeting will be held. The assistant must approximate the number of attendees in order to secure an adequate meeting room. Facilities should provide adequate, comfortable seating within view of the speaker. Also, the assistant must determine whether the attendees will be seated all the time or whether additional room will be necessary for the participants to stand or move around.

Number of Meeting Attendees. Certainly, the number of people affects many of the considerations for the meeting. Room size, refreshments, and the need for printed materials will be influenced by the number of attendees. Often, when planning for refreshments for a large group (more than 10 people), it is a good idea to ask participants to RSVP. This will help avoid overspending for refreshments.

Equipment Needed. The speaker may need an overhead, screen, or computer setup. Considerations as simple as where outlets are located to plug in equipment must be taken into account. If the room is large, a microphone may be needed so that audience members can ask questions.

Refreshments. As mentioned previously, an RSVP will help the assistant plan for an expected number of people. The assistant must consult with the physician and other necessary personnel to determine what type of refreshments are desired for the meeting. Depending on the meeting needs, catering services are an excellent resource for planning. They offer many suggestions and can provide an appropriate amount of refreshments for the expected amount of participants. If money is an issue, many grocery vendors provide box lunches, fruit trays, bakery goods, and paper goods at no extra charge to the customer. This will require the assistant to be more involved in the planning, however. When planning for refreshments, an assistant should not forget to include all the extras, such as plates, napkins, silverware, and sugar and cream for coffee.

Notification of Participants. Once the meeting date has been determined, participants should be invited to attend. Depending on the size of the facility reserved, the meeting may be limited to a specific number of participants. The meeting notice should include date, time, location, topic, and RSVP information (if applicable).

Not all meetings require every item mentioned in the list, but the list gives the essential requirements that need to be taken into consideration when planning an event. Depending on the nature of the meeting, the assistant may need to adjust the planning necessary to conduct a successful meeting.

Travel Planning

From time to time, the physician or some of the office staff may need to travel to attend a conference or other event away from the office. Very often, the cost of professional conferences is covered by the practice. It may be the responsibility of the assistant to make travel arrangements for the office staff.

Perhaps the easiest way to make travel arrangements is to have someone who is an expert do the work. Travel agents can make all reservations needed for a trip, such as air, rental cars, and hotel. Very often, even dinner arrangements and recreational outings can be scheduled in advance. Travel agents may or may not charge for their services, but agents are usually aware of the best fares available for travel and accommodations. Even if a rate may be slightly higher with use of a travel agent, the service may be well worth the money to save the assistant some time in the office.

If an assistant does take the time to do the travel planning, many airlines, rental agencies, and hotel chains have information available on the Internet and toll-free telephone numbers for inquiries about arrangements. There is usually no charge for reservations made over the Internet, although time spent researching fares and accommodations might be better spent on other tasks in the office.

Once the travel plans are set, it is important for the assistant to prepare an itinerary for the trip (Fig. 12–8). An itinerary is a complete schedule of the trip from beginning to end and should include the following information:

Figure 12–8. A travel itinerary summarizes important information regarding an individual's travel arrangements.

Travel Itinerary for Dr. Timothy I. Marks
National Medical Conference
Newark, NJ
November 9–11, 2001

November 9, 2001

Depart:	**1:01 p.m.**	E-ticket #384029476SLK Fairair Airlines Flight #6510–Coach Farmington National Airport Farmington, ND
Arrive:	**4:44 p.m.**	Newark International Airport Newark, NJ

Rental Car: Confirmation #XTD383501
Reliable Rent-a-Car
Rental agency will have directions to hotel.

Hotel: Parkside Inn, 1751 Lake Street, Newark, NJ
Phone 000-555-1111
1 room with king-size bed
Confirmation # GH40892

7:00–9:00   Early conference registration and social hour
Eagle Room, Parkside Inn

November 10, 2001

8:00–9:00   Continental breakfast
Eagle Room, Parkside Inn

9:00–5:00   Conference agenda

5:00–6:00   Social hour
Meadow Terrace, Parkside Inn

6:00–9:00   Dinner
Plains Room, Parkside Inn

November 11, 2001

8:00–9:00   Continental breakfast
Eagle Room, Parkside Inn

9:00–3:00   Conference agenda

3:30   Leave for airport

Depart:	**6:30 p.m.**	Fairair Airlines Flight #648–Coach Newark International Airport Newark, NJ
Arrive:	**8:48 p.m.**	Farmington National Airport Farmington, ND

- Dates and times of arrivals and departures.
- Name of airline or train service.
- Hotel accommodations.
- Rental car.
- Confirmation numbers for travel and hotel.
- Telephone numbers for airline, hotel, rental agency, and any other necessary numbers.
- Schedule of events.

Once the itinerary is prepared, two copies should be given to the individual traveling (one for the traveler and one for spouse or family members), and a copy should be retained at the office. The office copy will enable the practice to easily locate the traveler if necessary (Procedure Box 12–3).

SUMMARY

Many of the topics discussed in this chapter are "behind-the-scenes" functions that are necessary for the office to operate efficiently. Many individuals in the office may not realize the importance of each of these topics until a situation arises to bring the topic to their attention. Even then, it may be difficult for some individuals to understand why some things are done the way they are—either because of legal issues or other considerations. A complete understanding of the operations of the medical office enables a medical administrative assistant to understand why things are done a certain way and aids the assistant in providing optimal support to the physician and the medical practice.

PROCEDURE 12–3 *Prepare a Travel Itinerary*

Materials Needed
- Information regarding travel plans
- Computer

1. Obtain information on air or ground transportation. Identify the name of the transportation provider, departure and arrival locations, and travel confirmation numbers.
2. Obtain information on hotel accommodations. Identify the name, address, telephone number, and confirmation numbers.
3. Obtain information on any meetings, conferences, or other activities that will be attended. Identify the name, address, and telephone numbers when possible.
*4. Prepare an itinerary listing all the information obtained in chronological order.
5. Distribute two copies of the itinerary to the traveler (one for the traveler and one for the traveler's family) and retain one copy for the office.

Denotes crucial step in procedure. Student must complete this step satisfactorily in order to complete the procedure satisfactorily.

YOU ARE THE MEDICAL ADMINISTRATIVE ASSISTANT

You are the office supervisor in a medical office. The staff physicians have just informed you that the office will be extending its office hours from 9 AM to 6 PM Monday through Friday to 9 AM to 8 PM Monday through Friday and to 9 AM to 3 PM on Saturday. This change will affect the hours that the current medical administrative assistants will be scheduled to work and will require an additional assistant to be hired. What would be the best way to communicate this change to current employees?

Bibliography

Kinn ME, Woods MA: The Medical Assistant, Administrative and Clinical, 8th ed. Philadelphia, WB Saunders, 1999.

Internet Resources

Bureau of Labor Statistics, Safety and Health Statistics.
Joint Commission on Accreditation of Healthcare Organizations.
Occupational Safety and Health Administration (The Occupational Safety and Health Act of 1970).

Exercise 12–1 TRUE OR FALSE

Read each statement and determine whether the statement is true or false. Record the answer in the blank provided. T = true; F = false.

_____ 1. It is against the law for physicians to own pharmacies associated with the medical office.

_____ 2. A physician may select the pharmacy to fill a patient's prescription.

_____ 3. A board of directors is usually responsible for overall management of a large health care corporation.

_____ 4. An assistant does not have to be concerned about the chain of command in any situation.

_____ 5. JCAHO accreditation is required for all medical offices.

_____ 6. Accreditation by independent accrediting organizations may fulfill licensing requirements in some states.

_____ 7. The JCAHO establishes standards that health care organizations are required to meet in order to receive accreditation.

_____ 8. Circumventing the chain of command may be necessary if a problem exists with a direct supervisor.

_____ 9. OSHA conducts workplace inspections to determine whether a safe work environment exists.

_____ 10. Employees can be required to purchase their own safety equipment for work.

_____ 11. An employer with an unsafe workplace may be fined by OSHA.

_____ 12. A work-related injury may develop over time, depending on the work environment.

_____ 13. Carpal tunnel syndrome can sometimes be a work-related injury.

_____ 14. The identity of an employee who files a complaint with OSHA cannot be kept confidential.

_____ 15. Because a medical administrative assistant does not draw blood, there is no reason for the assistant to be concerned about blood-borne pathogens.

_____ 16. A 6-month stock of every office supply should always be on hand.

_____ 17. CLIA certification is required for facilities conducting laboratory tests.

_____ 18. An interoffice memo is an effective way to communicate easily understood information instead of convening a meeting.

_____ 19. E-mail can be used to circulate an office memo quickly.

_____ 20. Complicated topics regarding the medical office are better explained in a memo than a meeting.

_____ 21. A meeting agenda informs the staff about what the meeting will cover.

_____ 22. Meeting minutes should be retained in the office for future reference.

_____ 23. Some travel agents charge for services.

_____ 24. An itinerary details what transpired at a meeting.

Exercise 12–2 CHAPTER CONCEPTS

Read each statement or question and choose the answer that best completes the statement or question. Record the answer in the blank provided.

_____ 1. An inventory of office supplies should be done
    (a) Daily.
    (b) Weekly.
    (c) Monthly.
    (d) Yearly.

_____ 2. The type of organizational structure in which two physicians share expenses and income.
   (a) Sole proprietorship
   (b) Corporation
   (c) Partnership

_____ 3. Organization in which ownership consists of stockholders or shareholders.
   (a) Sole proprietorship
   (b) Corporation
   (c) Partnership

_____ 4. Organization in which structure does not need to be reorganized as physicians come and go from the organization.
   (a) Sole proprietorship
   (b) Corporation
   (c) Partnership

_____ 5. A physician makes all decisions regarding operation of a medical office.
   (a) Sole proprietorship
   (b) Corporation
   (c) Partnership

_____ 6. To avoid work-related injury, a worker should do all of the following except
   (a) Have appropriate lighting for the task.
   (b) Use proper lifting techniques.
   (c) Use personal funds to purchase necessary protective equipment.
   (d) Use an adjustable chair when working at a desk.

_____ 7. Which of the following is not true about ordering supplies for a medical office?
   (a) Frequent ordering saves time in the long run.
   (b) Buying supplies from regular local suppliers reduces the risk of falling victim to a scam.
   (c) It is usually an assistant's responsibility to order office supplies.
   (d) Supply inventory should be done on a regular basis to determine how frequently a supply is used.

_____ 8. Which of the following is not true about office meetings?
   (a) Meetings can give a supervisor the chance to check for understanding of an important topic.
   (b) Meetings help keep communication open in the medical office.
   (c) Meetings should be held only to discuss a crucial situation.
   (d) Meetings provide a good opportunity for staff members to ask questions.

_____ 9. When hosting a meeting, an assistant will need to do all of the following except
   (a) Verify the number of persons attending.
   (b) Prepare the minutes before the meeting.
   (c) Invite necessary participants.
   (d) Determine what refreshments should be ordered.

_____ 10. When making travel arrangements for members of the office staff, an assistant may expect to do all of the following except
   (a) Prepare an itinerary.
   (b) Search for travel arrangements on the Internet.
   (c) Obtain confirmation numbers for travel arrangements.
   (d) Pay cash for arrangements made with a travel agent.

12
ACTIVITIES

ACTIVITY 12–1 Research JCAHO standards on the Internet at www.jcaho.org.

ACTIVITY 12–2 Research ergonomics on the Internet.

ACTIVITY 12–3 Research specifications of a safe work station for a computer-related position.

ACTIVITY 12–4 Research carpal tunnel syndrome.

ACTIVITY 12–5 Identify the following information from the MSDS pictured in Figure 12–3.
    (a) Product name.
    (b) Manufacturer.
    (c) Is the product flammable?
    (d) What may happen if the product is swallowed?
    (e) First aid for exposure to skin.

ACTIVITY 12–6 Prepare a meeting agenda for the following:
An all-staff meeting will be held on August 8, 2002, at 8 AM in the staff lounge. The following will be presented:
Change in employee parking areas.
Holiday hours for the office.
Employment openings.
Medicare workshop, August 30, 2002.

ACTIVITY 12–7 Attend a meeting of a local group and prepare minutes of that meeting following the format given in the chapter.

12
DISCUSSION

The following topics can be used for class discussion or for individual student essay.

DISCUSSION 12–1 Read the quotation at the beginning of the chapter. What is the significance of this quotation in relation to the subject matter of the chapter?

DISCUSSION 12–2 Three employees of a medical office with 20 employees have had persistent allergy problems within the past year. The employees have asked the employer to conduct an inspection of the ventilation systems in the building. Is this the responsibility of the employer?

CHAPTER OUTLINE

LEARNING OUTCOMES

On successful completion of this chapter, the student will be able to

1. Demonstrate accounts receivable procedures and associated banking practices.
2. Demonstrate accounts payable procedures and associated banking practices.
3. Explain use of change funds.
4. Demonstrate use of petty cash funds.
5. Describe bookkeeping and accounting procedures and financial record retention.

CMA COMPETENCIES

1. Prepare a bank deposit.
2. Reconcile a bank statement.
3. Perform accounts receivable procedures.
4. Perform accounts payable procedures.
5. Prepare a check.
6. Establish and maintain a petty cash fund.
7. Process credit balance.
8. Process refunds.
9. Post nonsufficient funds checks.
10. Post collection agency payments.
11. Utilize computer software to maintain office systems.

RMA COMPETENCIES

1. Process insurance payments.
2. Know terminology associated with financial bookkeeping in the medical office.
3. Collect and post payments; manage patient ledgers.

4. Employ appropriate accounting procedures (e.g., pegboard).
5. Employ daily balancing procedures.
6. Prepare monthly trial balance.
7. Know accounts payable/receivable procedures.
8. Manage petty cash.
9. Prepare and make bank deposits.
10. Reconcile bank statements.
11. Use and process checks appropriately (including nonsufficient funds and endorsement requirements).
12. Maintain checking account.
13. Process payables (office bills).
14. Perform calculations related to patient and practice accounts.
15. Use computer for billing and financial transactions.

VOCABULARY

accounts payable
accounts receivable
purchase order
reconciling
restrictive endorsement
vendor

FINANCIAL MANAGEMENT

Money never starts an idea; it is the idea that starts the money.

—*W. J. Cameron*

BOOKKEEPING AND ACCOUNTING PROCEDURES IN A MEDICAL OFFICE

The past 20 years has brought about tremendous change in the financial operations of a medical office. Although computers were used in billing 20 years ago, the incorporation of computer systems throughout the office has made billing functions more streamlined in the office. Today, even very small offices usually use some type of computer software that tracks the financial transactions of the business.

No matter what the size of the practice, professional accounting services should always be retained by a medical practice. Large practices usually employ accountants to oversee all financial operations of the practice, and smaller practices typically hire accountants on a consultant basis to work with the financial information that is provided by a medical administrative assistant. The law pertaining to taxes and other parts of the financial operations of a medical practice is so complex that physicians are wise to use experts to oversee this part of a practice.

Although an assistant may not be solely responsible for the bookkeeping and accounting procedures, it is important to understand an assistant's part in the financial transactions of a practice. *Bookkeeping* refers to the recording of business transactions, whereas *accounting* includes developing reports from those financial transactions and analyzing those reports. Periodic financial reports are done to reveal the financial condition of a medical practice.

Bookkeeping can be done in one of two ways: single-entry bookkeeping or double-entry bookkeeping. *Single-entry* refers to systems such as the pegboard system mentioned in Chapter 10 and illustrated in Figure 10–7. The pegboard or "write-it-once" type of system is a simplified system, whereas double-entry requires that when an entry is made affecting one or more accounts, an equal entry or entries are made affecting other accounts. In *double-entry*

bookkeeping, transactions that affect accounts are entered as a debit or a credit to the account. Whenever one or more accounts are debited for a particular amount, one or more accounts will be credited for an equal amount. This system provides a system of checks and balances, can be done manually or electronically, and is an accurate way of tracking the financial transactions of the business.

Financial Reports

Computerizing the financial transactions of a medical office saves a tremendous amount of time in keeping track of the practice's finances. Imagine what it might be like to gather the total of outstanding balances on patients' accounts if the accounts were kept manually. The balance of every account would need to be entered into a calculator. With use of a computer program, a few buttons are clicked and the entire balance of patients' accounts can be ascertained.

Computer programs allow many different types of reports to be generated to give a picture of the financial health of the office. Reports can usually be run that will give the practice practically any information that is desired, such as the number of certain procedures done within a specific time period, the number of patients treated with a particular diagnosis, and the number of patients served on a particular day or during a month or year. Such reports (Fig. 13–1) are helpful in planning. For example, if several people with a particular diagnosis are treated monthly by a practice, it may be prudent to buy new or additional equipment to treat those patients. Likewise, if few patients are treated, it may be prudent to make arrangements for patients to receive treatment elsewhere.

An income statement, also called a profit and loss statement, identifies profit earned during a specific period of time. Income statements are often done monthly. Income received for a particular period less expenses paid during that period demonstrate either a profit or loss for the period.

Practice Analysis – Charges

Horizons Healthcare Center
October 31, 2002

Code	Description	GL Account	Amount	% Total	Count
99212	Office visit, est. pt.–focused		265.00	100.00%	6
Provider Totals					
Timothy I. Marks, M.D.			130.00	49.06%	3
Kristine G. O'Brian			90.00	33.96%	2
Mary M. Sanchez, M.D.			45.00	16.98%	1
Total Charges			265.00	100.00%	6

A

Figure 13–1. Financial reports can be used to analyze the business activities of a practice. *A*, a Practice Analysis of Charges; *B*, a Diagnosis Code Analysis; *C*, a Patient Balance Report.

Diagnosis Code Analysis

Horizons Healthcare Center
October 31, 2002

372.30 (CONJUNCTIVITIS NOS)

Chart	Name	First Date	Last Date	Procedure	Description	Units	Charges
647932	Tara D Olson	10/07/2002		99212	Office visit, est. pt.-foc	1.00	$45.00
Diagnosis Total				**Patients: 1**		**1.00**	**$45.00**

382.9 (OTITIS MEDIA NOS)

Chart	Name	First Date	Last Date	Procedure	Description	Units	Charges
689723	Evan D Stevens	10/08/2002		99212	Office visit, est. pt.-foc	1.00	$45.00
691124	Erin D Olson	04/01/2001		99212	Office visit, est. pt.-foc	1.00	$45.00
Diagnosis Total				**Patients: 2**		**2.00**	**$90.00**

473.9 (SINUSITIS)

Chart	Name	First Date	Last Date	Procedure	Description	Units	Charges
641030	Kirsten M French	10/07/2002		99212	Office visit, est. pt.-foc	1.00	$45.00
Diagnosis Total				**Patients: 1**		**1.00**	**$45.00**

786.2 (COUGH)

Chart	Name	First Date	Last Date	Procedure	Description	Units	Charges
691124	Erin D Olson	05/14/2001		99212	Office visit, est. pt.-foc	1.00	$45.00
Diagnosis Total				**Patients: 1**		**1.00**	**$45.00**

914.4 (INSECT BITE HAND)

Chart	Name	First Date	Last Date	Procedure	Description	Units	Charges
75600	Jeanne N Breckman	06/12/2001		99212	Office visit, est. pt.-foc	1.00	$40.00
Diagnosis Total				**Patients: 1**		**1.00**	**$40.00**

Report Totals						**6.00**	**$265.00**

B

Patient Balances

Horizons Healthcare Center
October 31, 2002

Chart	Name	Address	Phone	Balance
641030	Kirsten M French	2031 South 10th Street Farmington ND 58000	(012) 555-2458	45.00
647932	Tara D Olson	1452 Pleasant View Road Harvester MN 55555	(010) 555-9887	45.00
689723	Evan D Stevens	2414 South 10th Street Farmington ND 58000	(012) 555-3456	45.00
691124	Erin D Olson	1452 Pleasant View Road Harvester MN 55555	(010) 555-9887	90.00
75600	Jeanne N Breckman	514 East Oak Street Farmington ND 58000	(012) 555-3647	40.00
			Total Balance	265.00

C

Figure 13–1. *Continued*

A balance sheet reveals a practice's financial condition. Income statements may look good or bad for a particular period, but a balance sheet shows the true financial health of a practice. A balance sheet lists the amount of assets, liabilities, and owners' equity of the practice. Assets are items of value, such as banking accounts, furniture, or equipment, whereas liabilities are debts (accounts payable) or something that is owed by the practice, and capital consists of the investment of the owners of the practice. When a balance sheet is prepared, the following equation is always true: ASSETS = LIABILITIES + CAPITAL. Two practices might have similar amounts of assets, but if one practice has far more liabilities, the practice with fewer liabilities may be more financially healthy.

A cash flow statement gives a picture of the cash transactions of a practice. The cash balance at the beginning of the month, cash received during the month, cash disbursed during the month, and ending cash balance are identified.

Although most offices have computerized their financial recordkeeping, a fundamental understanding of the financial operations of a medical office helps an assistant understand how occurrences in the office can have an impact on an office's finances. For example, accounts receivable may get behind and bills entered for patients and subsequent insurance claims are not generated. Such activity will have a great impact on the financial picture of the practice because accounts receivable for that month may be greatly reduced and that will be reflected on the monthly income statement. Although the practice may have generated lots of revenue in a particular month, if the claims are not filed and patients are not billed, the practice's finances may look bleak.

ACCOUNTS RECEIVABLE

Chapter 10 conveys how accounts receivable balances can be determined using a computerized accounts system such as Lytec Medical 2001 or a pegboard system. Both systems can provide a total of patients' charges and payments for a period of time, whether that might be a day, week, or even a month. Every medical practice uses some method of tracking charges and payments for the accounts receivable of the office. In a smaller office, a physician may expect a medical administrative assistant to handle the accounts receivable and to report a balance of accounts to a bookkeeper or accountant at the end of the month.

In larger offices with many physicians, a separate billing department is typically responsible for managing the accounts receivable for the practice. Billing staff may be assigned to handle specific patient accounts or specific functions within the billing department, such as patient payments, insurance payments, and charges from certain areas of the practice. Because of the various procedures followed for different types of insurance plans or government benefit programs, some practices might assign specific personnel to handle payments for each plan. For instance, one individual could be responsible for Medicare accounts, another for Medicaid, another for Blue Cross/Blue Shield, and so on.

Given the complexity of the financial management of businesses today, a medical administrative assistant usually plays a supporting role in the financial management of the practice. It is often an assistant's responsibility to collect data and to then report the data to a financial expert who is either employed by the office or who is hired as an outside consultant to the office.

Receiving Payments on Account

Every medical office needs some cash on hand to conduct the daily business of the practice. A change fund of approximately $100 to $200 should be sufficient for most medical practices and is necessary to have on hand for those patients who pay their charges on the day the charges are incurred. Some patients prefer to pay their bill immediately after their visit, and cash is necessary to make change. Also, some offices require that patients outside the immediate vicinity of the office pay for their visit on the day they are seen. A practice may require all patients living out of state to pay their bill immediately after the visit. This requirement may be instituted to prevent any future problems collecting a bill from a patient who lives far away. In addition to receiving payments of cash or by check, an office may also allow patients to pay their bills using a major credit card, and an assistant may be required to process the payment using the card.

When a patient makes a payment in person, a receipt should be completed for the patient as proof of the payment (Fig. 13–2) (Procedure Box 13–1). The following items should be identified on a receipt:

- Amount of the payment.
- Who made the payment.
- How the payment was made (check, cash, credit card).
- Account number on which to apply the payment.
- Date of the payment.

All of the items mentioned must appear on a receipt in order to have enough information to process or track (or both) the payment internally. A copy of the receipt should always be retained by the practice because a receipt provides written documentation to enter a payment into a computer

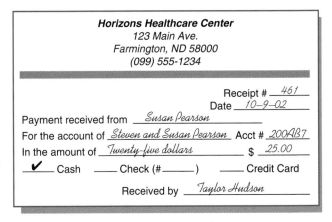

Figure 13–2. A receipt should be issued whenever a patient pays for services while in the office.

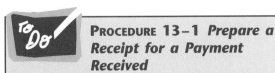

PROCEDURE 13–1 *Prepare a Receipt for a Payment Received*

Materials Needed
- Receipts
- Payments received
- Pen

1. Using the receipts in number order, enter the date the payment is received.
2. Enter the name of the payee.
3. Specify the method of payment (check or cash).
4. Enter the amount of the payment both numerically and descriptively in the spaces provided.*
5. Identify the account on which the payment should be applied.*
6. Enter the account balances if known.
7. Sign the receipt.*

Denotes crucial step in procedure. Student must complete this step satisfactorily in order to complete the procedure satisfactorily.

system at a later time if necessary. A receipt and bank deposit can be completed and the payment can be recorded on a daily banking sheet all in one step as shown in Figure 10–7. When a daily banking journal is completed, it can be used to enter payments in a computer system. The associated deposit slip can be removed and used to accompany checks, cash, and credit card charges to the bank. Payments may be processed where the payment is received, or payments may be forwarded to a central office for processing.

When a check is received, it should be endorsed immediately with a **restrictive endorsement** on the reverse of the check. A restrictive endorsement, as shown in Figure 13–3, allows the check to be deposited only in the account of Horizons Healthcare Center. If a check were either lost or stolen, a check with a restrictive endorsement would not be able to be cashed by anyone else. A check should always be stamped with an endorsement as soon as it is received. It is not enough to

sign or stamp the name of the party to whom the check was written, such as "Horizons Healthcare Center," because such an endorsement entitles whoever has the check to cash it.

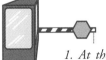

CHECKPOINT

1. At the end of many workdays, your coworkers comment that there is "too much to be done" to get ready for patients the next day and that the receipts of the day should be handled when the office atmosphere is less hectic—maybe at the end of the week or the next week. What is your response?

2. One of the assistants in the office proposes that receipts should no longer be written for payments received in person in the office, citing that patients who send checks in the mail do not get a receipt. What is your response?

Preparing a Bank Deposit

At the end of the day, the cash and checks received are totaled, and a deposit slip such as the one shown in Figure 10–7 is prepared to accompany the checks to the bank. Deposits to a practice's bank account should be made daily to ensure that there is a minimal amount of cash on hand when the office is closed (Fig. 13–4). Before depositing a check, the check must be logged in a receipts journal or must be entered into a computer system to ensure that the guarantor's account is properly credited. The checks and the deposit slip should each be totaled to verify the amount that will be deposited in the practice's account (Procedure Box 13–2).

Refunding Overpayment of a Patient's Account

If a guarantor has a credit or negative balance on account, the amount may be refunded to the guarantor. A negative balance can result from a patient paying for a service and an insurance company paying for the same service. An unexpected discount might have also been applied to the account.

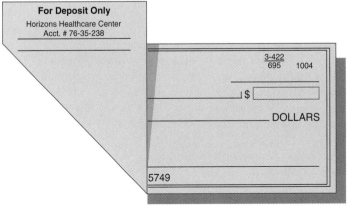

Figure 13–3. A restrictive endorsement can be used to limit where a check is deposited. (Modified from Chester GA: Modern Medical Assisting. Philadelphia, WB Saunders, 1998, p. 146.)

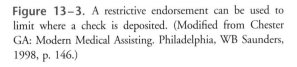

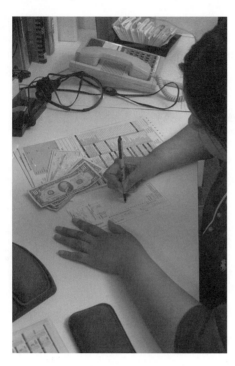

Figure 13–4. Deposits should be made daily to an office's bank account.

When money must be refunded to a guarantor, a check is written in the amount of the credit balance. The check is issued from the practice's account to the guarantor and is posted as a charge to the guarantor's account. This procedure should bring the account to zero. If patients on the guarantor's account are seen in the office frequently, a note may be included with the account statement that the credit balance will be applied to any future balances instead of a check written for the credit balance.

Processing Returned Checks

Occasionally, a check may be received from a patient or other payer for which there are nonsufficient funds in the payer's checking account to pay the check. When the office presents the check to the bank for payment, the payer's bank may refuse to pay the check, will return the check to the office, and will identify that there are nonsufficient funds to pay the check. This is also known as an *NSF check.*

When a check for a patient is deposited, the amount of the check is subtracted from the patient's balance. If a practice is unable to receive payment for a check, an assistant can call to notify the patient that the check was returned. The returned check should then be listed as a charge to the patient's account, and the explanation should be something similar to "NSF check."

A check may also be returned because a payer's account has been closed. This should be handled in the same way as an NSF check: the payer should be notified and the amount charged back to the patient's account.

PETTY CASH

From time to time, small amounts of cash are needed to purchase incidental items for use in a medical office. These types of expenses (often $10 or less) are generally too small to require a check to be written to pay for the item and should be paid for with cash. Examples of expenditures from a petty cash fund are batteries for a physician's tape recorder or coffee for the employee lounge. Cash for items such as these can be available in a petty cash fund that is kept in the office.

Physicians should communicate to their staff what type of expenses are allowed to be paid out of the petty cash fund. The following are examples of the various types of expenses that may be allowed:

- Pastries for a special office visitor.
- Inexpensive office supplies (usually under $10 to $20).
- Small donations.
- Postage due.
- Parking fees.
- Any other approved item costing $10 or less.

The petty cash fund is separate from the change fund that the medical office needs to process patient payments. The fund should be kept in a location separate from the change fund or should be in a separate container to distinguish it from the change fund in order to not confuse the funds. One individual should be responsible for disbursing cash from the petty cash fund, receiving the receipt and any change for the items purchased, and maintaining the petty

PROCEDURE 13–2 *Prepare a Bank Deposit*

Materials Needed
- Checks and currency to be deposited
- Deposit slip
- Pen

1. Enter the date of the deposit on the deposit slip.
2. Count the currency to be deposited. Enter the amount after "currency" on the deposit slip.
3. Count the coins to be deposited. Enter the amount after "coins" on the deposit slip.
4. Individually write the amount of each check to be deposited in the "checks" portion of the deposit slip.
5. Calculate the total of currency, coin, and checks to be deposited and enter the amount under "total."
6. Verify that the deposit is correct by adding currency, coin, and the amount of each check.*
7. Record the deposit in the check register.

Denotes crucial step in procedure. Student must complete this step satisfactorily in order to complete the procedure satisfactorily.

Petty Cash Log

date	description	amount	balance
10-1-0x	balance		$100.00
10-1-0x	AA batteries	$4.59	$95.41
10-4-0x	postage due	0.35	$95.06
10-4-0x	parking	$6	$89.06
10-8-0x	staples	$2.26	$86.80
10-15-0x	cleaning supplies	$10.72	$76.08
10-16-0x	refreshments for staff meeting	$16.83	$59.25

Figure 13–5. A petty cash log should be maintained to track disbursements and deposits into the fund.

cash log (Fig. 13–5). That individual should also be responsible for reconciling the fund when the fund is replenished (Procedure Box 13–3). At any time, the amount of the fund can be checked by adding all receipts since the last time the fund was replenished to any remaining cash. That amount should equal the original amount of the fund.

ACCOUNTS PAYABLE

The accounts payable functions of a practice include paying for items purchased for use by the practice and expenses incurred by the practice. When an invoice or bill is received for payment, the invoice may be due immediately or at a specific time. If the invoice is not due immediately, it may be filed in a folder designated for payment at a later date.

Purchase Orders

Supplies, equipment, and other items purchased for use in the medical office are frequently ordered using a purchase order (Fig. 13–6). A **purchase order** (PO) is a request to purchase merchandise from an identified supplier. A PO specifies certain items to be purchased as well as the quantity and price of the items.

A PO can be originated by anyone in an organization as long as that individual has the authority to purchase items. After a PO is written, it can be mailed or faxed to the **vendor** (business or supplier from which merchandise is being purchased), or someone from the office may take the PO directly to the vendor when the merchandise is picked up.

A PO signifies to a vendor that purchase of the identified merchandise has been authorized for the items listed on the order. POs are also signed by someone in the medical office. Using a PO gives a vendor the assurance that when a bill is sent for the purchased items, the bill will be paid.

PROCEDURE 13–3 Maintain a Petty Cash Fund

Materials Needed
- Petty cash record
- Receipts for expenditures
- Pen/pencil

1. A cash fund of a predetermined amount, possibly $100, is placed in a secure location in a locked, zippered bank bag.
2. When an approved purchase must be made, cash is removed from the bag that will cover the purchase and an employee makes the purchase.
3. When the employee returns, a receipt for the item and change (if any) is placed in the bag. *The receipt and change should total the amount that was removed to make the purchase.*
4. The item purchased is written in a petty cash log (see Fig. 13–5).*
5. When the fund becomes depleted, the expenses from the petty cash log are totaled and the log and receipts are kept as proof of expenses. A check is then written to "Petty Cash" for the amount of the expenses.
6. The check is cashed by the employee responsible for the fund, and the fund is replenished by placing the check proceeds in the bank bag. A new log sheet is started.
7. After the fund is replenished, the cash in the bank bag should equal the original amount of the petty cash fund.*

Denotes crucial step in procedure. Student must complete this step satisfactorily in order to complete the procedure satisfactorily.

Banking Procedures for Accounts Payable

If a medical administrative assistant is responsible for processing payments to pay bills that the practice has incurred, a record of payments can be easily logged in a check writing system like the one shown in Figure 13–7. This check writing system allows an assistant to write checks for either payment of bills or payroll. If the check is not used for payroll, the payroll stub is removed before sending to the payee. This system includes a carbon strip on the back of the check that allows for the check information to be transferred onto the Record of Checks Drawn. Checks may also be generated by computer, with the accounting transactions being performed by the computer.

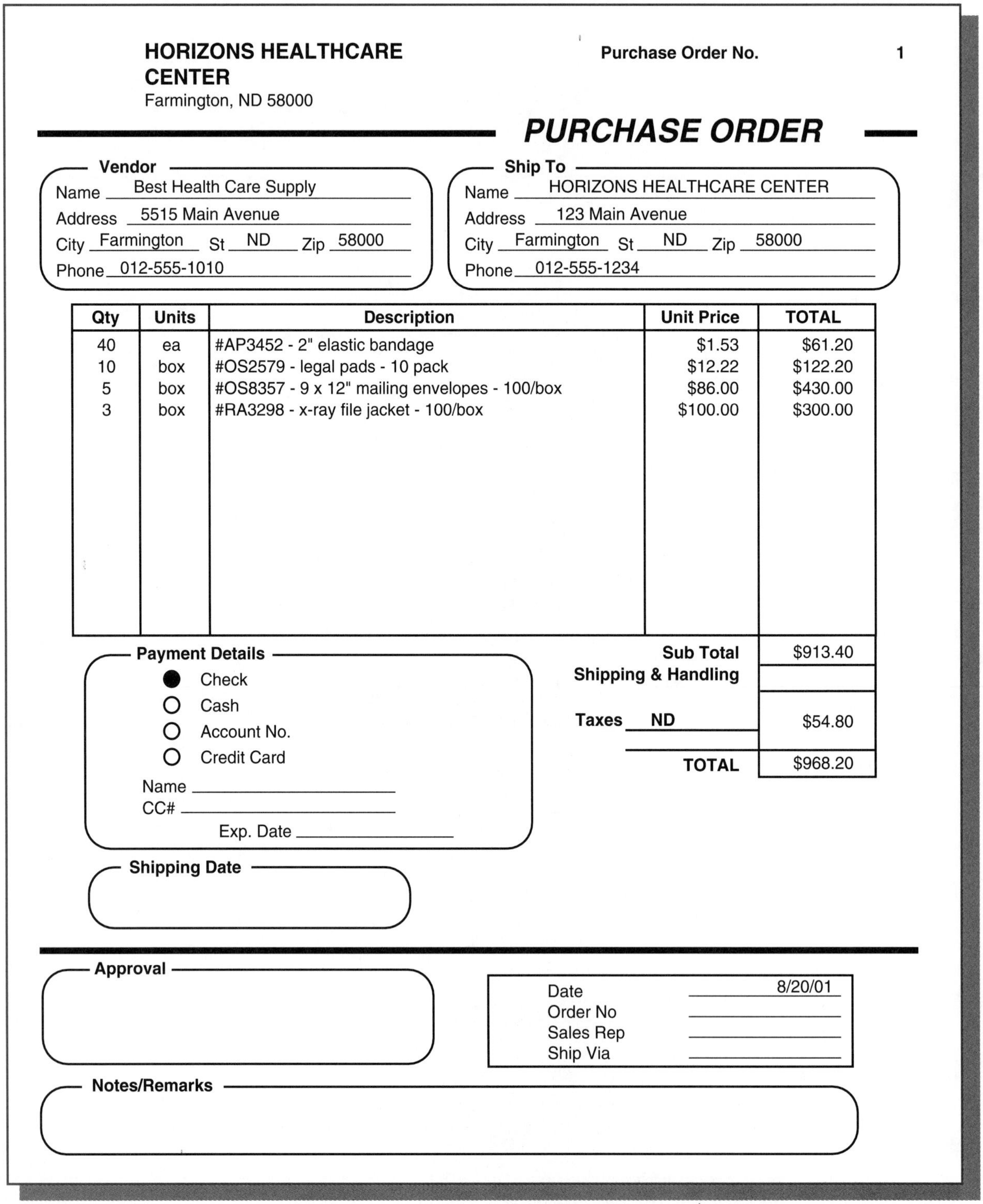

HORIZONS HEALTHCARE CENTER
Farmington, ND 58000

Purchase Order No.   1

PURCHASE ORDER

Vendor

Name: Best Health Care Supply
Address: 5515 Main Avenue
City: Farmington   St: ND   Zip: 58000
Phone: 012-555-1010

Ship To

Name: HORIZONS HEALTHCARE CENTER
Address: 123 Main Avenue
City: Farmington   St: ND   Zip: 58000
Phone: 012-555-1234

Qty	Units	Description	Unit Price	TOTAL
40	ea	#AP3452 - 2" elastic bandage	$1.53	$61.20
10	box	#OS2579 - legal pads - 10 pack	$12.22	$122.20
5	box	#OS8357 - 9 x 12" mailing envelopes - 100/box	$86.00	$430.00
3	box	#RA3298 - x-ray file jacket - 100/box	$100.00	$300.00

Payment Details

● Check
○ Cash
○ Account No.
○ Credit Card

Name _____
CC# _____
Exp. Date _____

Shipping Date

Sub Total	$913.40
Shipping & Handling	
Taxes ND	$54.80
TOTAL	$968.20

Approval

Date _____ 8/20/01
Order No _____
Sales Rep _____
Ship Via _____

Notes/Remarks

Figure 13–6. A purchase order is used to authorize purchases from a vendor.

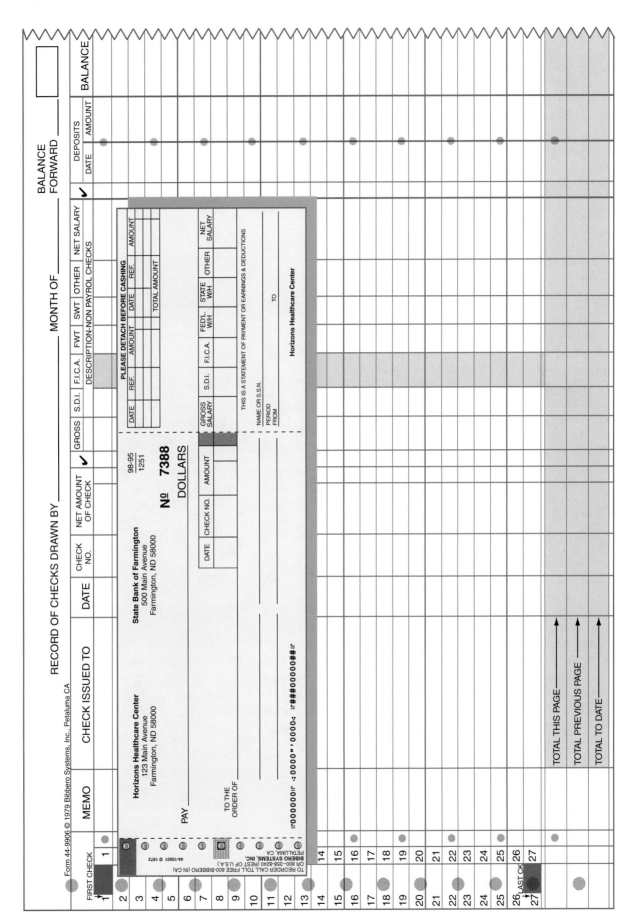

Figure 13–7. Some type of check writing system must be used to track checks written on a practice's account. (Form courtesy of Bibbero Systems, Inc., Petaluma, California, 800-242-2376. Fax 800-242-9330. www.bibbero.com.)

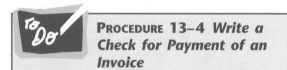

| HORIZONS HEALTHCARE CENTER | 18270 |

HORIZONS HEALTHCARE CENTER   18270
123 Main Avenue
Farmington, ND 58000

                                                    Oct. 19 20 *02*
PAY TO THE
ORDER OF____*Harmon Medical*_____ $ *3456.46*____

____*Three thousand four hundred fifty six and 46/100*_____ dollars

STATE BANK OF FARMINGTON
500 Main Avenue
Farmington, ND 58000

FOR _____   *Taylor Hudson*
        : #####: ########:

Figure 13–8. Correct format must be followed for checks written on account.

Writing Checks

Writing checks and authorizing payment are considerable responsibilities. Great care should be taken to make certain that the charges are truly owed by the practice. There are several different types of check writing systems available. Books with carbons or computer-generated checks might be used. Whatever type of checkwriting system is used, the following features should be included on each check:
- Payer of check is identified.
- Check is listed in numerical order to account for all checks.
- Date check was written is listed.
- Amount of check is subtracted from the account balance.
- Amount of check is assigned to an account for accounting purposes.

When writing a check, an assistant should be careful to write legibly. There should never be a question as to what was written on the check. If a mistake is made, the check should be voided. Information should not be crossed out. No information on the check should be able to be erased. Information regarding the amount of the check should not be able to be altered in any way (Fig. 13–8) (Procedure Box 13–4).

Reconciling the Bank Account

If maintaining the check register is the responsibility of an assistant, each month the account will need to be reconciled to ensure that no clerical errors have been made when entering checks. Each month, the bank sends a statement of account (Fig. 13–9) to the office that lists the checks, deposits, and other charges that have been incurred by the account as well as any bank charges to the account.

When the monthly statement arrives, the statement has to be reconciled with the office's check register (Procedure Box 13–5). This is necessary to ensure that the checkbook balance

---

TO DO

PROCEDURE 13–4 *Write a Check for Payment of an Invoice*

Materials Needed
- Check register with checks
- Invoices to be paid
- Pen

1. Complete the check stub, subtracting the amount of the check from the current balance of the account.
2. Complete the check using a pen.* Use checks in numerical order.
3. Enter the current date on the check.
4. On the "PAY TO THE ORDER OF" line, enter the payee's name.*
5. Enter the amount of the check numerically in the blank provided after the "$." Begin entering the amount immediately after the "$" to prevent anything from being added to the check amount.*
6. Enter the amount of the check in words in the line below the "PAY TO THE ORDER OF" line. If the entire line is not used, use dashes or a solid line to cross out the remainder of the line.*
7. The check is signed by an individual who has been authorized to sign checks for the account. The check can then be placed in a window envelope for mailing to the payee if necessary.*

Denotes crucial step in procedure. Student must complete this step satisfactorily in order to complete the procedure satisfactorily.

State Bank of Farmington
500 Main Avenue
Farmington, ND 58000
012-555-5000

Statement of Account for:
Horizons Healthcare Center
123 Main Avenue
Farmington, ND 58000

Date: 11-30-02
Account number: 76-375-238

Previous Balance:	5,012.45
Deposits/credits:	10,347.78
Checks/debits:	9,385.13
Service charges:	0.00
Ending Balance:	5,975.10

Deposits:

Date	Amount
11-5	2,305.46
11-8	456.38
11-9	235.90
11-15	4038.98
11-21	2972.00
11-28	339.06

Checks drawn on account:

Check No.	Date	Amount	Check No.	Date	Amount
18275	11-1	493.47	18285	11-16	890.56
18276	11-2	50.00	18286	11-16	1500.00
18277	11-2	37.50	18288*	11-19	234.34
18278	11-6	395.00	18289	11-21	470.00
18279	11-5	500.00	18290	11-21	3310.00
18280	11-9	40.00	18291	11-26	500.00
18281	11-8	120.00	18292	11-28	39.46
18282	11-8	324.52	18294*	11-29	109.78
18283	11-9	35.50			
18284	11-14	335.00			

Figure 13–9. A bank sends a monthly statement identifying checks, deposits, and other charges made to an account.

and bank balance are in agreement. Again, the responsibility of maintaining the checkbook for a practice is an important one, and the account should never go unreconciled any month. One mistake in the check register might cause the embarrassment of checks being returned to payers.

BUSINESS RECORD RETENTION

In the course of business in the medical office, many important documents are received. Insurance policies for property liability and malpractice insurance should be re-tained by the practice until the statutes of limitations have expired for any potential liability. In the case of malpractice policies for physicians who treat children, remember that the statute of limitations does not begin until the patient is 18 years of age.

All office documents relating to the business practices of the office should be retained until all statutes of limitations have expired. The statute of limitations varies from state to state, and an assistant should verify the statute of limitations for the state in which the medical office does business. Financial records must be retained until they are no longer needed according to the applicable statute of limitations.

PROCEDURE 13–5 *Reconcile a Bank Statement*

Materials Needed

- Current month's bank statement
- Record of checks drawn or check register
- Calculator
- Pen/pencil

1. All checks that have been paid by the bank should be checked on the record of checks drawn or the check register.
2. Any charges applied to the account by the bank should be listed on the record/register and subtracted from the balance.
3. Any interest deposits from the bank should be listed on the record/register and added to the balance.
4. Take the ending monthly balance on the account and do the following:
   (a) Add any deposits made by the practice that are not included on the statement.
   (b) Subtract any checks written by the practice that have not been paid by the bank.
   The total should then equal the ending balance in the RECORD. If the total in 4C does not equal the balance in the RECORD, you should look for errors in addition and subtraction when figuring the ending balance, as well as any other errors that may be present in the record/register.*

*Denotes crucial step in procedure. Student must complete this step satisfactorily in order to complete the procedure satisfactorily.

SUMMARY

The size of the practice and the scope of the responsibilities of the medical administrative assistant dictate whether an assistant is responsible for handling the financial operations of the practice. As mentioned previously, in many large offices today, professionals may be hired or contracted by the practice to perform many of the financial functions of the practice. Whether an assistant has a small or a large role, an understanding of the financial operations of the practice will give an assistant a greater appreciation for how office activities impact the finances of the office.

Bibliography

Fordney MT, Follis JJ: Administrative Medical Assisting, 4th ed. Albany, NY, Delmar, 1998.

Kinn ME, Woods MA: The Medical Assistant: Administrative and Clinical, 8th ed. Philadelphia, WB Saunders, 1999.

Palko T, Palko H: Q&A Review for the Medical Assistant. Upper Saddle River, NJ, Prentice Hall, 2001.

REVIEW EXERCISES

Exercise 13–1 TRUE OR FALSE

Read each statement and determine whether the statement is true or false. Record the answer in the blank provided. T = true; F = false.

_____ 1. A change fund is used to pay for small expenditures such as supplies used in the office.

_____ 2. It is best if several people are responsible for the petty cash fund to reduce the chance of mistakes with the fund.

_____ 3. Reports generated from a computer billing system provide detail on the financial health of the practice.

_____ 4. It is common for a medical administrative assistant to have the sole responsibility of managing the financial operations of a medical practice.

_____ 5. A medical practice must be ready to accept cash, checks, or credit cards in payment of patients' account balances.

_____ 6. Because medical charges are billed directly to insurance companies, a medical office has no need to have cash on hand.

_____ 7. A receipt provides proof of payment on a patient's account.

_____ 8. A restrictive endorsement limits where a check can be deposited.

_____ 9. A negative balance on a patient's account is an amount that is owed to the practice.

_____ 10. NSF and returned checks should be subtracted from a patient's account balance.

_____ 11. All business records should be kept for a period of 5 years.

_____ 12. If a bank refuses to pay a check, this is known as a restrictive endorsement.

_____ 13. Reconciling a checking account ensures that the check register agrees with the bank's balance of a checking account.

_____ 14. Once a checking account has been reconciled and the check register agrees with the bank statement, the bank statement can be shredded.

_____ 15. A credit balance on an account may be applied to future charges on an account.

_____ 16. Patients living outside the vicinity of a medical practice may be expected to pay their bill on the date of an office visit because it may be difficult to collect a bill if it goes unpaid at a later date.

Exercise 13–2 CHAPTER CONCEPTS

Read the following statements or questions and choose the answer that best completes each statement or question. Record the answer in the blank provided.

_____ 1. Identifies profit earned over a period of time.
  (a) Transaction journal
  (b) Check register
  (c) Income statement
  (d) Balance sheet

_____ 2. Identifies the amount of assets, liabilities, and owners' equity of a medical practice.
  (a) Cash flow statement
  (b) Balance sheet
  (c) Check register
  (d) Accounts payable

_____ 3. Which of the following is not true about a petty cash account?
   (a) Petty cash is used to purchase small items for use in a medical office.
   (b) Receipts should be kept for petty cash expenditures.
   (c) A petty cash fund is different from a change fund.
   (d) Petty cash is normally used to cover expenditures of more than $100.

_____ 4. All of the following are true about writing checks except
   (a) Some practices may use computer-generated checks.
   (b) Checks should be used in numerical order.
   (c) When entering the amount on a check, care should be taken to eliminate the possibility of alteration of the amount.
   (d) Mistakes on a check can be crossed out with a single line and corrected with red ink.

_____ 5. All of the following can be found on a purchase order except
   (a) Name of vendor.
   (b) Listing of items purchased.
   (c) Balance of the account to which the purchase will be charged.
   (d) Name of person authorizing the purchase.

_____ 6. Accounts payable is an example of
   (a) An asset.
   (b) A liability.
   (c) Owners' equity.

_____ 7. Cash is an example of
   (a) An asset.
   (b) A liability.
   (c) Owners' equity.

_____ 8. Deposits to a practice's bank account should be made
   (a) When there is time.
   (b) Weekly.
   (c) Daily.
   (d) After each check is received.

_____ 9. Which of the following is not included on a receipt?
   (a) Date of the patient's visit.
   (b) Name of the person who made the payment.
   (c) Method of payment.
   (d) Name of person who received the payment.

_____ 10. All of the following are true about bookkeeping and accounting in a medical office except
   (a) An assistant can expect to play a supporting role in the financial management of a practice.
   (b) Computer systems can provide important financial data needed for planning in a matter of seconds.
   (c) An assistant should expect to be responsible for analyzing financial reports to plan for future expansion of a practice.
   (d) Office documents should be retained until applicable statutes of limitations have expired.

13

ACTIVITIES

ACTIVITY 13–1 Using the purchase order in Figure 13–6, identify the following:
- Vendor.
- Date of PO.
- How many different items are going to be purchased.
- Total amount of PO.

ACTIVITY 13–2 Research computer programs such as Peachtree Accounting and Quicken to determine what types of features are included in such a program.

ACTIVITY 13–3 Following Procedure Box 13–2, prepare the deposit slip here for the checks listed in Activity 13–9.

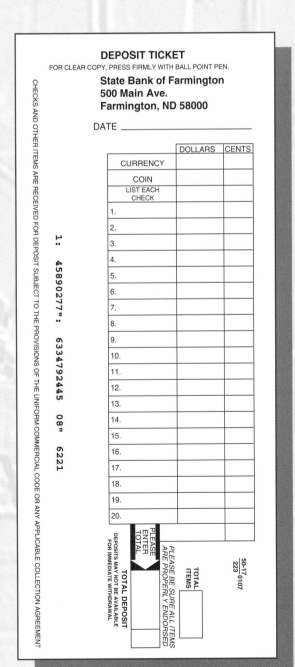

ACTIVITY 13–4 Reconcile a bank account using the check register and form here and the statement pictured in Figure 13–9.

Check Register

Number	Date	Description	Payment/debit	Ref	Deposit/credit	Balance
						9703.63
18270	10/19/02	Harmon Medical	3465.46	X		6238.17
18271	10/22/02	Acme Rental	789.00	X		5449.17
18272	10/22/02	Custodial Suppliers	46.72	X		5402.45
18273	10/24/02	Taylor Hudson	50.00	X		5352.45
18274	10/24/02	Bob Smith	340.00	X		5012.45
18275	10/25/02	Timothy Marks	493.47			4518.98
18276	10/25/02	GM Supply	50.00			4468.98
18277	10/30/02	Hearty Bakery	37.50			4431.48
18278	10/31/02	Palm Tree Inn	395.00			4036.48
18279	11/1/02	Lincoln Mutual	500.00			3536.48
	11/5/02	deposit			2305.46	5841.94
18280	11/5/02	BAP Printing	40.00			5801.94
18281	11/5/02	NT Phone Services	120.00			5681.94
18282	11/5/02	Custodial Suppliers	324.52			5357.42
18283	11/5/02	Office Suppliers Inc	35.50			5321.92
18284	11/6/02	Electric Co-op	335.00			4986.92
18285	11/7/02	Harmon Medical	890.56			4096.36
	11/8/02	deposit			456.38	4552.74
	11/9/02	deposit			235.90	4788.64
18286	11/12/02	TMI Leasing	1500.00			3288.64
18287	11/12/02	Mary Sanchez	573.00			2715.64
	11/15/02	deposit			4038.98	6754.62
18288	11/15/02	French Pharmaceuticals	234.34			6520.28
18289	11/15/02	Goodwin Oil	470.00			6050.28
18290	11/17/02	Payroll Account	3310.00			2740.28
18291	11/19/02	GM Supply	500.00			2240.28
18292	11/20/02	Hearty Bakery	39.46			2200.82
	11/21/02	deposit			2972.00	5172.82
18293	11/23/02	BAP Printing	100.00			5072.82
18294	11/23/02	ABC plumbing	109.78			4963.04
	11/28/02	deposit			339.06	5302.10
18295	11/28/02	Furniture Outlet Inc	50.00			5252.10
	11/29/02	deposit			585.00	5837.10
18296	11/29/02	Federated Delivery	23.00			5814.10
18297	11/29/02	Vision Security Services	420.00			5394.10
18298	11/29/02	United Supply	34.00			5360.10
18299	11/29/02	U S Postmaster	375.00			4985.10
18300	11/29/02	Custodial Suppliers	180.50			4804.60

X = check received

Bank reconciliation

Ending balance per statement $ _____

Plus deposits not included on statement   + _____

Subtotal $ _____

Minus outstanding checks   − _____

Total $ _____

ACTIVITY 13–5 Using the petty cash log pictured here, enter the following transactions to the log using Procedure Box 13–3 as a guide.

Petty Cash Log

Date	Description	Amount	Balance

Petty Cash Log

10-17-0x spent $3.52 for pens for the front office.

10-19-0x paid $1.21 for postage due.

10-23-0x purchased coffee and filters for employee lounge—$6.73.

10-24-0x purchased new surge protector for computer—$9.95.

10-26-0x paid $15.00 for cab fare for visiting physician.

On 10-26-0x, a check was written to replenish the petty cash fund to the original amount of $100. The amount of the check was $_____.

ACTIVITY 13-6 Write a receipt for each of the following payments:

1. On 10-19-02, Ann Walker paid $25.00 on her account (check #654).

Horizons Healthcare Center
123 Main Ave.
Farmington, ND 58000
(099) 555-1234

Receipt # _____
Date _____
Payment received from _____
For the account of _____ Acct # _____
In the amount of _____ $ _____
_____ Cash _____ Check (#_____) _____ Credit Card
Received by _____

2. On 10-09-02, Susan Pearson paid a $10.00 co-payment (in cash) for her office visit.

Horizons Healthcare Center
123 Main Ave.
Farmington, ND 58000
(099) 555-1234

Receipt # _____
Date _____
Payment received from _____
For the account of _____ Acct # _____
In the amount of _____ $ _____
_____ Cash _____ Check (#_____) _____ Credit Card
Received by _____

ACTIVITY 13–7 Following Procedure Box 13–4, prepare a check for check #18300 as listed in the check register in Activity 13–4.

```
┌────────────────────────────────────────────────────────────────┐
│ HORIZONS HEALTHCARE CENTER                              18300    │
│ 123 Main Avenue                                                  │
│ Farmington, ND 58000                                             │
│                                                                  │
│ PAY TO THE                              _____ 20 _____         │
│ ORDER OF_____  $ _____         │
│                                                                  │
│ _____  dollars               │
│                                                                  │
│ STATE BANK OF FARMINGTON                                         │
│ 500 Main Avenue                                                  │
│ Farmington, ND 58000                                             │
│                                                                  │
│ FOR _____      _____           │
│          : #####: ########:                                      │
└────────────────────────────────────────────────────────────────┘
```

ACTIVITY 13–8 Design a spreadsheet that would keep track of expenditures from a petty cash account. Enter the amounts identified in Figure 13–5 and add the expenses identified in Activity 13–5. The spreadsheet should automatically calculate the fund balance. Print two copies of the spreadsheet—one showing the amounts and the other showing the formulas used to calculate the amounts.

ACTIVITY 13–9 **PAYMENTS ON ACCOUNT**

Using Lytec Medical 2001, record the following payments on account. Instructions for recording a patient payment and insurance payment are given here. Follow the instructions to process all payments.

Posting Patient Payments

1. Open Lytec Medical 2001. At the main menu, click file, then *Horizons Healthcare Center.*
2. Click *Billing* then *Apply patient payment.*
3. Enter the appropriate information in the identified blanks.
   Patient or guarantor: Identify who made the payment. Click on the button before patient or guarantor, then select the appropriate name from the patient and guarantor list.
   Payment date: Date payment was received.
   Reference: Check number.
   Payment amount: The amount of the payment.
   Codes—Patient payment: Identify the patient's method of payment (cash, check, or credit card. For this exercise, all payments are checks.) PWO should be listed in the *Write off* box. (No amounts will be written off in this exercise.)
4. Click *Next* to move to the next screen.

5. Apply all payments at the billing level. Enter the amount of the payment to be applied in the *Apply* box pertaining to the bill. Click on the *Apply* box and type in the payment amount in the following format: 20.00. Press Enter key after amount is entered. If the patient is making a payment for more than one billing, enter the appropriate payment amount for each specific bill item. Keep applying amounts until the entire payment item has been applied. Note that the amount of the check appears in the upper portion of the window and the amount of the check that is unapplied also appears.

   NOTE: At any time during this process, the back button can be clicked to revert to previous screens and wipe out any mistakes.

6. After all of the check has been applied, click *Close* to post the payment to the account.

7. To post a new payment from a patient, begin again at Step 2.

Date payment received	Payer	Check reference #	Amount	Comments
11-30-02	Brian Stevens	#3247	$20.00	Partial payment for 10-08-02 charges for Evan Stevens
11-30-02	Jeanne Breckman	#4328	$25.00	Partial payment for 10-07-02 services
11-30-02	Ann Walker	#193	$25.00	Partial payment for 10-07-02 services

Posting Insurance Payments

1. Open Lytec Medical 2001. At the main menu, click file, then *Horizons Health-care Center*.

2. Click *Billing*, then *Apply insurance payment*.

3. Enter the appropriate information in the identified blanks.
   Payment date: Date payment was received.
   Reference: Check number.
   Check amount: The amount of the check.
   Chargebacks: Any amounts that were previously overpaid by the insurance company. (For the purposes of this exercise, there are no chargebacks.)
   The codes on the right of the window should appear automatically.

4. Click *Next* to move to the next screen.

5. Identify the patient by clicking on the magnifying glass next to the *Please select a patient* box.

6. Identify the insurance company that has sent the check by clicking the magnifying glass next to the *Please select an insurance* box.

7. Apply all payments at the billing level. Enter the amount of the payment to be applied in the *Apply* box pertaining to the bill. If the insurance company is making payments for more than one patient, click *Next* after you have applied the appropriate portion of the payment to the correct patient. Keep entering payment amounts until all patients have received credit for benefits paid. Note that the amount of the check appears in the upper right-hand corner of the window and that the amount of the check that is unapplied also appears.

   NOTE: At any time during this process, the back button can be clicked to revert to previous screens and wipe out any mistakes.

8. After all of the check has been applied, click *Close* to post the payment to all patients' accounts.

Date payment received	Payer	Check reference #	Amount	Comments
11-30-02	Medicare	#126583	$125.00	Payment in full for 10-08-02 charges for Marge Armstrong
11-30-02	Hert Inc.	#47586	$35.00	Payment in full for 10-07-02 charges for Tara Olson
11-30-02	Hert Inc.	#192845	$70.00	Payment in full for 10-07-02 charges for Kirsten French, 10-07-02 charges for Deanne Olson

ACTIVITY 13–10 *FINANCIAL REPORTS*

Open Lytec Medical 2001. At the main menu, click *Horizons Healthcare Center.* Follow the instructions listed to print the identified reports.

Patient Account Balances

1. Click *Reports,* then move down to *Patient,* then click *Patient balances.*
2. Click *Total balance* and *Greater than or equal to.*
3. In the *This amount* box, enter 0.01.
4. Click *Sort by name* in order to display the results alphabetically.
5. Click *Preview.* Patients with balances of greater than zero should be displayed.
6. Click the *Print* icon in the preview window.

Monthly Summary Report

1. Click *Reports,* then click *Monthly summary.*
2. In the *Month* and *Year* boxes, enter October and 2002.
3. Click *Preview.* The monthly summary for October 2002 should be displayed in the open window. If the display is correct, click the *Print* icon.

Practice Analysis

1. Click *Reports,* then click *Practice analysis.*
2. The box before *Subtotal by provider* should be checked.
3. Click *Preview.* The practice analysis should display in the open window. If the display is correct, click the *Print* icon.

Procedure Code Analysis

1. Click *Reports,* then click *Procedure code analysis.*
2. Remove the check in the box before *Subtotal by provider.*
3. Click *Preview.* The procedure code analysis should display in the open window. If the display is correct, click the *Print* icon.

Patient Ledger Balances

1. Click *Reports,* then move down to *Patient,* then click *Patient ledger.*
2. The following boxes should be checked: *Include paid billings; Show billing detail; Include transactions—active.*
3. The following buttons should be selected: *Amounts—debit/credit; Sort patients by—name; Reference—do not print references.*
4. Click *Preview.*
5. If the display appears correct, click the *Print* icon in the preview window.

13

DISCUSSION

The following topics can be used for class discussion or for individual student essay.

DISCUSSION 13–1 Read the quotation at the beginning of the chapter. What is the significance of this quotation?

DISCUSSION 13–2 Explain why it is important that the services of a financial professional, such as an accountant, be used to monitor the financial operations of a medical practice.

DISCUSSION 13–3 Explain how financial software can aid in financial planning for a medical practice.

CHAPTER OUTLINE

LEARNING OUTCOMES

On completing this chapter, the student will be able to

1. Describe a management style that can help create an efficient, yet effective office environment for patients.
2. Explain components of the employee selection process.
3. Explain policy and procedure manuals.
4. Prepare payroll.
5. Identify components of employee records.
6. Identify essentials of employee discipline and termination.
7. Describe labor laws and legal issues related to human resources.
8. Describe employee health issues.

RMA COMPETENCIES

1. Prepare employee payroll.
2. Maintain payroll tax deduction records, prepare employee tax forms, and prepare payroll tax deduction reports.
3. Know terminology pertaining to payroll and taxes.

VOCABULARY

employee compensation record
employer identification number (EIN)
empower, empowerment
human resources
job description
participatory management
performance review
policy manual
probationary period
procedure manual
sexual harassment

HUMAN RESOURCE MANAGEMENT

The first and perhaps greatest lesson I learned from the Mayos was that of teamwork. For "my brother and I" was no mere convenient term of reference, but rather the expression of a basic, indivisible philosophy of life.

—Harry Harwick, who worked 31 years with the Mayo brothers

Perhaps the most vital component in the operation of any organization is the people who are employed by or who represent the organization—the **human resources** of the organization. All staff members of a medical office are vital to a practice's success. No practice would function efficiently or effectively without all groups working together, complimenting one another's efforts. Creating a harmonious work environment in which all employees truly value and support each other is perhaps the greatest challenge for many managers, but such an environment promotes the growth and stability of the practice.

In this chapter, components of human resource management are introduced along with fundamental legal topics pertinent to human resource management. Even if an assistant is not employed as a manager, knowledge of human resource management helps an assistant recognize the various human resource components that enter into creating an optimal work environment in which all staff members work together to provide optimal service for all patients.

PARTICIPATORY MANAGEMENT STYLE

The atmosphere of the medical office is influenced by variables such as the size of the office staff, the facility itself, what type of patients are served, and the management style that is inherent in the operation of the office. Physicians and associated staff who manage the day-to-day operations of the office significantly influence the atmosphere of the office by the type of management style they use (Fig. 14–1). Management style is an integral part of a practice's success.

A common trend in management of employees today is to **empower** all employees to become involved with how

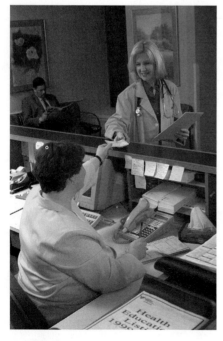

Figure 14–1. Management style greatly influences the environment of the medical office.

they contribute to the overall goals or mission of an organization. In a medical office, a typical mission statement would likely include a declaration about supporting one another as a team in providing the finest quality health care and service to all patients. A mission statement might appear as the following:

The mission of Horizons Healthcare Center is to provide an atmosphere of caring and compassion for all patients while offering state-of-the-art health care services. This is accomplished through the selection, hiring, and training of the best-qualified staff available.

To contribute to the mission, the input of staff members is gathered for organizational planning involving finances, staffing, and strategic planning. The front office staff members plan, organize, and perform their work to match the mission of the organization.

When **empowerment** is applied to a medical practice, all employees are given some degree of responsibility in achieving the mission within their area of expertise. To demonstrate how employees are empowered in a medical office, consider the following example:

All office staff members can be given a authority to organize and coordinate their work to meet the mission of the practice and to support the other work groups of the practice. The groups or departments within the practice collaborate with one another to determine staffing needs from the start to the end of the day.

The front office staff can provide feedback to meet the staffing needs of the physicians and other support staff. Of course, the staffing may have some budgeting constraints, but in general, the front office staff members in association with management can assist with decisions as to how the staffing needs will be met. They may work 8-hour days 5 days a week or 10-hour days 4 days a week, depending on which best meets the needs of the practice. The physicians or other management depend on the front office staff to meet the day-to-day scheduling needs of the practice, and they appreciate a smooth flow of operations that allows them to practice medicine and see patients.

The type of empowerment environment mentioned is usually well received by office staff. Many people, when given the chance, welcome the opportunity to decide what type of schedule works best for them. People, in general, appreciate opportunities to be in charge of their surroundings. There may be a few individuals who wish to be told what to do, but in an empowered environment, these individuals will be encouraged to join in the decision-making.

The concept of empowerment is present in what is frequently called a **participatory management** style (Box 14–1). This type of style works well in a medical office for the following reasons:

• A medical office is usually a very fast-paced environment, and empowering employees to make decisions allows employees to serve patients more efficiently.
• Empowered employees are happy employees, and a medical office with happy employees attracts and retains more patients.

Box 14-1 Characteristics of a Participatory Management Style

A manager
- Communicates openly and honestly.
- Is team oriented.
- Encourages employees to grow.
- Presents clear guidelines to let employees know what is expected of them.
- Recognizes quality work; gives staff credit and positive feedback.
- Informs employees what is expected of them.
- Does not have hidden agendas.
- Delegates work.
- Welcomes new ideas or suggestions from staff.
- Does not micromanage or make every decision.
- Is a mentor, role model, and leader.

- Employees who have input into the decisions of the medical office are more dedicated to the practice; thus, employee turnover is reduced.

Depending on the size of the organization, the front office staff may consist of one, several, or many assistants. If there are many assistants and a participatory management style is used, the management of the practice must identify individual positions, such as office manager or supervisor, to facilitate communication among the various groups of the organization and to define the delegation of duties and tasks. As both a supervisor and coordinator of office operations, the manager serves as a communication link among physicians, the front office staff, and other groups within the organization. When performing job duties, the office manager gathers input from the front office staff, yet he or she is ultimately responsible for making and implementing decisions that are consistent with the mission and goals of the organization.

Empowerment is a new trend and may not be the management style present in many offices around the country. Some offices may still have a management that is dictated from the top down. Some physicians or office managers may wish to make most of the decisions that affect their practice. If this is the case, an assistant must respect the wishes of the office's management. An assistant should always work for the good of the patients and the organization.

THE EMPLOYMENT PROCESS

Posting an Open Position

Suppose there is an opening in the office, and people in the office are commenting that the "right" person is needed to fill the position. What constitutes the "right" person? Of course, it is the person with the qualifications—education or experience (or both)—to fill the position. Any other requirements could cause the office to lose patients or to be sued.

When listing the necessary qualifications for a position, it is important to include only those items that are related to and necessary to perform the job. A **job description** identifies

what a person employed in a particular position will be required to do in that position (Fig. 14-2). A job description usually also identifies who supervises the position and the wage range for the position. The job description serves as the basis for the qualifications that are identified in an advertisement for a position.

Generally, objective criteria, or those items that can be measured, should be listed as qualifications for a position. Examples of these include a certain level of education (e.g., diploma, Associate's degree, Bachelor's degree), a certain type of skill or knowledge (e.g., typing, knowledge of medical terminology, billing and coding, proficiency using certain types of computer software), or a certain number of years of experience in a similar position in a medical office.

Subjective criteria, or soft skills, can be qualifications for a position, but these skills are often hard to measure. Soft skills are related to a person's attitude or behavior and include such attributes as motivation and enthusiasm, enjoying working with people, or being a team player.

The objective and subjective criteria listed for the position and application of the criteria when interviewing each candidate must be equal. For instance, when advertising an opening for a medical administrative assistant, objective criteria might include computer skill at a certain level, such as typing 45 words per minute, knowledge of a particular computer software, medical administrative assistant education or experience in a medical office, or both. The ability to lift 100 pounds or run a marathon would not be the qualifications

Horizons Healthcare Center Job Description

Position title: Medical Administrative Assistant

Reports to: Office Manager

Payroll rate: 10.36–14.32/hour

Responsibilities:

- maintain appointment schedule
- release medical records
- process telephone calls
- transcribe medical dictation
- maintain patient's registration/insurance information
- process patient billing
- prepare insurance claims

Revised: July 2001

Figure 14-2. A job description identifies responsibilities of a position.

Help Wanted – Health

Medical Administrative Assistant

Full-time opening in our family practice clinic working 8-5 Monday through Friday. Position requires excellent communication skills, medical transcription proficiency and knowledge of medical office procedures such as appointment scheduling, registration, billing, coding, and insurance. Applicants must possess a working knowledge of XYZ Office software.

Interested applicants should apply in person to Human Resources at Horizons Medical Center, 123 Main Ave, Farmington, ND 58000.

Figure 14–3. Employment openings in a medical office are advertised in a variety of locations.

necessary to perform the job and obviously could not be considered during the selection process.

Once the qualifications for a position have been determined, the position is advertised (Fig. 14–3) or published in a variety of sources. Openings can be posted within a medical office, state employment services, school placement services, Internet listings, employment agencies, newspapers, and even professional publications. Job postings should list deadlines by which resumés or applications should be submitted for consideration.

When the deadline for the position has passed, the resumés that have been submitted for consideration are reviewed. After applications or resumés from individuals interested in a position are received, candidates for interviewing can be selected from the applicants. If at all possible, a committee should be formed that will be involved in all aspects of the selection process. Using the committee selection process helps eliminate potential biases and future conflicts. Sometimes this is not possible, and the applicants are interviewed by only one individual. Whether a committee or an individual does the interviewing, there should always be more than one interview. A second interview insures proper selection of the most qualified candidate.

The committee or interviewer should establish a list of evaluation criteria necessary for the position and should assign points to each of the criteria. After all resumés are received, copies of each are evaluated by the committee members and points are assigned for each candidate's qualifications. Point assignments are totaled and reviewed by the committee. The candidates with the most points are invited to come to the office for an interview (Procedure Box 14–1).

The Interview

After the resumés have been reviewed and candidates selected for interviewing, appropriate questions must be selected for the interviews. It is of the utmost importance to keep the

questions related to the position available and to the person's qualifications for the position. Questions regarding marital status or whether or not the candidate owns a home or has a car to drive to work cannot be asked. Questions cannot be asked about a person's family or plans to have a family nor can questions be asked about a person's age, race, or religion. Such questions may bring a lawsuit for discrimination.

All applicants should be asked the same questions to allow each applicant the same interview opportunities and to assure that equal opportunity standards are being followed. Female applicants cannot be asked additional questions that may appear related to their gender, such as "Will you be able to make daycare arrangements for your children?" Instead of asking "Will children make it difficult to get to work at a certain hour?", ask the applicant if he or she will be able to work the designated hours for the job and if there is flexibility in case of office hours change or unexpected needs arise. Employers are allowed to ask such questions as "Will you be able to work flexible hours?" (if needed for the job) or "Will you have any problems getting to work?" All applicants, regardless of gender, race, age, or religion, should receive equal opportunity to respond to all questions and should not be discriminated against. Most interview questions should be centered around the applicant's ability to perform job requirements.

Questions for the interview should be prepared and a separate copy of the questions should be available for every

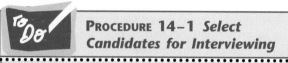

PROCEDURE 14–1 *Select Candidates for Interviewing*

Materials Needed
- Resumés or job applications
- Selection criteria
- Pen or pencil

1. If possible, form a committee that will be involved in all aspects of the selection process. Using the committee selection process helps eliminate potential biases and future conflicts. (Sometimes this is not possible, and the applicants will be interviewed by only one individual.) However, there should always be more than one interview. A second interview insures proper selection of the most qualified candidate.
2. The committee or interviewer should establish a list of criteria necessary for the position and assign points to each of those criteria.
3. After all resumés have been received, give copies of each resumé to each member on the committee.
4. Resumés are evaluated by each member and points are assigned for each candidate's qualifications.*
5. Point assignments are totaled and reviewed by the committee. The candidates with the most points are invited for an interview.

Denotes crucial step in procedure. Student must complete this step satisfactorily in order to complete the procedure satisfactorily.

interview. The interviewer can then refer to the sheet during the interview. Some interviewers choose to rate each candidate's answer on a scale, such as from 1 to 5, with 1 being poor or no answer and 5 being an excellent answer. At the end of all interviews, the interviewer can then add up the total points for each applicant. The applicant with the highest score should be the best candidate for the position (Fig. 14–4).

When possible, the top two or three candidates should be chosen for the position. References listed by each candidate are then checked. During a reference check, the previous employer is asked questions about when the applicant worked with the organization and what type of work was performed, as well as other questions related to the applicant's position, such as about production and attendance. Concerns about giving references are identified later in this chapter, and those concerns may influence the responses obtained during a reference check.

If the references support the selection of a top candidate, the interviewer should contact the top candidate and offer the position to that candidate. If the top candidate declines the offer (for whatever reason), the interviewer can offer the position to the next best qualified candidate, provided that candidate's references "check out." After the position has been accepted, the interviewer should notify all remaining candidates by telephone or mail to thank them for applying and to inform them that someone else has been selected for the position. Notification of all applicants helps maintain a positive public image for the practice.

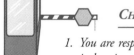

CHECKPOINT

1. *You are responsible for hiring an additional medical assistant to work in the office. A physician in the practice has asked you to find an older woman whose children are grown so that she will be able to stay late if necessary. How do you reply?*
2. *You are working for a pediatric practice. When hiring, the pediatricians have asked you to screen for an assistant who likes children. Would this be acceptable in an interview?*

Employee Training and Probationary Period

Once an employee is selected, orientation and training sessions are arranged to familiarize the employee with the specific expectations and operations of the office. Even if an employee has formal education in medical administrative assisting, each office has specific ways to perform tasks in the office. A training period allows the new employee to become familiar with specific office procedures. During this period, it is most beneficial if a new employee works alongside other members of the staff in addition to a senior employee. The senior employee may serve as a mentor, guiding the new employee in the philosophy, policies, and procedures of the organization. In addition, working alongside the other employees helps the new employee acclimate as a team member.

New employees are usually subject to a **probationary period,** which is a specific amount of time such as 90 days or 6 months in which the employee is working under a temporary employment arrangement. This is a "no strings attached" type of arrangement; shortly before the end of the probationary period, the employer meets with the employee and decides whether the employment arrangement should continue, and the employee evaluates whether or not to stay in the position permanently. This period gives both the employee and employer a chance to measure performance and observe if the employer/employee arrangement is compatible.

POLICY MANUALS

When an employee is newly hired, one of the first documents the employee receives is a **policy manual** detailing the practice's policies on various human resource–related topics.

Policy manuals, or employee handbooks, contain information on matters such as vacation, sick leave, personal leave, holidays, retirement plans, dress codes, and confidentiality (Box 14–2). Basically, anything an employee would want to know about working in an organization should be included in the policy manual. The manual may apply to all employees in the organization or just a specific group of employees. In large organizations, it is common to have a separate policy manual for professional staff such as physicians and executive staff. Because they may be under a contractual arrangement with the organization, different standards may be established as a condition of their employment.

Box 14–2 Sample of Policy Manual Components

The following topics are usually found in a policy manual or employee handbook. This list is not inclusive.
- Payroll periods.
- Performance reviews.
- Work schedule.
- Overtime.
- Dress code.
- Absence from work.
- Sick leave.
- Maternity/paternity leave.
- Vacation leave.
- Holiday pay.
- Religious holidays.
- Bereavement leave.
- Jury/legal leave.
- Military leave.
- Educational leave.
- Health insurance.
- Dental insurance.
- Life insurance.
- Retirement plans.
- Work-related injuries and OSHA requirements.
- Confidentiality.
- Employee reprimand.
- Employee dismissal.

SUMMARY OF EVALUATION	
POINTS FROM APPLICATION AND INTERVIEW	
POINTS FROM REFERENCES	
TOTAL POINTS	
OVERALL IMPRESSION	

INTERVIEW EVALUATION AND REFERENCE INVESTIGATION FORM, MEDICAL or DENTAL OFFICE

NAME OF APPLICANT

DATE

RATING: GOOD - 2 POINTS FAIR - 1 POINT POOR - 0 POINTS

POSITION APPLIED FOR:

FROM APPLICATION FOR POSITION, GAUGE APPLICANT IN FOLLOWING AREAS	GOOD	FAIR	POOR
1. STABILITY (REMAINED IN ONE PLACE OF RESIDENCE AND ONE JOB FOR A REASONABLE LENGTH OF TIME)?			
2. HEALTH?			
3. THE PROPER EDUCATIONAL BACKGROUND TO FILL THE POSITION?			
4. LEGIBLE HANDWRITING?			
5. AN EMPLOYMENT HISTORY THAT POINTS TOWARD DEPENDABILITY?			
6. LIMITATION ON WORKING HOURS?			
7. THE PROPER EXPERIENCE AND / OR SKILLS TO FILL THE POSITION?			
8. SALARY REQUIREMENT COMMENSURATE WITH POSITION?			
FROM THE PERSONAL INTERVIEW - (SHOULD BE SPECIFIC QUALITIES - OBJECTIVE)			
9. SUFFICIENT CAPABILITY TO HANDLE ANY SITUATION THAT MAY ARISE WHEN ALONE IN OFFICE?			
10. AN APPROPRIATE ATTITUDE TOWARD WORK?			
11. AN APPROPRIATE VOICE, DICTION, GRAMMAR?			
12. POISE?			
13. SELF CONFIDENCE (NOT OVER-CONFIDENCE)?			
14. TACT?			
15. SUFFICIENT MATURITY FOR JOB?			
16. AN ABILITY TO EXPRESS ONESELF WELL?			
17. AN INITIATIVE OR INTEREST IN LEARNING?			
18. ABILITY TO WORK WITH OTHERS IN OFFICE?			
19. APPROPRIATE APPEARANCE (NEAT, CLEAN; SUITABLE TO BUSINESS)?			
20. ENERGY, VITALITY, AND PERCEIVED ABILITY TO HANDLE PRESSURE OF POSITION?			
21. EAGERNESS TO OBTAIN THE POSITION IN QUESTION?			
COLUMNAR TOTALS			
GRAND TOTAL			

DIRECTIONS FOR USE OF FORM:
1. Look over your ratings. A zero score on any one VITAL question should automatically eliminate applicant. Add up the total rating points and enter in the SUMMARY OF EVALUATION BLOCK in the upper right-hand corner of this page.
2. After finishing all interviews, choose the "best bets" and check their references using the reverse side of this form.
3. Enter, as above, the results of your reference check and then your overall impression. (E - Excellent, G - Good, F - Fair, P - Poor)

ORDER # 72-120 • BIBBERO SYSTEMS, INC. • PETALUMA, CA.
TO REORDER CALL TOLL FREE: (800) BIBBERO (800-242-2376) OR FAX (800) 242-9330   M FG IN U.S.A.   (PLEASE TURN OVER)

Figure 14–4. An interview form helps objectively identify the best candidates for an office position. (Form courtesy of Bibbero Systems, Inc., Petaluma, California, 800-242-2376. Fax 800-242-9330. www.bibbero.com)

NOTES:

REFERENCE INVESTIGATION

1. OFFICE CONTACTED   PHONE: (   )   DATE

PERSON CONTACTED

HOW LONG HAVE YOU KNOWN THIS PERSON ?

BETWEEN WHAT DATES WAS THIS PERSON EMPLOYED BY YOU?   FROM   TO

WHAT TYPE OF WORK DID THIS PERSON DO FOR YOU?   TITLE OF POSITION: SATISFACTORILY?

WAS THIS PERSON CONSISTENTLY COOPERATIVE?   WHAT WERE SHORTCOMINGS?

DID THIS PERSON GET ALONG WELL WITH OTHERS?

WAS THIS PERSON TRUSTWORTHY / DEPENDABLE?   ATTENDANCE RECORD:

WHY DID THIS PERSON LEAVE YOUR EMPLOY?   SALARY LEVEL:

WOULD YOU REHIRE THIS PERSON?

NOTES:

RATING:

2. OFFICE CONTACTED   PHONE: (   )   DATE

PERSON CONTACTED

HOW LONG HAVE YOU KNOWN THIS PERSON ?

BETWEEN WHAT DATES WAS THIS PERSON EMPLOYED BY YOU?   FROM   TO

WHAT TYPE OF WORK DID THIS PERSON DO FOR YOU?   TITLE OF POSITION: SATISFACTORILY?

WAS THIS PERSON CONSISTENTLY COOPERATIVE?   WHAT WERE SHORTCOMINGS?

DID THIS PERSON GET ALONG WELL WITH OTHERS?

WAS THIS PERSON TRUSTWORTHY / DEPENDABLE?   ATTENDANCE RECORD:

WHY DID THIS PERSON LEAVE YOUR EMPLOY?   SALARY LEVEL:

WOULD YOU REHIRE THIS PERSON?

NOTES:

RATING:

3. OFFICE CONTACTED   PHONE: (   )   DATE

PERSON CONTACTED

HOW LONG HAVE YOU KNOWN THIS PERSON ?

BETWEEN WHAT DATES WAS THIS PERSON EMPLOYED BY YOU?   FROM   TO

WHAT TYPE OF WORK DID THIS PERSON DO FOR YOU?   TITLE OF POSITION: SATISFACTORILY?

WAS THIS PERSON CONSISTENTLY COOPERATIVE?   WHAT WERE SHORTCOMINGS?

DID THIS PERSON GET ALONG WELL WITH OTHERS?

WAS THIS PERSON TRUSTWORTHY / DEPENDABLE?   ATTENDANCE RECORD:

WHY DID THIS PERSON LEAVE YOUR EMPLOY?   SALARY LEVEL:

WOULD YOU REHIRE THIS PERSON?

NOTES:

RATING:

INTERVIEWER _____   DATE: _____

Figure 14–4. *Continued*

Box 14-3 Sample Dress Code for Office Staff

1. Clothing must be clean and pressed.
2. A name tag must be worn at all times while on duty.
3. Hosiery must be worn at all times.
4. Hair should be neat and trimmed.
5. Perfume or cologne is not allowed because patients and other employees may be sensitive.
6. Tennis shoes may be worn only with uniforms.
7. Use of cosmetics and jewelry should be conservative.
8. Crop top, tank top, backless, or low-cut apparel is not acceptable.
9. Shorts of any kind are not allowed.
10. Jeans (any color) are not allowed.

Employees in violation of the dress code will be asked to leave and to remedy the situation on their own time.

The items included in a policy manual detail the organization's guidelines or rules on certain behavior or actions. A sample policy regarding sick leave might appear as follows:

Employees shall be granted 40 hours of sick leave on the day employment begins. For every 80 hours worked, the employee shall earn an additional 4 hours of sick leave. Employees may accumulate sick leave to a maximum of 800 hours.

Sick leave may be used for personal illness or injury; illness or injury of employee's dependent, spouse, or parent; or medical or dental appointments of the employee, employee's dependent, spouse, or parent. Sick leave used for medical and dental appointments may be used in 1-hour increments. Sick leave used for other reasons is used in half-day increments.

Sick leave may be used in accordance with the Family and Medical Leave Act.

A dress code is often developed to ensure that standards of professional dress are established and followed. Dress codes may vary for different positions within an organization. Office staff may have a certain dress code, and the clinical staff may have another. An example of a dress code for office staff is included in Box 14–3.

PROCEDURE MANUALS

What is the standard procedure for business activities in the medical office? Just as this text details procedures on how the medical administrative assistant would accomplish a given task, a **procedure manual** gives specific instructions for procedures, guidelines, and protocols in a medical office. A procedure manual can be developed with input from all staff members. The manual can include existing procedures, and new procedures can be added as they are incorporated into the office activities. A procedure manual serves as a guide to both new and established employees.

PAYROLL

Payroll is a major responsibility of individuals responsible for human resource management. Processing of payroll can be quite an involved process. There are many components in payroll processing: gathering salary and withholding information for each employee; calculating the amount due each pay period; and depositing, reporting, and paying payroll taxes and other withholding amounts (Procedure Box 14–2).

The practice determines at what intervals payroll processing will be done. Employees may be paid on a weekly, biweekly, bimonthly, or monthly basis.

PROCEDURE 14–2 *Prepare Payroll*

Materials Needed
- Time cards
- Tax tables or percentages
- Calculator

1. Calculate wages earned by multiplying hours worked by hourly rate. If the employee has worked overtime, the overtime hours worked will be multiplied by 1.5 times the employee's hourly rate.*
2. Enter the total wages earned for the period in the gross (earnings) column.*
3. Enter Social Security and Medicare tax in the FICA column. Refer to the employee's form W-4 to obtain his or her marital status and withholding allowances. Note any additional amount the employee wishes to have withheld.*
4. Determine the amount of federal tax to be withheld by referring to the employee's wages and withholding allowance amounts. Enter the federal income tax in the FWT column.*
5. Determine the amount of state tax to be withheld by referring to the employee's wages and withholding allowance amounts. Enter the state tax in the SWT column.*
6. Enter the total of other deductions in another column or in columns on the right.*
7. To figure the employee's net earnings, subtract the total deductions from their gross earnings.*
8. Enter the payroll amounts in the employee compensation record.*
9. Prepare payroll checks listing all payroll amounts in the check summary on the right.*

*Denotes crucial step in procedure. Student must complete this step satisfactorily in order to complete the procedure satisfactorily.

Computerized software can be used to calculate payroll and generate payroll checks. This type of software tracks all employee data related to payroll and can oftentimes be used to predict turnover. Payroll software can be a timesaver when completing the various reports that are required for payroll purposes. Some small offices choose to hire an outside payroll service that eliminates many tax issues and problems because payroll services are done by experts.

Time Cards

Depending on the employment arrangements of the medical office staff, time cards (Fig. 14–5) may be used to account for the hours a staff member works. The time card is inserted into a time clock and imprinted with the correct time and date. Some larger organizations are now tracking employee hours electronically. Employees may be issued a name badge with a magnetic strip on the reverse of the badge. The employee swipes the badge through an electronic time clock that will record when the employee enters and leaves the office.

Smaller practices with few employees may decide to forgo the use of a time clock. Practices in which the same people work every day, all day long, may decide not to use a time clock to track hours. When a time clock is not used, work hours may be written by the employee on a time card.

In the example pictured in Figure 14–5, the employee either punches a time clock or writes in the time next to the corresponding date of the month. The reverse of the card contains boxes for the 8th to the 15th and the 24th to the 31st of the month. This type of card works well for a 2-week or bimonthly pay period. The employee or supervisor totals the hours worked for each day and enters the total in the left-hand column of the card. At the end of the week, the total hours worked for that week are written on the time card. The time card then serves to document the hours worked when payroll is calculated.

All employees should be taught how to complete a time card. Cards should be filled out consistently, using the same formats for numbers. A half hour is usually documented using .50 instead of 1/2 because .50 is the format in which a half hour is entered into a computer. Using consistent numbering helps eliminate potential mistakes.

Employee Compensation Record

At the end of each payroll period, every employee is paid wages earned during that period. Employees may be paid an hourly wage or a salary. At an hourly wage, the employee's hourly rate is multiplied by the number of hours worked in the pay period. Overtime hours, usually those hours worked in excess of 8 hours per day or 40 hours per week, are usually paid at 1.5 times the hourly rate.

A salaried employee is paid a specific amount each pay period. Salaried employees usually are not paid overtime and may not even be required to punch a time clock.

The **employee compensation record** (Fig. 14–6) keeps the payroll data for each individual employee. Amounts paid and deducted from each check as well as year-to-date totals are available on this record. At the end of the year, this record provides documentation to prepare a form W-2 for the employee.

Payroll Deductions

Many deductions are subtracted from an employee's paycheck. Some deductions are mandatory; some are optional. Federal and state income taxes and Social Security and Medicare taxes are mandatory (with very few exceptions). Optional deductions may include premiums for health or dental insurance (or both), retirement contributions, and even deductions for medical or child care expenses (see Fig. 14–6).

Some employers offer pre-tax plans for employees who have medical or child care expenses. Pre-tax plans can save money for an employee. With a pre-tax arrangement, health and dental insurance premiums, child care, or other medical expenses may be deducted from the gross salary. For medical and child care expenses, employees enroll in a pre-tax plan and specify the amount they want subtracted from each paycheck (throughout the year) for those expenses. Taxes are then computed on the amount left after the pretax deductions. To be reimbursed for the amounts withheld from each paycheck, the employee must submit a written request or claim with receipts for the expenses to a plan administrator. A separate check for the claim is then written from the plan to the employee.

Premiums for health, dental, and life insurance may be all or partly the employee's responsibility. Employees may also have the option to make retirement contributions in addition to what their employer may provide. These deductions should be detailed on the employee's paycheck and listed on the employee's compensation record (Fig. 14–7; see Fig. 14–6).

Occasionally, an employee may have court-ordered deductions subtracted from each paycheck. This practice is known as garnishing wages and is not optional for an employee. Wages may be garnished for child support payments to ensure that the money is given to a child.

Payroll Taxes

Employers must withhold federal income tax, state income tax (if any), social security tax, and Medicare tax from employee paychecks. There are few exceptions to this requirement. Under special circumstances, some people may be exempt from federal income tax withholding. Otherwise, employers are required to withhold taxes and pay appropriate taxes for all employees of an organization. An individual is deemed to be an employee if the employer controls what work will be done and how it will be done.

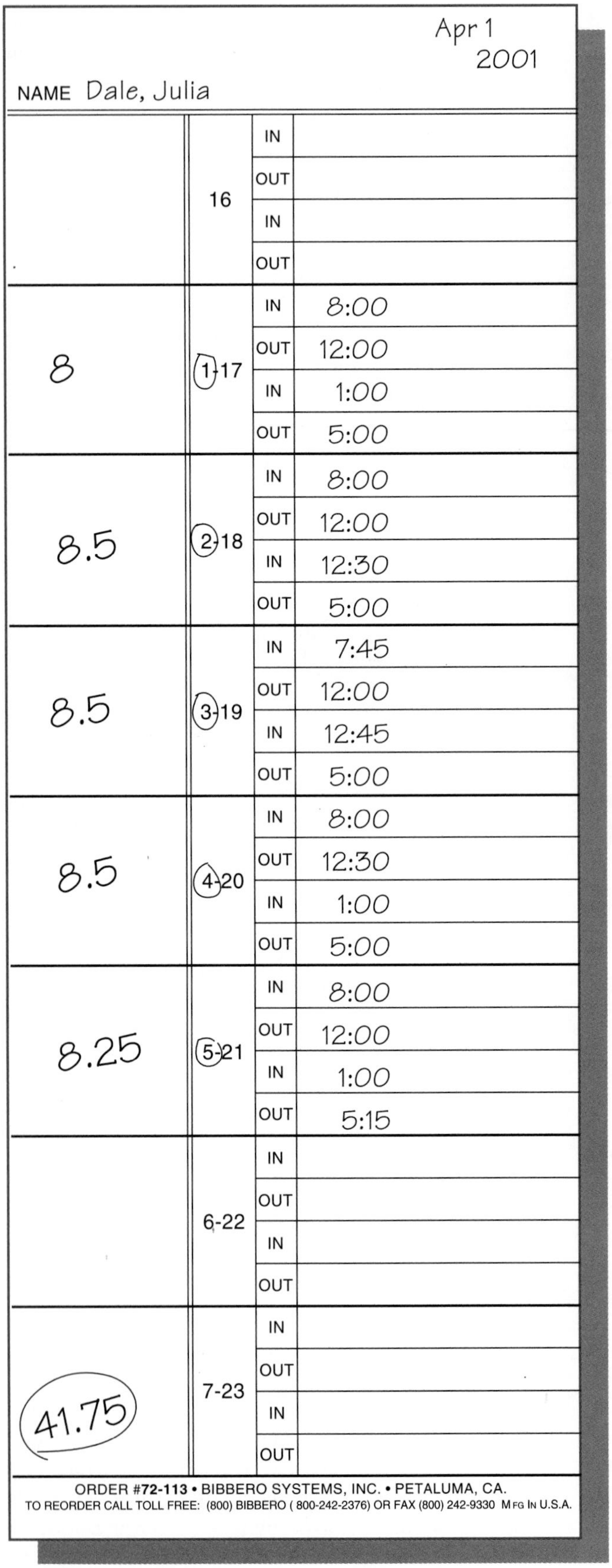

		Apr 1		
		2001		
NAME Dale, Julia				

	16	IN	
		OUT	
		IN	
		OUT	
8	(1) 17	IN	8:00
		OUT	12:00
		IN	1:00
		OUT	5:00
8.5	(2) 18	IN	8:00
		OUT	12:00
		IN	12:30
		OUT	5:00
8.5	(3) 19	IN	7:45
		OUT	12:00
		IN	12:45
		OUT	5:00
8.5	(4) 20	IN	8:00
		OUT	12:30
		IN	1:00
		OUT	5:00
8.25	(5) 21	IN	8:00
		OUT	12:00
		IN	1:00
		OUT	5:15
	6-22	IN	
		OUT	
		IN	
		OUT	
(41.75)	7-23	IN	
		OUT	
		IN	
		OUT	

ORDER #72-113 • BIBBERO SYSTEMS, INC. • PETALUMA, CA.
TO REORDER CALL TOLL FREE: (800) BIBBERO (800-242-2376) OR FAX (800) 242-9330 M FG In U.S.A.

Figure 14–5. Time cards are used to document an employee's hours worked. (Form courtesy of Bibbero Systems, Inc., Petaluma, California, 800-242-2376. Fax 800-242-9330. www.bibbero.com)

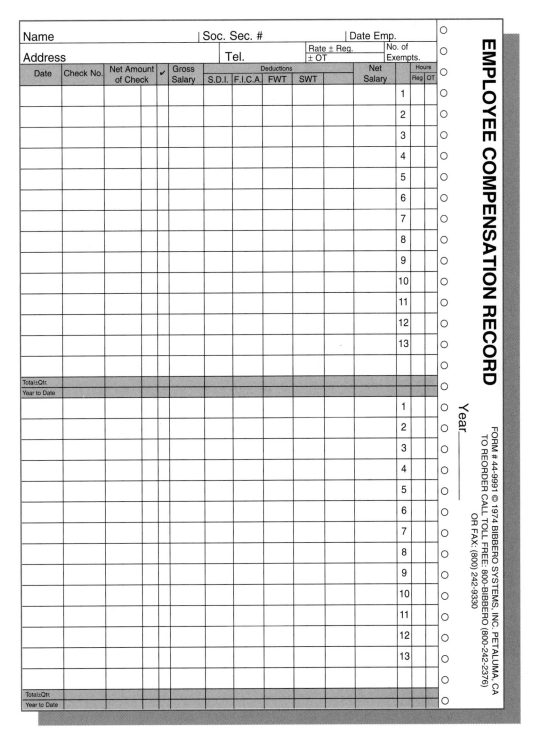

Figure 14–6. A compensation record tracks an employee's earnings. (Form courtesy of Bibbero Systems, Inc., Petaluma, California, 800-242-2376. Fax 800-242-9330. www.bibbero.com)

Federal Income Tax

All wages paid to employees are subject to federal income tax. Wages may be cash or other compensation, such as daycare assistance, stock options, bonuses, or educational assistance. The amount of tax on wages earned is determined by the amount of wages the employee earned during that specific payroll period and the information the employee has provided on the form W-4. The tax due is calculated by using the tax table applicable to the length of the payroll period. Tables for single or married individuals in a biweekly payroll are shown in Figure 14–8. If an employer's payroll period is every 2 weeks, the employer uses the tax table for a biweekly payroll period, looking up the amount of wages earned and the number of exemptions listed. Even if an employee does not work the entire payroll period, the employer should use the table for the established length of the payroll period.

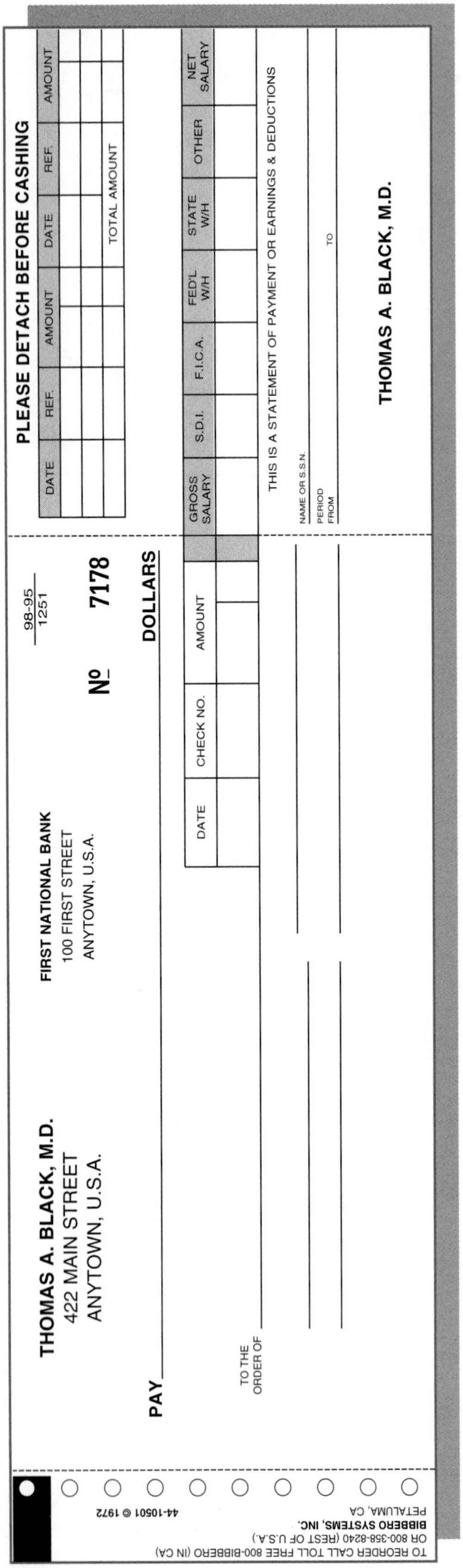
THOMAS A. BLACK, M.D.
422 MAIN STREET
ANYTOWN, U.S.A.

FIRST NATIONAL BANK
100 FIRST STREET
ANYTOWN, U.S.A.

98-95/1251

№ 7178

PAY ______ DOLLARS

TO THE ORDER OF

DATE	CHECK NO.	AMOUNT

THOMAS A. BLACK, M.D.

PLEASE DETACH BEFORE CASHING

DATE	REF.	AMOUNT	DATE	REF.	AMOUNT
			TOTAL AMOUNT		

GROSS SALARY	S.D.I.	F.I.C.A.	FED'L W/H	STATE W/H	OTHER	NET SALARY

THIS IS A STATEMENT OF PAYMENT OR EARNINGS & DEDUCTIONS

NAME OR S.S.N.

PERIOD FROM ______ TO ______

TO REORDER CALL TOLL FREE 800-BIBBERO (IN CA) OR 800-358-8240 (REST OF U.S.A.)
BIBBERO SYSTEMS, INC.
PETALUMA, CA

44-10501 © 1972

Figure 14–7. Every payroll check identifies the earnings and deductions for an employee. (Form courtesy of Bibbero Systems, Inc., Petaluma, California, 800-242-2376. Fax 800-242-9330. www.bibbero.com)

Form W-4

All new employees should be asked to complete a form W-4 (Fig. 14–9) when they begin work. The W-4 identifies the employee's name, address, social security number, and marital status, as well as the number of exemptions he or she wishes to take for tax purposes. A personal allowances worksheet is available at the top of form W-4 to help the employee determine the number of exemptions that should be claimed. If an employee is married, an allowance cannot be claimed if the allowance is already claimed by the employee's spouse. The more exemptions an employee claims, the less tax will be withheld from the employee's paycheck.

Employees should take only those exemptions to which they are entitled, or they may be underwithheld and owe significant tax at the end of the year. If an employee is grossly underwithheld, a penalty may be assessed to the employee for failure to pay enough tax. Employees may wish to claim fewer exemptions than those to which they are entitled to ensure that they have enough tax withheld throughout the year. If an employee believes he or she will owe significant tax at the end of the year, the employee may authorize additional tax to be withheld, as listed on line 6 of form W-4.

If an employee wishes to change the amount of tax withholding, the employee is required to complete a new form W-4. The new W-4 does not take effect until the date the employee lists on the form.

A form W-4 must be signed by an employee in order to be valid. The language on a form W-4 may not be altered by an employee. If an employee fails to turn in a form W-4, if the form is altered or if it is otherwise not completed correctly, taxes should be withheld as though the employee were single with no dependents—this would be withholding at the highest rate possible.

FICA Tax

The Federal Insurance Contributions Act (FICA) includes provisions for Social Security tax and Medicare tax. Employees must pay these taxes, and an employer must match an employee's contribution. Tax rates and wages limits are identified in Figure 14–10. Using the amounts shown in Figure 14–10, employees who earn more than $76,200 in one calendar year would not have Social Security tax withheld on any earned amounts more than $76,200, although Medicare tax would still be owed on all wages earned for that calendar year.

State Income Tax

Depending on the state in which the employee works or resides, state income tax may also be required to be withheld from an employee's wages. Employees who reside in a different state from the one in which they work may need to file an exemption from tax in the employer's state. Depending on arrangements between neighboring states, employers may be able to withhold taxes from other states for employees who reside out of state. A few states do not have any state income tax.

SINGLE Persons—BIWEEKLY Payroll Period
(For Wages Paid in July–Dec 2001)

If the wages are—		And the number of withholding allowances claimed is—										
At least	But less than	0	1	2	3	4	5	6	7	8	9	10
		The amount of income tax to be withheld is—										
$400	$410	45	29	12	0	0	0	0	0	0	0	0
410	420	47	30	14	0	0	0	0	0	0	0	0
420	430	48	32	15	0	0	0	0	0	0	0	0
430	440	50	33	17	0	0	0	0	0	0	0	0
440	450	51	35	18	1	0	0	0	0	0	0	0
450	460	53	36	20	3	0	0	0	0	0	0	0
460	470	54	38	21	4	0	0	0	0	0	0	0
470	480	56	39	23	6	0	0	0	0	0	0	0
480	490	57	41	24	7	0	0	0	0	0	0	0
490	500	59	42	26	9	0	0	0	0	0	0	0

A

MARRIED Persons—BIWEEKLY Payroll Period
(For Wages Paid in July–Dec 2001)

If the wages are—		And the number of withholding allowances claimed is—										
At least	But less than	0	1	2	3	4	5	6	7	8	9	10
		The amount of income tax to be withheld is—										
$390	$400	22	5	0	0	0	0	0	0	0	0	0
400	410	24	7	0	0	0	0	0	0	0	0	0
410	420	25	8	0	0	0	0	0	0	0	0	0
420	430	27	10	0	0	0	0	0	0	0	0	0
430	440	28	11	0	0	0	0	0	0	0	0	0
440	450	30	13	0	0	0	0	0	0	0	0	0
450	460	31	14	0	0	0	0	0	0	0	0	0
460	470	33	16	0	0	0	0	0	0	0	0	0
470	480	34	17	1	0	0	0	0	0	0	0	0
480	490	36	19	2	0	0	0	0	0	0	0	0

B

Figure 14–8. Sample of tax tables for a biweekly payroll. *A,* Single persons. *B,* Married persons. (From Department of the Treasury, Internal Revenue Service, Washington, DC, 2001.)

Tax Reports and Deposits

All employers are required to file tax reports to the government and to make deposits for payroll taxes withheld. Each employer is assigned a unique **employer identification number** (EIN) to use when reporting employment taxes or when giving tax statements to employees. This number is used to identify the tax account of the employer. An EIN is a nine-digit number (00-0000000) issued by the Internal Revenue Service (IRS).

Employers are required to deposit the employee's and employer's portion of income tax, Social Security, and Medicare tax either monthly or semimonthly. The deposit schedule is determined by the amount of taxes previously reported by the employer in a four-quarter lookback period. Employers are required to deposit all of the taxes owed on or before the deposit due date. Depending on the amount of taxes owed, deposits can be made by using deposit coupons or by means of electronic deposit.

Form 941, Employer's Quarterly Federal Tax Return (Fig. 14–11), and Form 941-V are used when reporting and depositing taxes owed. All employers (with a few exceptions) are required to file Form 941. Employers should file only one Form 941 per quarter and should include only one quarter of wages on a return. Employers who fail to pay all of the tax due will face a penalty.

Federal Unemployment Tax

Employees who lose their jobs are often paid unemployment compensation that is funded in part by the federal unemployment (FUTA) tax. Employers, not employees, pay FUTA tax. Generally, employers are required to pay FUTA tax if they pay more than $1500 in wages to nonfarm or nonhousehold employees. In 2000, the FUTA tax rate was 6.2% of the first $7000 in wages paid to each employee during the year. The employer may also be required to pay

Form W-4 (2001)

Purpose. Complete Form W-4 so your employer can withhold the correct Federal income tax from your pay. Because your tax situation may change, you may want to refigure your withholding each year.

Exemption from withholding. If you are exempt, complete only lines 1, 2, 3, 4, and 7, and sign the form to validate it. Your exemption for 2001 expires February 18, 2002.

Note: *You cannot claim exemption from withholding if (1) your income exceeds $750 and includes more than $250 of unearned income (e.g., interest and dividends) and (2) another person can claim you as a dependent on their tax return.*

Basic instructions. If you are not exempt, complete the **Personal Allowances Worksheet** below. The worksheets on page 2 adjust your withholding allowances based on itemized deductions, certain credits, adjustments to income, or two-earner/two-job situations. Complete all worksheets that apply. They will help you figure the number of withholding allowances you are entitled to claim. **However, you may claim fewer (or zero) allowances.**

Head of household. Generally, you may claim head of household filing status on your tax return only if you are unmarried and pay more than 50% of the costs of keeping up a home for yourself and your dependent(s) or other qualifying individuals. See line **E** below.

Tax credits. You can take projected tax credits into account in figuring your allowable number of withholding allowances. Credits for child or dependent care expenses and the child tax credit may be claimed using the **Personal Allowances Worksheet** below. See **Pub. 919,** How Do I Adjust My Tax Withholding? for information on converting your other credits into withholding allowances.

Nonwage income. If you have a large amount of nonwage income, such as interest or dividends, consider making estimated tax payments using **Form 1040-ES,** Estimated Tax for Individuals. Otherwise, you may owe additional tax.

Two earners/two jobs. If you have a working spouse or more than one job, figure the total number of allowances you are entitled to claim on all jobs using worksheets from only one Form W-4. Your withholding usually will be most accurate when all allowances are claimed on the Form W-4 for the highest paying job and zero allowances are claimed on the others.

Check your withholding. After your Form W-4 takes effect, use Pub. 919 to see how the dollar amount you are having withheld compares to your projected total tax for 2001. Get Pub. 919 especially if you used the **Two-Earner/Two-Job Worksheet** on page 2 and your earnings exceed $150,000 (Single) or $200,000 (Married).

Recent name change? If your name on line 1 differs from that shown on your social security card, call 1-800-772-1213 for a new social security card.

Personal Allowances Worksheet (Keep for your records.)

A Enter "1" for **yourself** if no one else can claim you as a dependent . . . . **A** _____

B Enter "1" if:
- You are single and have only one job; or
- You are married, have only one job, and your spouse does not work; or
- Your wages from a second job or your spouse's wages (or the total of both) are $1,000 or less.

. . **B** _____

C Enter "1" for your **spouse.** But, you may choose to enter -0- if you are married and have either a working spouse or more than one job. (Entering -0- may help you avoid having too little tax withheld.) . . . . **C** _____

D Enter number of **dependents** (other than your spouse or yourself) you will claim on your tax return . . . . **D** _____

E Enter "1" if you will file as **head of household** on your tax return (see conditions under **Head of household** above) . **E** _____

F Enter "1" if you have at least $1,500 of **child or dependent care expenses** for which you plan to claim a credit . . **F** _____

    (**Note:** *Do not include child support payments. See **Pub. 503,** Child and Dependent Care Expenses, for details.*)

G **Child Tax Credit** (including additional child tax credit):
- If your total income will be between $18,000 and $50,000 ($23,000 and $63,000 if married), enter "1" for each eligible child.
- If your total income will be between $50,000 and $80,000 ($63,000 and $115,000 if married), enter "1" if you have two eligible children, enter "2" if you have three or four eligible children, or enter "3" if you have five or more eligible children. **G** _____

H Add lines A through G and enter total here. (**Note:** *This may be different from the number of exemptions you claim on your tax return.*) ▶ **H** _____

For accuracy, complete all worksheets that apply.
- If you plan to **itemize or claim adjustments to income** and want to reduce your withholding, see the **Deductions and Adjustments Worksheet** on page 2.
- If you are **single,** have **more than one job** and your combined earnings from all jobs exceed $35,000, **or** if you are **married** and have a **working spouse or more than one job** and the combined earnings from all jobs exceed $60,000, see the **Two-Earner/Two-Job Worksheet** on page 2 to avoid having too little tax withheld.
- If **neither** of the above situations applies, **stop here** and enter the number from line H on line 5 of Form W-4 below.

---------- **Cut here and give Form W-4 to your employer. Keep the top part for your records.** ----------

Form W-4

Department of the Treasury
Internal Revenue Service

Employee's Withholding Allowance Certificate

▶ **For Privacy Act and Paperwork Reduction Act Notice, see page 2.**

OMB No. 1545-0010

2001

1	Type or print your first name and middle initial Last name		2 Your social security number

Home address (number and street or rural route)	**3** ☐ Single ☐ Married ☐ Married, but withhold at higher Single rate.

    Note: If married, but legally separated, or spouse is a nonresident alien, check the Single box.

City or town, state, and ZIP code	**4** If your last name differs from that on your social security card, check here. You must call 1-800-772-1213 for a new card. ▶ ☐

5 Total number of allowances you are claiming (from line **H** above **or** from the applicable worksheet on page 2)   **5** _____

6 Additional amount, if any, you want withheld from each paycheck . . . . **6** $ _____

7 I claim exemption from withholding for 2001, and I certify that I meet **both** of the following conditions for exemption:
- Last year I had a right to a refund of **all** Federal income tax withheld because I had **no** tax liability **and**
- This year I expect a refund of **all** Federal income tax withheld because I expect to have **no** tax liability.

If you meet both conditions, write "Exempt" here . . . . ▶ **7** _____

Under penalties of perjury, I certify that I am entitled to the number of withholding allowances claimed on this certificate, or I am entitled to claim exempt status.

Employee's signature
(Form is not valid
unless you sign it.) ▶

Date ▶

8 Employer's name and address (Employer: Complete lines 8 and 10 only if sending to the IRS.)	9 Office code (optional)	10 Employer identification number

Cat. No. 10220Q

Figure 14–9. Form W-4 identifies an employee's exemptions for tax purposes. (From Department of the Treasury, Internal Revenue Service, Washington, DC, 2001.)

Deductions and Adjustments Worksheet

Note: *Use this worksheet only if you plan to itemize deductions, claim certain credits, or claim adjustments to income on your 2001 tax return.*

1 Enter an estimate of your 2001 itemized deductions. These include qualifying home mortgage interest, charitable contributions, state and local taxes, medical expenses in excess of 7.5% of your income, and miscellaneous deductions. (For 2001, you may have to reduce your itemized deductions if your income is over $132,950 ($66,475 if married filing separately). See **Worksheet 3** in Pub. 919 for details.) . . . **1** $ _____

2 Enter:
- $7,600 if married filing jointly or qualifying widow(er)
- $6,650 if head of household
- $4,550 if single
- $3,800 if married filing separately

. . . . **2** $ _____

3 **Subtract** line 2 from line 1. If line 2 is greater than line 1, enter -0- . . . . **3** $ _____

4 Enter an estimate of your 2001 adjustments to income, including alimony, deductible IRA contributions, and student loan interest **4** $ _____

5 **Add** lines 3 and 4 and enter the total (Include any amount for credits from **Worksheet 7** in Pub. 919.) . **5** $ _____

6 Enter an estimate of your 2001 nonwage income (such as dividends or interest) . . . . **6** $ _____

7 **Subtract** line 6 from line 5. Enter the result, but not less than -0- . . . . **7** $ _____

8 **Divide** the amount on line 7 by $3,000 and enter the result here. Drop any fraction . . . . . . **8** _____

9 Enter the number from the **Personal Allowances Worksheet,** line H, page 1 . . . . **9** _____

10 **Add** lines 8 and 9 and enter the total here. If you plan to use the **Two-Earner/Two-Job Worksheet,** also enter this total on line 1 below. Otherwise, **stop here** and enter this total on Form W-4, line 5, page 1 . **10** _____

Two-Earner/Two-Job Worksheet

Note: *Use this worksheet only if the instructions under line H on page 1 direct you here.*

1 Enter the number from line H, page 1 (or from line 10 above if you used the **Deductions and Adjustments Worksheet**) **1** _____

2 Find the number in **Table 1** below that applies to the **lowest** paying job and enter it here . . . . . **2** _____

3 If line 1 is **more than or equal to** line 2, subtract line 2 from line 1. Enter the result here (if zero, enter -0-) and on Form W-4, line 5, page 1. **Do not** use the rest of this worksheet . . . . **3** _____

Note: *If line 1 is **less than** line 2, enter -0- on Form W-4, line 5, page 1. Complete lines 4–9 below to calculate the additional withholding amount necessary to avoid a year end tax bill.*

4 Enter the number from line 2 of this worksheet . . . . **4** _____

5 Enter the number from line 1 of this worksheet . . . . **5** _____

6 **Subtract** line 5 from line 4 . . . . **6** _____

7 Find the amount in **Table 2** below that applies to the **highest** paying job and enter it here . . . . . **7** $ _____

8 **Multiply** line 7 by line 6 and enter the result here. This is the additional annual withholding needed . . **8** $ _____

9 Divide line 8 by the number of pay periods remaining in 2001. For example, divide by 26 if you are paid every two weeks and you complete this form in December 2000. Enter the result here and on Form W-4, line 6, page 1. This is the additional amount to be withheld from each paycheck . . . . **9** $ _____

Table 1: Two-Earner/Two-Job Worksheet

Married Filing Jointly				All Others			
If wages from **LOWEST** paying job are—	Enter on line 2 above	If wages from **LOWEST** paying job are—	Enter on line 2 above	If wages from **LOWEST** paying job are—	Enter on line 2 above	If wages from **LOWEST** paying job are—	Enter on line 2 above
$0 - $4,000	0	42,001 - 47,000	8	$0 - $6,000	0	65,001 - 80,000	8
4,001 - 8,000	1	47,001 - 55,000	9	6,001 - 12,000	1	80,001 - 105,000	9
8,001 - 14,000	2	55,001 - 65,000	10	12,001 - 17,000	2	105,001 and over	10
14,001 - 19,000	3	65,001 - 70,000	11	17,001 - 22,000	3		
19,001 - 25,000	4	70,001 - 90,000	12	22,001 - 28,000	4		
25,001 - 32,000	5	90,001 - 105,000	13	28,001 - 40,000	5		
32,001 - 38,000	6	105,001 - 115,000	14	40,001 - 50,000	6		
38,001 - 42,000	7	115,001 and over	15	50,001 - 65,000	7		

Table 2: Two-Earner/Two-Job Worksheet

Married Filing Jointly		All Others	
If wages from **HIGHEST** paying job are—	Enter on line 7 above	If wages from **HIGHEST** paying job are—	Enter on line 7 above
$0 - $50,000	$440	$0 - $30,000	$440
50,001 - 100,000	800	30,001 - 60,000	800
100,001 - 130,000	900	60,001 - 120,000	900
130,001 - 250,000	1,000	120,001 - 270,000	1,000
250,001 and over	1,100	270,001 and over	1,100

Figure 14–9. *Continued*

Social Security and Medicare tax limits and rates

Type of tax	Wage base limit for year 2000	Employee rate	Employer rate
Social Security	$76,200	6.2% of wages	6.2% of wages
Medicare	No wage limit; all wages subject to tax	1.45% of wages	1.45% of wages

Figure 14–10. 2000 Social Security and Medicare tax limits and rates. (From Department of the Treasury, Internal Revenue Service, Washington, DC.)

state unemployment tax. Certain types of employees may be exempt from this tax. FUTA tax is calculated quarterly, and, depending on the amount owed, deposits may be due quarterly. FUTA tax is reported using Form 940 (Fig. 14–12) or 940-EZ.

Depending on state requirements, the employer may also be required to pay taxes to a state unemployment fund. Employers should check with individual state agencies to determine what state unemployment taxes may be due.

Form W-2

Employers are required to retain each employee's name, social security number (SSN), wages earned, and taxes paid each year. The W-2 form is a federal form that summarizes the employee's payroll record for the year (Fig. 14–13). Employers should ask for the employee's Social Security card, and the name of the employee should be entered on the W-2 exactly as it appears on the card. If the name on the card is not the same as the employee's current name (as in cases of marriage or divorce), the employee should be instructed to obtain a new card from the Social Security Administration. If an employer wishes to verify an employee's SSN as listed on a W-2, they may verify up to 50 names by calling their local social security office.

HUMAN RESOURCE RECORDS

Personnel files should only contain information that is objective and well-substantiated. Items such as the employee's application, resumé, form W-4, records of employee evaluations, and any written reprimands are kept in the employee's human resource file. Subjective information and items that are not substantiated do not belong in an employee's file.

Employee Evaluation

As mentioned previously, many employees when initially hired serve a probationary period of 3 to 6 months. Within

that time, the employee has a chance to become familiar with the procedures of the office. Before the end of the probationary period, a preliminary review of the employee's performance is conducted, and the employer ascertains whether the employee should remain permanently.

A **performance review** should be conducted on a regular basis. No more than 1 year should pass between reviews. A schedule for employee reviews should be included in the policy manual. In addition to receiving feedback on individual performance, the review is also the time that an employee usually receives a pay increase based on performance. This evaluation gives the employee and employer a chance to set some goals for performance in the coming year. The evaluation process also gives an employee the opportunity to offer suggestions and feedback.

All employees should be given a performance review. Reviews should not be conducted only for employees who need to improve job skills. A review gives an employer the chance to notify the employee as regards any behavior that needs correction or modification as well as to give the employer a chance to praise an employee for a job well done.

Performance reviews should always be objective and honest. Employees should not be given false praise if performance is less than acceptable. Problems may result if a long-time employee is suddenly discharged after receiving exceptional reviews throughout the years. An employee's file should contain all documentation about the employee, whether positive or negative. Repeated insubordinate behavior must be noted.

Essentials of a Performance Review

When conducting an employee performance review, the evaluation (Fig. 14–14) should be based on objective criteria that can be evidenced by action on the job. On the evaluation form itself, such information as the employee's name, date of hire, and current position with the organization is included.

The employee's direct supervisor then ranks the employee's performance on several criteria, such as quality and quantity of work, judgment, and other items as listed in

Form **941**
(Rev. October 2000)
Department of the Treasury
Internal Revenue Service

Employer's Quarterly Federal Tax Return

▶ See separate instructions for information on completing this return.

Please type or print.

Enter state code for state in which deposits were made ONLY if different from state in address to the right ▶ ⬚⬚
(see page 2 of instructions).

Name (as distinguished from trade name)	Date quarter ended
Trade name, if any	Employer identification number
Address (number and street)	City, state, and ZIP code

OMB No. 1545-0029

| T |
| FF |
| FD |
| FP |
| I |
| T |

If address is different from prior return, check here ▶ ⬚

IRS Use

| 1 | 1 | 1 | 1 | 1 | 1 | 1 | 1 | 1 | 1 | 2 | | 3 | 3 | 3 | 3 | 3 | 3 | 3 | | 4 | 4 | 4 | | 5 | 5 | 5 |
| 6 | 7 | | 8 | 8 | 8 | 8 | 8 | 8 | 8 | | 9 | 9 | 9 | 9 | 9 | | 10 | 10 | 10 | 10 | 10 | 10 | 10 | 10 | 10 |

If you do not have to file returns in the future, check here ▶ ⬚ and enter date final wages paid ▶ ⬚

If you are a seasonal employer, see **Seasonal employers** on page 1 of the instructions and check here ▶ ⬚

1	Number of employees in the pay period that includes March 12th . ▶	1		
2	Total wages and tips, plus other compensation		2	
3	Total income tax withheld from wages, tips, and sick pay		3	
4	Adjustment of withheld income tax for preceding quarters of calendar year		4	
5	Adjusted total of income tax withheld (line 3 as adjusted by line 4—see instructions) . . .		5	

6	Taxable social security wages	6a		× 12.4% (.124) =	6b	
	Taxable social security tips	6c		× 12.4% (.124) =	6d	
7	Taxable Medicare wages and tips . . .	7a		× 2.9% (.029) =	7b	

8	Total social security and Medicare taxes (add lines 6b, 6d, and 7b). Check here if wages are not subject to social security and/or Medicare tax . . . . ▶ ⬚	8	
9	Adjustment of social security and Medicare taxes (see instructions for required explanation) Sick Pay $ _____ ± Fractions of Cents $ _____ ± Other $ _____ =	9	
10	Adjusted total of social security and Medicare taxes (line 8 as adjusted by line 9—see instructions)	10	
11	**Total taxes** (add lines 5 and 10)	11	
12	Advance earned income credit (EIC) payments made to employees	12	
13	Net taxes (subtract line 12 from line 11). **If $1,000 or more, this must equal line 17, column (d) below (or line D of Schedule B (Form 941))**	13	
14	Total deposits for quarter, including overpayment applied from a prior quarter	14	
15	**Balance due** (subtract line 14 from line 13). See instructions	15	

16 **Overpayment.** If line 14 is more than line 13, enter excess here ▶ $ _____
and check if to be: ⬚ Applied to next return **OR** ⬚ Refunded.

- **All filers:** If line 13 is less than $1,000, you need not complete line 17 or Schedule B (Form 941).
- **Semiweekly schedule depositors:** Complete Schedule B (Form 941) and check here . . . . ▶ ⬚
- **Monthly schedule depositors:** Complete line 17, columns (a) through (d), and check here. . . . . ▶ ⬚

17	**Monthly Summary of Federal Tax Liability.** Do not complete if you were a semiweekly schedule depositor.			
(a) First month liability	**(b)** Second month liability	**(c)** Third month liability	**(d)** Total liability for quarter

Sign Here

Under penalties of perjury, I declare that I have examined this return, including accompanying schedules and statements, and to the best of my knowledge and belief, it is true, correct, and complete.

Signature ▶ | Print Your Name and Title ▶ | Date ▶

For Privacy Act and Paperwork Reduction Act Notice, see back of Payment Voucher. Cat. No. 17001Z Form **941** (Rev. 10-2000)

Figure 14–11. Form 941, Employer's Quarterly Federal Tax Return, is used for reporting taxes owed. (From Department of the Treasury, Internal Revenue Service, Washington, DC, 2000.)

Form 941
Payment Voucher

Purpose of Form

Complete Form 941-V if you are making a payment with **Form 941,** Employer's Quarterly Federal Tax Return. We will use the completed voucher to credit your payment more promptly and accurately, and to improve our service to you.

If you have your return prepared by a third party and make a payment with that return, please provide this payment voucher to the return preparer.

Making Payments With Form 941

Make payments with Form 941 only if:

1. Your net taxes for the quarter (line 13 on Form 941) are less than $1,000 or

2. You are a monthly schedule depositor making a payment in accordance with the **accuracy of deposits** rule. (See section 11 of **Circular E,** Employer's Tax Guide, for details.) This amount may be $1,000 or more.

Otherwise, you must deposit the amount at an authorized financial institution or by electronic funds transfer. (See section 11 of Circular E for deposit instructions.) Do not use the Form 941-V payment voucher to make Federal tax deposits.

Caution: *If you pay amounts with Form 941 that should have been deposited, you may be subject to a penalty. See Circular E.*

Specific Instructions

Box 1. Enter the first four characters of your name as follows:

● **Individuals (sole proprietors, estates).** Use the first four letters of your last name (as shown in box 5).

● **Corporations.** Use the first four characters (letters or numbers) of your business name (as shown in box 5). Omit "The" if followed by more than one word.

● **Partnerships.** Use the first four characters of your trade name. If no trade name, enter the first four letters of the last name of the first listed partner.

Box 2—Employer identification number (EIN). If you do not have an EIN, apply for one on **Form SS-4,** Application for Employer Identification Number, and write "Applied for" and the date you applied in this entry space.

Box 3—Amount paid. Enter the amount paid with Form 941.

Box 4—Tax period. Darken the capsule identifying the quarter for which the payment is made. Darken only one capsule.

Box 5—Name and address. Enter your name and address as shown on Form 941.

● Make your check or money order payable to the United States Treasury. Be sure to enter your EIN, "Form 941," and the tax period on your check or money order. Do not send cash. Please do not staple this voucher or your payment to the return or to each other.

● Detach the completed voucher and send it with your payment and Form 941 to the address provided on the back of Form 941.

▼ **DETACH HERE AND MAIL WITH YOUR PAYMENT** ▼   Form **941-V** (2000)

Form **941-V** Department of the Treasury Internal Revenue Service (99)	**Payment Voucher** ▶ **Do not staple or attach this voucher to your payment.**	OMB No. 1545-0074 20**00**

1 Enter the first four letters of your last name (business name if corporation or partnership)	**2** Enter your employer identification number	**3** **Enter the amount of the payment** $.

4 Tax period		**5** Enter your business name (individual name if sole proprietor)
⟋ 1st Quarter	⟋ 3rd Quarter	───────────────────── Enter your address
⟋ 2nd Quarter	⟋ 4th Quarter	───────────────────── Enter your city, state, and ZIP code

Figure 14–11. *Continued*

Form 940

Department of the Treasury
Internal Revenue Service (99)

Employer's Annual Federal Unemployment (FUTA) Tax Return

OMB No. 1545-0028

2000

▶ **See separate Instructions for Form 940 for information on completing this form.**

T	
FF	
FD	
FP	
I	
T	

Name (as distinguished from trade name)   Calendar year

Trade name, if any

Address and ZIP code   Employer identification number

A Are you required to pay unemployment contributions to only one state? (If "No," skip questions B and C.) . ☐ Yes ☐ No

B Did you pay all state unemployment contributions by January 31, 2001? ((1) If you deposited your total FUTA tax when due, check "Yes" if you paid all state unemployment contributions by February 12, 2001. (2) If a 0% experience rate is granted, check "Yes." (3) If "No," skip question C.) . . . . ☐ Yes ☐ No

C Were all wages that were taxable for FUTA tax also taxable for your state's unemployment tax? . . . . . ☐ Yes ☐ No

If you answered "No" to any of these questions, you must file Form 940. If you answered "Yes" to all the questions, you may file Form 940-EZ, which is a simplified version of Form 940. (Successor employers see **Special credit for successor employers** on page 3 of the instructions.) You can get Form 940-EZ by calling 1-800-TAX-FORM (1-800-829-3676) or from the IRS Web Site at **www.irs.gov**.

If you will not have to file returns in the future, check here (see **Who Must File** in separate instructions), **and complete and sign the return** . . . . ▶ ☐

If this is an Amended Return, check here. . . . . ▶ ☐

Part I	**Computation of Taxable Wages**

1 Total payments (including payments shown on lines 2 and 3) during the calendar year for services of employees **1**

2 Exempt payments. (Explain all exempt payments, attaching additional sheets if necessary.) ▶ ------------------------------------- ------------------------------------- **2**

3 Payments of more than $7,000 for services. Enter only amounts over the first $7,000 paid to each employee. (See separate instructions.) Do not include any exempt payments from line 2. The $7,000 amount is the Federal wage base. Your state wage base may be different. **Do not use your state wage limitation**. **3**

4 Total exempt payments (add lines 2 and 3) **4**

5 **Total taxable wages** (subtract line 4 from line 1) . . . . ▶ **5**

Be sure to complete both sides of this form, and sign in the space provided on the back.

For Privacy Act and Paperwork Reduction Act Notice, see separate instructions.   Cat. No. 11234O   Form **940** (2000)

DETACH HERE

Form 940-V

Department of the Treasury
Internal Revenue Service

Form 940 Payment Voucher

Use this voucher only when making a payment with your return.

OMB No. 1545-0028

2000

Complete boxes 1, 2, 3, and 4. Do not send cash, and do not staple your payment to this voucher. Make your check or money order payable to the **"United States Treasury"**. Be sure to enter your employer identification number, "Form 940", and "2000" on your payment.

1 Enter the first four letters of your last name (business name if partnership or corporation).

2 Enter your employer identification number.

3 Enter the amount of your payment.

$.

Instructions for Box 1

—Individuals (sole proprietors, trusts, and estates)— Enter the first four letters of your last name.

—Corporations and partnerships—Enter the first four characters of your business name (omit "The" if followed by more than one word).

4 Enter your business name (individual name for sole proprietors)

Enter your address

Enter your city, state, and ZIP code

Figure 14–12. Federal form 940 is used to report federal unemployment tax. (From Department of the Treasury, Internal Revenue Service, Washington, DC, 2000.)

Form 940 (2000)   Page **2**

Part II   **Tax Due or Refund**

1	Gross FUTA tax. Multiply the wages from Part I, line 5, by .062	**1**
2	Maximum credit. Multiply the wages from Part I, line 5, by .054 . . | **2** |	
3	Computation of tentative credit (**Note:** *All taxpayers must complete the applicable columns.*)	

(a) Name of state	(b) State reporting number(s) as shown on employer's state contribution returns	(c) Taxable payroll (as defined in state act)	(d) State experience rate period From / To	(e) State ex- perience rate	(f) Contributions if rate had been 5.4% (col. (c) x .054)	(g) Contributions payable at experience rate (col. (c) x col. (e))	(h) Additional credit (col. (f) minus col.(g)). If 0 or less, enter -0-.	(i) Contributions paid to state by 940 due date

3a	Totals . . . ▶	
3b	**Total tentative credit** (add line 3a, columns (h) and (i) only—for late payments also see the instructions for Part II, line 6 . . . . ▶	**3b**
4		
5		
6	**Credit:** Enter the smaller of the amount from Part II, line 2 or line 3b; or the amount from the worksheet in the Part II, line 6 instructions	**6**
7	**Total FUTA tax** (subtract line 6 from line 1). If the result is over $100, also complete Part III . .	**7**
8	Total FUTA tax deposited for the year, including any overpayment applied from a prior year . .	**8**
9	**Balance due** (subtract line 8 from line 7). Pay to the "United States Treasury". If you owe more than $100, see **Depositing FUTA Tax** on page 3 of the separate instructions . . . . . . ▶	**9**
10	**Overpayment** (subtract line 7 from line 8). Check if it is to be: ☐ **Applied to next return** or ☐ **Refunded** . . . . ▶	**10**

Part III   **Record of Quarterly Federal Unemployment Tax Liability** (Do not include state liability.) **Complete only if line 7 is over $100.** See page 6 of the separate instructions.

Quarter	First (Jan. 1–Mar. 31)	Second (Apr. 1–June 30)	Third (July 1–Sept. 30)	Fourth (Oct. 1–Dec. 31)	Total for year
Liability for quarter					

Under penalties of perjury, I declare that I have examined this return, including accompanying schedules and statements, and, to the best of my knowledge and belief, it is true, correct, and complete, and that no part of any payment made to a state unemployment fund claimed as a credit was, or is to be, deducted from the payments to employees.

Signature ▶   Title (Owner, etc.) ▶   Date ▶

✪   Form **940** (2000)

Figure 14–12. *Continued*

Figure 14–14. The supervisor should rate the employee objectively, based on the criteria specified, and should be very careful not to include any personal bias. The example in Figure 14–14 allows for detailed assessment of an employee's performance. It allows the employer to address concerns and provides an opportunity to document the employee's plan for personal growth. In some instances, the performance review is conducted by more than one reviewer to ensure that no misunderstanding occurs.

Employee Discipline or Termination

One of the more difficult situations in office management is dealing with an employee who is performing poorly in the workplace. Most employees do not want to perform poorly, but owing to a variety of personal, work, or educational circumstances, their work may not be adequate.

The first instinct for some managers may be to say to an employee, "Shape up!" A good manager, however, investigates the situation thoroughly. When dealing with an employee

problem, a manager must be sure to consider all parties involved and should act in a way that is best for all concerned.

If an employee problem exists, the employee should be notified that there is a problem with job performance and should be given an adequate opportunity to respond to and correct the problem. Tips on dealing with employee problems are shown in Box 14–4. Significant employee problems—ones that could possibly warrant future termination—should be objectively and adequately documented and should be included in the employee's human resource file.

Separation of Employment

If an employee must be discharged, firing should never be a surprise. An employee who is not performing properly should be given sufficient warning that a problem with performance exists. A "paper trail" must be kept to demonstrate that the employee has been notified about poor performance. Well-documented evidence of reprimands and the reasons for reprimands as well as evidence of any suspensions

a Control number 22222	Void ☐	For Official Use Only ▶ OMB No. 1545-0008	

b Employer identification number ##00000		1 Wages, tips, other compensation $ 25764.20	2 Federal income tax withheld $ 2112.66
c Employer's name, address, and ZIP code Horizons Healthcare Center 123 Main Ave. Farmington, ND 58000		3 Social security wages $ 25764.20	4 Social security tax withheld $ 1597.38
		5 Medicare wages and tips $ 25764.20	6 Medicare tax withheld $ 373.58
		7 Social security tips $	8 Allocated tips $
d Employee's social security number ##1-00-11##		9 Advance EIC payment $	10 Dependent care benefits $
e Employee's first name and initial Amy G	Last name Dixon	11 Nonqualified plans $	12a See instructions for box 12 $ $
1567 Meadow Valley Rd. Farmington, ND 58000		13 Statutory employee ☐ Retirement plan ☐ Third-party sick pay ☐	12b Code $
		14 Other	12c Code $
			12d Code $
f Employee's address and ZIP code			

15 State ND	Employer's state ID number ##0011	16 State wages, tips, etc. $ 25764.20	17 State income tax $ 296.29	18 Local wages, tips, etc. $	19 Local income tax $	20 Locality name
		$	$	$	$	

Form **W-2** Wage and Tax Statement **2001** Department of the Treasury–Internal Revenue Service

Copy A For Social Security Administration–Send this entire page with Form W-3 to the Social Security Administration; photocopies are **not** acceptable.

Cat. No. 10134D

For Privacy Act and Paperwork Reduction Act Notice, see separate instructions.

Do Not Cut, Fold, or Staple Forms on This Page – Do Not Cut, Fold, or Staple Forms on This Page

Figure 14–13. Portion of a W-2 form, which summarizes an employee's payroll information for a specific year. (From Department of the Treasury, Internal Revenue Service, Washington, DC, 2001.)

must be included in the employee's file. It is critical to cover issues at the time of release from employment. Failure to do so may invite a discrimination suit against the employer.

If it has been decided that an employee should be discharged, the employer should carefully document the reason for termination. All reasons for termination must have been applied to all employees equally. For example, if an employee was discharged because the employee was late for work five times in a month and other employees were late that many times or more, a lawsuit may ensue because office policy was not consistently applied to all individuals in the office, which means discrimination has occurred.

A breach of patient confidentiality would likely warrant an immediate termination from employment. The office's policy manual should contain a clear statement about confidentiality and the consequences of violating confidentiality. A confidentiality statement similar to the one shown in Figure 4–3 should be signed by every employee at the time of hire and at each performance review. In very obvious instances of violation, an employee would be terminated immediately and the reasons clearly documented in the employee's file.

References for Former Employees

When an employee leaves the job under good terms, he or she may request a reference from the office when applying for employment elsewhere. Giving references can be a potentially "sticky" legal situation and must be handled with care.

Many defamation lawsuits have been pursued by former employees who received unfavorable references from former employers. A defamation lawsuit may be initiated and won against an employer who gives detrimental information and does not have records to substantiate the information. Even the simple act of saying a former employee was fired may bring a lawsuit because the employee may have to reveal damaging information about the release from employment.

Because of the concern about legal entanglements, employers may decide to give references only for good employees. If a positive recommendation cannot be made, an employer may choose to not comment. An employer should refrain from giving good references for employees that do not deserve them because this can create other problems. Not all employees deserve good references, and by giving everyone a good reference, the employer may lose the respect of peers in the community and may actually support the hiring of a person wrong for a position.

A safe approach to handling references is to give only limited information about the employee, such as the dates of employment, salary information, and the type of position held. Such references are unfavorable to employees who have performed well on the job, however, and a quality reference should be given for an employee for work well done.

Text continued on page 320

PERFORMANCE EVALUATION AND DEVELOPMENT PLAN
(OFFICE AND CLERICAL)

NAME: _____   DATE OF EVALUATION: _____

DATE OF HIRE: _____   DEPARTMENT: _____

JOB TITLE: _____   SUPERVISOR: _____

DATE APPOINTED THIS JOB: _____   MANAGER: _____

LAST REVIEW DATE: _____   LAST REVIEW RATING: _____

NEXT REVIEW DATE: _____   CURRENT REVIEW RATING: _____

PURPOSE

The purpose of this evaluation is to:

1. SET GOALS WITHIN SCOPE OF PRESENT JOB.
2. COMMUNICATE OPENLY ABOUT PERFORMANCE.
3. EVALUATE PAST PERFORMANCE.
4. DISCUSS FUTURE DEVELOPMENT PLANS FOR GROWTH.

INSTRUCTIONS

1. Supervisor to review form prior to completion. If specific items are not applicable they should be left blank.

2. Supervisor and employee to review job description prior to review.

3. In "COMMENTS" section supervisor may indicate which factors should be more heavily weighted in this particular evaluation.

4. Comments should be specific and job-related. All appropriate evaluation factors should be commented on to some degree.

I. POSITION OBJECTIVES AND MAJOR RESPONSIBILITIES. Summarize specific responsibilities of the job.

_____

_____

_____

II. ACCOMPLISHMENTS AND/OR IMPROVEMENTS. What specific accomplishments and/or improvements has employee made since last review with respect to set goals?

_____

_____

_____

PLEASE CONSIDER THE EMPLOYEE'S DEMONSTRATED PERFORMANCE AND MARK THE CIRCLE WHICH MOST CLOSELY DESCRIBES THAT PERFORMANCE.

4 - Performance consistently far exceeds expectations and requirements.
3 - Performance consistently exceeds normal expectations and job requirements.
2 - Performance consistently meets expectations and job requirements
1 - Performance usually meets expectations and minimum job requirements.
0 - Performance does not meet job requirements.

— CONTINUED, NEXT PAGE —

FORM # 72-119 ' 1987 BIBBERO SYSTEMS, INC. PETALUMA, CA

TO REORDER CALL TOLL FREE:
800-BIBBERO /(800 242-2376) OR
FAX: (800) 242-9330 MFG IN U.S.A.

Figure 14–14. A performance review gives an employer and employee an opportunity to review past performance and to make plans for future growth. (Form courtesy of Bibbero Systems, Inc., Petaluma, California, 800-242-2376. Fax 800-242-9330. www.bibbero.com)

1. WORK QUALITY: CONSIDER COMPLETENESS, ACCURACY, NEATNESS AND RELIABILITY .

   ○ 0   ○ 1   ○ 2   ○ 3   ○ 4

   _____
   _____
   _____

2. WORK QUANTITY: CONSIDER ACCEPTABLE LEVEL EXPECTED AND TIME UTILIZATION.

   ○ 0   ○ 1   ○ 2   ○ 3   ○ 4

   _____
   _____
   _____

3. JUDGMENT: CONSIDER ABILITY TO MAKE WELL-REASONED, SOUND DECISIONS WHICH AFFECT WORK PERFORMANCE.

   ○ 0   ○ 1   ○ 2   ○ 3   ○ 4

   _____
   _____
   _____

4. INITIATIVE: CONSIDER JOB INTEREST, DEDICATION AND WILLINGNESS TO EXTEND ONESELF TO COMPLETE ASSIGNED TASKS. CONSIDER RESOURCEFULNESS.

   ○ 0   ○ 1   ○ 2   ○ 3   ○ 4

   _____
   _____
   _____

5. TEAMWORK: CONSIDER WORKING RELATIONSHIPS WITH FELLOW EMPLOYEES AND MANAGEMENT WITHIN THE WORK ENVIRONMENT .

   ○ 0   ○ 1   ○ 2   ○ 3   ○ 4

   _____
   _____
   _____

6. JOB UNDERSTANDING: CONSIDER KNOWLEDGE OF SPECIFIC JOB FUNCTION

   ○ 0   ○ 1   ○ 2   ○ 3   ○ 4

   _____
   _____
   _____

— CONTINUED, NEXT PAGE —

FORM # 72-119 ' 1987 BIBBERO SYSTEMS, INC. PETALUMA, CA

Figure 14–14. *Continued*

7. <u>DEPENDABILITY:</u> CONSIDER ATTENDANCE, PUNCTUALITY, IDLE TIME AND RELIANCE THAT CAN BE PLACED ON EMPLOYEE TO PERSEVERE AND CARRY THROUGH TO COMPLETION ALL ASSIGNED TASKS

    ○ 0   ○ 1   ○ 2   ○ 3   ○ 4

_____

_____

_____

8. <u>COMPLIANCE WITH COMPANY POLICIES:</u> DOES THE EMPLOYEE COMPLY WITH RULES AND REGULATIONS THAT APPLY TO SAFETY, FAIR EMPLOYMENT PRACTICES AND GENERAL ADMINISTRATIVE PROCEDURE.

    ○ 0   ○ 1   ○ 2   ○ 3   ○ 4

_____

_____

_____

SPECIFIC PERFORMANCE	1	2	3	4	COMMENTS
A. Ability to handle scheduling:					
B. Willingness to work OT when necessary:					
C. Handling of calls and follow-up:					
D. Maintenance of equipment:					
E. Ability to handle patient complaints:					
F. Tact in dealing with patients:					
G. Speed (in specific technical procedures):					
H. Secretarial accuracy:					
I. Professional terminology:					
J. Assisting procedures:					
K. Laboratory techniques:					
L. X-ray techniques:					
M. Physical therapy:					
N. Collections:					
O. Medical Insurance:					
P. Bookkeeping:					

10. PERSONAL	1	2	3	4	COMMENTS
A. Grooming:					
B. Professional conduct:					
C. Energy, enthusiasm:					
D. Ability to handle stress:					

ADDITIONAL COMMENTS: _____

_____

_____

_____

_____

_____

— CONTINUED, NEXT PAGE —

FORM # 72-119 ' 1987 BIBBERO SYSTEMS, INC. PETALUMA, CA

Figure 14–14. *Continued*

III. AREAS OF CONCERN: SPECIFY, IF ANY, PROBLEM AREAS:

_____

_____

_____

IV. DEVELOPMENT PLANS: WHAT SPECIFIC ACTION CAN YOU SUGGEST TO HELP THE
EMPLOYEE IMPROVE PERFORMANCE? HOW CAN YOU, AS THE
SUPERVISOR, HELP?

_____

_____

_____

_____

☐ Promotable with additional training and experience.
☐ Promotable now   ☐ Properly placed   ☐ Not properly placed.

V. GOAL STATEMENT FOR NEXT REVIEW PERIOD: WITH THE EMPLOYEE, ESTABLISH
GOALS WHICH MAY INCLUDE NEW AND BETTER WAYS TO CARRY OUT JOB RESPONSIBIL-
ITIES, AS WELL AS PLANS FOR PERSONAL DEVELOPMENT. STATED GOALS SHOULD BE
CONSIDERED THE BASIS FOR THE NEXT FORMAL PERFORMANCE EVALUATION.

_____

_____

_____

_____

_____

_____

VI. EMPLOYEE COMMENTS:

_____

_____

_____

_____

I am signing this evaluation form to indicate that my supervisor and I have had a discussion of the
above comments and ratings. Signature does not imply agreement.

EMPLOYEE: _____   DATE: _____

NAME OF REVIEWER _____

SIGNATURE _____   DATE: _____

TO REORDER CALL TOLL FREE:
800-BIBBERO /(800 242-2376) OR
FAX: (800) 242-9330 MFG IN U.S.A.

FORM # 72-119 ' 1987 BIBBERO SYSTEMS, INC. PETALUMA, CA

Figure 14–14. *Continued*

Box 14–4 Helping with Poor Work Performance

When dealing with poor employee performance,

- Choose a private location for the discussion.
- Be calm and professional.
- Approach the employee in a positive manner. Negativity will help create a hostile atmosphere.
- Focus on the performance, not the person. Remain objective.
- Assume the employee wants to improve performance.
- Allow enough time to discuss the employee's performance.
- Describe what is acceptable performance. Describe the situation as you see it.
- Ask the employee how he/she sees it. Let the employee explain the situation in full without interruption. There are always two sides to a story.
- Keep the discussion on neutral ground.
- Check for understanding. Be sure the employee understands what is acceptable and not acceptable performance.
- Encourage the employee to develop a solution. Employee ownership in the solution goes a long way toward correcting poor performance.
- Try to arrive at a solution that is beneficial to both parties.
- Remember that the goal of the discussion is to improve performance.
- Establish a time to meet again and follow up on the situation.

Some employers elect to give no references after the employee is gone and will instead provide a written reference letter to an employee before the employee leaves. Such references may be addressed "To Whom It May Concern" and are given directly to the employee. The employee may make photocopies of the reference letter to give to prospective employers. The employee is then responsible for disclosure of the information in the letter. If a reference letter is given, a copy of the letter should be filed in the employee's personnel file. This may well be the best approach to take, because the employee controls whether information is given to potential employers.

EMPLOYEE HEALTH

Much time and effort goes into selecting the best candidate for a position in the medical office. Once good employees are selected, the organization should expend every effort to keep them. To reduce turnover of employees, the practice should pay particular attention to the work environment and the needs of the people who work there. Frequent turnover is costly to the practice because new employees

require training and adjustment to office staff. Frequent turnover can result in the loss of patients and referrals as a result of an inexperienced staff.

Creating a healthy work environment is not difficult. First and foremost, management sets the tone for the office atmosphere. A friendly, teamwork-type atmosphere helps to create an enjoyable place to work. Honest and open communication among all employees in the office contributes to a harmonious work environment. A medical office is no place for personal agendas or competitiveness that work against an atmosphere of teamwork. A health care organization requires an atmosphere of teamwork to effectively handle all patients served by the physicians and staff.

Occasionally, employees have personal problems that affect their job performance. Oftentimes when an employee is in a difficult situation, the productivity of the employee is diminished. Employee assistance programs provide counseling services for employees experiencing difficult situations at work or at home. Initial sessions with these types of programs are usually free to the employee. Employers who participate in such programs are aware that such participation goes a long way in heading off future difficulties at work. Happy, satisfied employees generally provide quality customer service. Disgruntled, troubled employees tend to reduce service.

Adapting to Change

It is often said that the only thing one can be sure of is that things will change. Certainly, change is inevitable in the health care industry. Constant advances in technology mean that employees must adapt to new systems, technologies, and procedures in the workplace. Only 15 years ago, for example, many medical offices used very little computer equipment in the front office. Today, the changes in the business office of a medical practice have been dramatic, with the addition of computerized systems to support everyday front office functions. The future will probably bring many more changes, and the skills learned by the medical office staff today will need to be continually updated to keep pace with these changes.

Dealing with change can be an ongoing concern in the medical office. Everyone reacts in his or her own way to change. Some people adapt to change quite well. Others may be very resistant and may find it difficult to cope with change. People may have this difficulty because of a variety of reasons.

Job Security. When any noticeable change is made in how an organization accomplishes its work, employees may be concerned that they are no longer needed in the office. A shift in the workload or in the organizational structure may produce anxiety in some employees. The addition of a new technology in the office may lead an employee to believe he or she will no longer be needed. Most employers take preventive action in assuring employees that layoffs will not occur because of a proposed change. The addition of technology does not have to be a threat in the workplace. In actuality, employee security may be more threatened if changes were not made. An office that fails to keep up with technology may soon find it will not be able to keep a quality level of service for existing customers and may risk losing them.

Resistance to Change. It is important for the office management to discuss the reasons for change with the office staff. Depending on the management style of the organization, the staff may even be asked to find solutions for addressing a problem. If it fits with the management style in the office, this tactic can help give employees ownership in the solution to a problem. When the staff has participated in a solution, the solution often becomes easier to implement.

New Technology. Sometimes office employees are intimidated by the new technology that may accompany change. When change is necessary, office management should provide the support to implement new technology. Training sessions on new equipment and offsite workshops provide an opportunity for employees to learn new technologies and to network with other professionals.

Whatever the reason for change, the transition will be smoother if employees are made aware of why change is necessary and how it will affect them.

Stress Management

Stress can be a serious problem in the workplace. There are good and bad types of stress. Good stress is the deadline that motivates someone to get a job done or an office environment that may be busy with activity. Examples of bad stress are constant deadlines that can almost never be met or being the only assistant available to answer eight incoming phone lines.

Sometimes stress is a result of conditions at work, and sometimes individuals are under stress because of situations in their personal lives. Whatever the case, it is important for the management of the medical office to be aware of employee behaviors that can be signals of bad stress.

- Frequent absenteeism or illness.
- Tension at work.
- Crying spells.
- Acting "out of character," "spacey," daydreaming.
- Poor work quality, frequent mistakes.
- Feeling unappreciated or picked on.

Employers should be aware of the effects of stress and take the following measures to reduce or prevent work-related stress:

- Establish reasonable work expectations.
- Give employees reasonable break time during the workday.
- Provide a comfortable work environment.
- Solicit employees' input on work-related matters and incorporate input whenever possible.
- Give employees adequate time to complete job tasks.

Working to reduce or prevent employee stress can go a long way toward creating a pleasing environment not only for employees but also for patients. Employees who are satisfied and comfortable in their work environment will convey that feeling to the patients of the practice.

LABOR LAWS AND LEGAL ISSUES

At the beginning of the 20th century, the world of work was a dangerous and difficult place. Workers had little legal protection in various cases of work-related matters. As more and more people left family farm employment and began to work in an industrial setting, the need for legal protection for workers became apparent. Throughout the past century, great strides have occurred in developing laws that protect employees in the workplace. Following are a few of the major legislative enactments affecting the workplace today.

Labor Law Enforcement

A federal agency within the U.S. Department of Labor, the Employment Standards Administration (ESA) enforces many laws and regulations pertaining to working conditions. Within the ESA, agencies have been established to enforce specific groups of laws and regulations pertaining to labor. The Wage and Hour Division, a division within the ESA, is responsible for protecting workers against unfair labor practices.

Fair Labor Standards Act

In 1938, the Fair Labor Standards Act (FLSA), which included provisions for minimum wage, overtime pay, and child labor, was passed. Certain groups of individuals are exempt from overtime pay and minimum wage requirements. The FLSA also sets standards for hiring youth workers, such as work time restrictions and separate minimum wage requirements. Currently, the FLSA protects approximately 114 million government and private sector workers throughout the United States.

Family and Medical Leave Act

Promoting family stability is one of the chief purposes of the Family and Medical Leave Act of 1993 (FMLA). The Family and Medical Leave Act applies to all public sector employers and private sector employers who employ 50 or more workers and who are engaged in any activity that affects commerce.

The FMLA provides up to 12 weeks of leave during any 12-month period for the following reasons:

- Birth and care of an employee's child or placement of an adopted or foster care child with the employee.
- Care of an immediate family member (spouse, child, parent) who has a serious health condition.

- Care of an employee's own serious health condition.

During a leave, the employee is entitled to health insurance benefits that the employee was receiving at the time the leave began. Employees may be required by their employer to take any accrued paid leave, such as sick or vacation pay, while on an FMLA leave.

When returning to work after taking a leave under the FMLA, employees are entitled to their previous job or a job of equal status. If an employee takes a leave for reasons of personal illness, an employer may require that an employee provide certification from a physician that the employee is able to return to work.

No state law can supersede the FMLA, but if a state law is more beneficial to an employee, the employer must abide by the more beneficial law. The specifics of the FMLA are available from the U.S. Department of Labor at the United States Department of Justice Web site, www.dol.gov.

Americans with Disabilities Act

What are an employer's responsibilities in hiring or employing individuals who are disabled? Federal law does provide protection against discrimination toward disabled individuals. Enacted in 1990, the Americans with Disabilities Act (ADA) prohibits discrimination on the basis of a disability in employment practices. The ADA also prohibits discrimination in commercial facilities and requires governmental agencies to provide access to programs offered to the public.

This law states that reasonable accommodations must be made for disabled individuals when policies or procedures may be discriminatory. An accommodation is a modification in a structure or process to help a disabled individual. Included in this legislation are provisions for improving access for disabled individuals to new construction and existing buildings that provide goods and services to the public. New construction accommodations include ramps for individuals who use wheelchairs, automatic door openers, and Braille signage.

In the medical office, the ADA might apply in the following ways: (1) An employee who has a musculoskeletal injury may need a special chair in which to sit while working, (2) a diabetic employee may be given time to monitor blood sugar levels and administer insulin during the workday, or (3) an employee who cannot hear may be given a special hearing device.

The application of ADA requirements is often a gray area. The ADA requires only that an employer make reasonable accommodations; it does not require an employer to make all possible accommodations. The employer must decide what is reasonable and what is not. The U.S. Department of Justice does provide technical assistance with ADA regulations and is responsible for enforcing the regulations. However, the department is very strict when cases are reported regarding the apparent lack of effort to accommodate the disabled.

Sexual Harassment

Fair treatment of everyone in the workplace is an issue affecting management today. In the interviewing section of this chapter, we learn that it is unlawful to discriminate against women or anyone else in employment practices.

Another issue that has grabbed many headlines in the past 20 years is the issue of sexual harassment in the workplace. Sexual harassment can be defined as unwelcome sexual behavior or innuendo. Sexual harassment can take the form of threats such as "If you don't give in to me, you'll be out of a job" or other activity that creates a hostile working environment, such as lewd jokes, foul language, or sexual comments.

Companies can be, and very often are, held responsible for the actions of their employees. If an individual in a position of authority uses that authority to coerce or intimidate an employee, the office management has a responsibility to protect the worker and must be vigilant in maintaining a work environment free of sexual harassment. A medical office should have established policy on sexual harassment as well as identified procedures on how to report incidents. Sexual harassment policy should be reviewed, and education about recognizing and dealing with sexual harassment should be presented on an annual basis (at a minimum) for all employees. Employees may be asked to sign a form acknowledging that such behavior is against office policy.

When hearing the term *sexual harassment*, people often think of women being harassed. Even though most legal cases involve women as the subject of harassment, it is important to note that men can be victims of sexual harassment too and are afforded the same rights as women as regards this subject.

Sexual harassment has been defined as unwelcome sexual behavior or innuendo, but what really is it? Sexual harassment may take the form of one of the following examples:

- Giving special treatment to a woman or man who is a sexual partner, even if the relationship is consensual.
- Using terms such as "honey" or "babe."
- Telling or displaying jokes of a sexual nature.
- Commenting on someone's physical appearance, such as "nice legs" or "that outfit is sexy."
- Touching, hugging, or bumping against someone.
- Whistling or winking suggestively.

These are only a few examples of what might constitute sexual harassment. What is important to remember is that sexual harassment is unwelcome sexual behavior or innuendo. An employee who is feeling harassed should notify the perpetrator that the actions are unwelcome. Such comments as "stop doing that" or "I find that offensive" communicate displeasure. An employee sometimes is unable to inform the perpetrator that the actions are unwelcome because the employee may fear retaliation from the perpetrator. Even in such a case, harassment has taken place. The employee may go directly to the supervisor, and the supervisor will be expected to address the unwanted behavior.

Once the incident is reported to the appropriate individual, an investigation of the allegations should be conducted. One incident, if severe enough, is sufficient to bring allegations of harassment. The office should have a well-defined investigative procedure that identifies a specific individual to whom allegations are given. Dealing with situations of harassment often requires specific training, and specific individuals are usually assigned to investigate such matters.

Workers' Compensation

Much is written in Chapters 11 and 12 about matters relating to workers' compensation. OSHA has specific guidelines for mandatory reporting of workplace injuries. When an employee is injured on the job, a report of injury must be completed as required by law. Timelines required for reporting vary from state to state. The state workers' compensation office or private workers' compensation carrier has specific information on when reports must be filed. Management should never discourage employees from seeking medical care or for filing reports for work-related injuries.

Information on Employment Matters

The information in this chapter is meant to serve as an introduction to the essentials of human resource management and to provide a basis for inquiry when consulting financial or legal counsel with regard to human resource issues. There is no substitute for prudent planning. Professional counsel is an essential component of planning when managing the human resources of an organization.

Experts in payroll accounting provide a valuable service when meeting the various requirements for processing payroll. The services of an accountant should be available for answers to specific questions and for legal and tax advice about payroll requirements.

Because the area of employment practices has such a potential for litigation, a medical practice is wise to retain the services of legal counsel before dealing with employment matters such as contracts, discipline, hiring, firing, and other potential litigious situations. A few dollars spent on legal counsel will potentially save thousands in future litigation.

Information on employment laws and regulations can also be obtained from the federal government on the U.S. Department of Labor and other Internet sites. Popular sites are listed in the bibliography section of this chapter.

SUMMARY

The human resources of the organization are vital to the longevity and effective operations of an organization. Appropriate management of a practice's human resources can keep a medical office growing and running smoothly. A medical administrative assistant, whether an office manager or staff member, should be aware of the various human resource issues affecting employment and compensation of employees. The assistant who is well informed will know how to facilitate a positive employer/employee relationship and can help alleviate any legal entanglements related to employment.

Bibliography

Coleman DL: What you must know before you hire or fire an employee. Phys Management: 60–70, May 1992.

Internal Revenue Service.

U.S. Department of Labor.

U.S. Office of Personnel Management, Federal Employees Health Benefits.

Weiss DH: Fair, Square and Legal: Safe Hiring, Managing, and Firing Practices to Keep You and Your Company Out of Court. New York, AMACOM, 1991.

State of Minnesota Department of Employee Relations: Your Health Your Choice, vol VIII. Kalamazoo, MI, Hope Publications, April 1997.

YOU ARE THE MEDICAL ADMINISTRATIVE ASSISTANT

Several of your coworkers comment that they are upset about a recent staff meeting in which they were asked for input regarding a specific situation but the office manager did not incorporate the input. Is management obligated to incorporate the input? How could this situation be better handled?

Exercise 14–1 TRUE OR FALSE

Read each statement and determine whether the statement is true or false. Record the answer in the blank provided. T = true; F = false.

_____ 1. The participatory management style works well in a fast-paced medical office because it allows employees some decision-making without always referring to a supervisor.

_____ 2. A chain of command is still necessary if a participatory management style is used in the medical office.

_____ 3. When reviewing applications for a position in the medical office, the best candidate from the resumés should be invited for an interview. If the interview goes well, no other candidates will need to be interviewed.

_____ 4. Inappropriate questions by an interviewer can bring about a lawsuit.

_____ 5. Employees are allowed to take as many exemptions as they want in order to reduce taxes.

_____ 6. If a W-4 is not completed by an employee, taxes at the lowest rate possible will be subtracted for the employee.

_____ 7. Social Security tax is withheld on all wages earned during a year.

_____ 8. Some employees may be exempt from federal income tax withholding.

_____ 9. The amount of taxes previously paid by an employer will determine how often the employer must make deposits of taxes that are withheld.

_____ 10. Employers should use an employee's name as it appears on the employee's Social Security card.

_____ 11. Anything that pertains to an employee, whether verified or not, should be included in the employee's file in order to avoid any future lawsuits.

_____ 12. Personal bias is acceptable and is expected on an employee's performance review.

_____ 13. Every employee should receive a performance review regardless of the quality of the employee's work.

_____ 14. Frequent employee turnover can be costly to a medical office.

_____ 15. When asked for a reference, an employer should tell everything about an employee, especially the negative points.

_____ 16. An employer should not give a positive job reference for an employee who does not deserve one.

_____ 17. Giving a reference letter to a previous employee is probably the safest way to give an employment reference.

_____ 18. Because change is so frequent in the workplace, it is easy for employees to handle.

_____ 19. Sexual harassment has not taken place if the perpetrator has not been told.

_____ 20. All allegations of sexual harassment must be investigated.

_____ 21. A medical office may be liable for the actions of an office manager if sexual harassment is alleged.

_____ 22. In some offices, employees may have to sign a form acknowledging understanding of a sexual harassment policy.

_____ 23. ADA may require an employer to adapt a work environment for an employee who needs it.

Exercise 14–2 CHAPTER CONCEPTS

Read the statement and determine the answer that best fits the statement. Record the answer in the blank provided.

_____ 1. Which of the following is a subjective criterion for a job opening?
   (a) Experience using word processing and spreadsheet software.
   (b) Works well under pressure.
   (c) Medical administrative assistant education.
   (d) Two years' previous experience working in a medical office.

_____ 2. Which of the following is not true about a probationary period?
   (a) Probationary periods are typically 90 to 180 days.
   (b) An employee's performance is measured during a probationary period.
   (c) If an employee leaves the job after a probationary period, severance must be paid by the employer.
   (d) An employer and employee meet at the end of a probationary period to determine whether the employment arrangement should continue.

_____ 3. Which of the following keeps a record of what an employee has earned over a year?
   (a) Policy manual.
   (b) Employee compensation record.
   (c) Payroll tax record.
   (d) Form W-4.

_____ 4. A change in income tax withholding must be reported using
   (a) Form W-2.
   (b) Form W-4.
   (c) An employee compensation record.
   (d) A written personal note from the employee.

_____ 5. Which of the following is an optional deduction from an employee's paycheck?
   (a) State income tax.
   (b) Medicare tax.
   (c) Dental insurance premium.
   (d) Federal income tax.
   (e) Court-ordered deduction.

_____ 6. Which of the following is a form used for reporting and depositing taxes owed to the federal government?
   (a) Form 941.   (b) Form 940.
   (c) Form W-2.   (d) Form W-4.

_____ 7. Which of the following is not true when discharging an employee?
   (a) Sufficient warning should be given to the employee that performance is not acceptable.
   (b) Reason(s) for termination should be well documented.
   (c) Office policies can be applied differently for every employee.
   (d) Failure to inform an employee of the reason that the employee is terminated could lead to a lawsuit.

_____ 8. All of the following could lead to work-related stress except
   (a) Adequate breaks during the day.
   (b) Not enough time to complete necessary work.
   (c) Hectic, tense work environment.
   (d) No opportunity to give input to office matters.

_____ 9. Which of the following is not correct about the FMLA?
   (a) The Act applies to both private and public sector employers of more than 50 persons.
   (b) Twelve weeks of leave is allowed for each 12-month period.
   (c) Leave can be used to care for certain ill family members.
   (d) The FMLA does not apply if the company has a sick leave policy that differs from the provisions of the Act.

_____ 10. Which of the following is not a likely example of sexual harassment?
   (a) Telling lewd jokes.   (b) Shaking hands.
   (c) Rubbing up against someone.   (d) Winking suggestively.

Exercise 14–3 PAYROLL CALCULATIONS

Determine the correct amounts for the situation given. Use the information in this chapter and the amounts listed here when figuring tax. Record the correct answer in the blank provided.

_____ 1. An employee earning $11.63 per hour working 40 hours per week using a biweekly pay period would have gross earnings of
(a) $465.20   (b) $930.40
(c) $1007.93   (d) None of the above

_____ 2. What are the gross monthly earnings of an employee hired at $24,000 per year?
(a) $2400   (b) $932.08
(c) $2000   (d) None of the above

_____ 3. Assuming that the employee mentioned in question 2 works 40 hours per week, what is the employee's hourly wage?
(a) $23.07   (b) $11.54
(c) $9.78   (d) None of the above

_____ 4. An employee works the following hours in a week: Monday, 6.75 hours; Tuesday, 4.5 hours; Wednesday, 8.25 hours; Thursday, 8 hours; Friday, 7.75 hours. What are the total hours worked during the week?
(a) 33.75   (b) 35
(c) 35.25   (d) None of the above

_____ 5. The amount of FUTA withheld from an employee who earned $1000 is
(a) $6.20   (b) $62.00
(c) $0.62   (d) None

_____ 6. An employee earning $24,000 per year will pay how much in Social Security tax?
(a) $348.00   (b) $1488.00
(c) $2184.00   (d) $2976.00

Exercise 14–4 PAYROLL PREPARATION

Compute the payroll amounts for a biweekly period using the information in this table. Use information given in the chapter and the amounts listed here when figuring tax. Complete the payroll record. (No employee has met the maximum amount for Social Security tax.) Procedure Box 14–2 can be used as a guide when completing this exercise.

Payroll Information

Employee Name	Hours Worked	Hourly Rate	Marital Status	Exemptions
Dixon, Amy	80	11.73	M	0
Dorland, Robert	75	11.40	M	2
Gordon, Margaret	48	11.80	S	1
Michaels, Connie	64	12.25	S	0
Scott, Patrick	80	12.02	M	3
Sears, Jackie	80	10.21	M	1

Payroll Record

Employee Name	Gross Earnings	FICA Tax	Federal Withholding Tax	State Income Tax (2% of gross earnings)	Total Deductions	Net Earnings
Dixon, Amy						
Dorland, Robert						
Gordon, Margaret						
Michaels, Connie						
Scott, Patrick						
Sears, Jackie						

ACTIVITY 14–1 Look up information pertaining to federal income taxes on the Internet and identify under which circumstances an individual is exempt from federal income tax.

ACTIVITY 14–2 Research the Family and Medical Leave Act.

ACTIVITY 14–3 Conduct research on the causes, signs, and symptoms of stress. Locate information on how to alleviate or reduce the effects of stress.

14
DISCUSSION

The following topics can be used for class discussion or for individual student essay.

DISCUSSION 14–1 Read the quotation at the beginning of the chapter. Relate this quotation to working in the medical office.

DISCUSSION 14–2 You are one of five assistants in the office. One of the assistants seems to have a persistently negative, down attitude. What should you do?

DISCUSSION 14–3 Discuss what causes stress for you and positive or negative ways that you handle it.

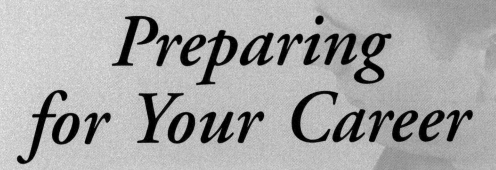

Preparing
for Your Career

CHAPTER OUTLINE

PREPARATION FOR EMPLOYMENT

APPLYING FOR A POSITION

DEVELOPING A WINNING RESUMÉ

COVER LETTER

FINDING OUT ABOUT JOB OPENINGS
 Networking
 Academic Placement Services
 Professional Employment Services
 Classified Ads
 Internet Job Search
 Professional Associations
 Cold Calls
 Internship Opportunities

AN APPLICATION FOR EMPLOYMENT

PREPARING FOR A GREAT INTERVIEW
 The Interview

CHOOSING THE RIGHT POSITION

SUMMARY

LEARNING OUTCOMES

On successful completion of this chapter, the student will be able to

1. Identify where job openings may be advertised.
2. Prepare a cover letter and resumé.
3. Complete an application for employment.
4. Identify successful interview techniques.

CMA COMPETENCIES

1. Project a professional manner and image.

VOCABULARY

internship
resumé
student portfolio

JOB SEARCH ESSENTIALS

Your daily agenda must be goal driven. If not, a task driven agenda will perpetuate.
—Glenn Crider

A medical administrative assistant must present to prospective employers his or her acquired skills, knowledge, and personal attributes in a professional manner. Following are some fundamental details an assistant should consider when seeking a position in a medical office.

PREPARATION FOR EMPLOYMENT

During the course of their education, students in a medical office–related program are exposed to many different subjects. Health sciences–related courses such as anatomy and physiology, medical terminology, and disease conditions as well as office–related courses such as bookkeeping, medical office procedures, and computer technology provide a well-rounded education for anyone wishing to work as a medical administrative assistant.

As mentioned in Chapter 1, however, a medical administrative assistant's formal education is just the beginning. Technologic advances in health care keep the industry moving at a fast pace. An assistant must learn to adapt to those changes and to implement new procedures in the medical office. Continuing education is necessary to keep pace with those changes. Opportunities for continuing education can be found in evening or weekend classes at a local college, distance education courses via the Internet, and workshops conducted by industry professionals, government agencies, and career development companies.

Throughout education and training, an assistant should work to gain as much exposure as possible to all aspects of the operation of the medical office. Courses in human relations, accounting, and management can enhance an assistant's education and increase his or her employability.

In preparation for employment, assistants should focus on their particular skills and interests. Not everyone is suited to the same type of position. Assistants should try to match their interests to a position that is well suited to them. By identifying their interests, assistants will be able to identify certain qualities they would be able to bring to a position.

For example, suppose that an assistant has identified excellent math skills as one of his or her strengths. Obviously, such skills would be a great asset in a position in which the assistant may be responsible for managing a practice's accounts receivable or accounts payable. Or maybe the assistant speaks a foreign language. In many locales, a bilingual assistant can be a tremendous asset when serving as an interpreter for patients.

APPLYING FOR A POSITION

When advertising an open position, medical offices may elect to gather interested applicants in a number of ways. They may choose to do the following:

- Have applicants telephone the medical office to inquire about the position.
- Ask interested applicants to send a resumé to the office or other location.
- Require interested applicants to come to the office to complete an application (Fig. 15–1).

Some employers may prefer to use an application; others may prefer to ask for a resumé. Regardless of how the medical office asks applicants to inquire, a well-prepared medical assistant will always bring along a resumé to give to the employer. Even if the medical office asks the assistant to complete an application, the assistant should give a resumé to the employer along with the application.

If the office asks an assistant to come to the office to pick up an application, the assistant should always go to the office dressed in attire that is suitable for an interview. "Stopping by" the office in a pair of jeans or the like is not appropriate and would probably create a bad first impression. When going into the office of a possible future employer, an assistant should dress as he or she would for an interview. You never know—the employer might decide to hold an interview right then and there!

DEVELOPING A WINNING RESUMÉ

As a medical administrative student prepares to enter the workforce, information should be gathered for compiling and producing a **resumé** (Fig. 15–2). A resumé documents the student's qualifications for a position. It provides a place for the student to highlight his or her education, work experience, personal achievements, strengths, and qualities.

The resumé is sometimes the first contact the student will have with the employer. Because first impressions are so important, much time and effort should go into creating a resumé. Tips for creating a great resumé are listed in Box 15–1.

Quite a collection of information is needed to complete an assistant's resumé. In preparing a resumé, it is a good idea to keep all gathered information in one place that is easy to access. Procedure Box 15–1 outlines how to prepare a resumé. Following is the basic information included within many resumes:

Career Objective. Usually listed first in the body of the resumé, the career objective identifies where the applicant hopes to go with his or her education and experience. It should have some connection with the position for which the assistant is applying.

Education. Information regarding the assistant's formal education is listed in this section. Education from high school to any and all post-secondary education at a business school, college, or university should be given to the prospective employer. Information regarding specific courses taken during post-secondary training and identification of any degree awarded or the highest grade completed can be listed in this section. If the student's grade point average was good, it should be specifically listed. If the employer requests a transcript of education, the grade point average will not be necessary, because it will be given on the transcript.

If an advertisement for a medical office position lists specific requirements, such as medical transcription, the assistant should mention specifically whether he or she has taken courses in that subject.

Work Experience or Work History. After education that may be preferred or even required for a position, employers often want to know the applicant's work history: whether it is related to the position for which the assistant has applied. Work experience is usually listed in reverse chronological order, that is, the most recent experience is listed first and the oldest experience is listed last. Volunteer experience can be listed in this section.

When listing work experience, the assistant should give specific information related to each position, such as

- Name and address of previous employer.
- Dates of employment.
- Position held.
- Job responsibilities.

The assistant may also choose to add other information, such as that he or she worked at the job while going to college. Applicants may or may not choose to give the reason for leaving previously held positions.

Applicants should never be embarrassed to list job experience that is entry level or unrelated to the position sought. Listing this previous experience gives applicants the chance to let employers know more about their work history. In the example provided in Figure 15–2, note how the assistant has mentioned specific duties that may enhance the ability to work in a medical office.

Achievements, Awards, Interests, or Skills. Students should keep track of achievements, awards, or other personal or professional accomplishments that might interest an employer (e.g., fluency in a language other than English). Membership in professional organizations should also be mentioned. Any personal interests can be listed at the applicant's discretion.

References. Some publications recommend that references be listed as "available on request." Why would an applicant make a potential employer work to get references? It would be much easier for the employer if the references were included with the resume. Before listing references on a resume, the applicant should obtain permission from each reference. This is done as a common courtesy and to alert the person that he or she may be receiving a call regarding a reference.

COVER LETTER

With each resume, a cover letter (Fig. 15–3) should be included to introduce the applicant to the interviewer or interview team. The cover letter highlights some of the best qualifications of the candidate and should get the reader's attention so that the applicant will be called for an interview.

The sample of the cover letter shown in Figure 15–3 identifies the applicant's interest in the position as well as chief qualifications for the position. The use of a cover letter is a good way to highlight an applicant's major qualifications for a position twice—once in the cover letter and once in the resume. Procedure Box 15–2 outlines how to prepare a cover letter.

FINDING OUT ABOUT JOB OPENINGS

Employment openings for individuals with training as medical administrative assistants occur in a variety of places (see Chapter 1 and Box 15–2).

How do employers advertise for open positions? There are a multitude of places in which positions are "advertised." When many people think of looking for a job, the first place they look is in the newspaper classified advertising section. It is sometimes said, however, that the best jobs never appear in a newspaper classified section. The newspaper classified ads should never be the sole method of locating a job; in fact, no method listed in this section should be the sole method of locating a position. An assistant should use a combination of sources to locate the desired opening.

Networking

It is often said "It's not what you know, it's who you know." Although having the right skills or qualifications is necessary to secure employment, information about job openings is often gathered casually from individuals with whom an assistant comes in contact. For instance, someone may mention at a professional meeting that an opening is becoming available in a physician's office. Assistants may hear the information directly, or the information may be given to them by someone they know. Assistants seeking employment should spread the word about the type of position they are looking for and should let people know of their search for employment. An acquaintance or close friend may be the lead to the ideal position.

Academic Placement Services

Educational institutions often provide assistance in helping their graduates obtain employment. Placement services offered by educational institutions are usually free to the graduate. Sometimes, many of the best jobs are found through an academic placement service. Many employers prefer to list openings with schools that they know provide top-quality training.

Educational placement services allow graduates to receive information on employment listings that are sent to the placement office. The placement service, in turn, sends information about employment listings to the graduate. Schools very often receive notice of job openings that may never appear in the newspaper. For this reason, the graduate may have an advantage over other job seekers who do not have access to a school's placement services.

APPLICATION FOR POSITION / Medical or Dental Office
AN EQUAL OPPORTUNITY EMPLOYER

(In answering questions, use extra blank sheet if necessary)

No employee, applicant, or candidate for promotion, training or other advantage shall be discriminated against (or given preference) because of race, color, religion, sex, age, physical handicap, veteran status, or national origin.

PLEASE READ CAREFULLY AND WRITE OR PRINT ANSWERS TO ALL QUESTIONS. DO NOT TYPE.

Date of Application

A. PERSONAL INFORMATION

| Name - Last | First | Middle | Social Security No. | Area Code/Phone No. ( ) |

| Present Address: - Street | (Apt #) | City | State | Zip | How Long At This Address? |

| Previous Address: - Street | City | State | Zip | Person to notify in case of Emergency or Accident - Name: |
| From: | To: | Address: | Telephone: |

B. EMPLOYMENT INFORMATION

| For What Position Are You Applying? | ☐ Full-Time ☐ Part-Time ☐ Either | Date Available For Employment? | Wage/Salary Expectations: |

| List Hrs./Days You Prefer To Work | List Any Hrs./Days You Are Not Available: (Except for times required for religious practices or observances) | Can You Work Overtime, If Necessary? ☐ Yes ☐ No |

| Are You Employed Now? ☐ Yes ☐ No | If So, May We Inquire Of Your Present Employer?: ☐ No ☐ Yes, If Yes: |
| | Name Of Employer: | Phone Number: ( ) |

| Have You Ever Been Bonded? ☐ Yes ☐ No | If Required For Position, Are You Bondable? ☐ Yes ☐ No ☐ Uncertain | Have You Applied For A Position With This Office Before? ☐ No ☐ Yes If Yes, When?: |

Referred By / Or Where Did You Learn Of This Job?:

| Can You, Upon Employment, Submit Verification Of Your Legal Right To Work In The United States?: ☐ Yes ☐ No Submit Proof That You Meet Legal Age Requirement For Employment? ☐ Yes ☐ No | Language(s) Applicant Speaks or Writes (If Use Of A Language Other Than English is Relevant To The Job For Which The Applicant Is Applying: |

C. EDUCATIONAL HISTORY

Name & Address Of Schools Attended (Include Current)	Dates From	Thru	Highest Grade/Level Completed	Diploma/Degree(s) Obtained/Areas of Study
High School				
College				Degree/Major
Post Graduate				Degree/Major
Other				Course/Diploma/License/Certificate

Specific Training, Education, Or Experiences Which Will Assist You In The Job For Which You Have Applied.

Future Educational Plans

D. SPECIAL SKILLS

CHECK BELOW THE KINDS OF WORK YOU HAVE DONE:

		☐ MEDICAL INSURANCE FORMS	☐ RECEPTIONIST
☐ BLOOD COUNTS	☐ DENTAL ASSISTANT	☐ MEDICAL TERMINOLOGY	☐ TELEPHONES
☐ BOOKKEEPING	☐ DENTAL HYGIENIST	☐ MEDICAL TRANSCRIPTION	☐ TYPING
☐ COLLECTIONS	☐ FILING	☐ NURSING	☐ STENOGRAPHY
☐ COMPOSING LETTERS	☐ INJECTIONS	☐ PHLEBOTOMY (Draw Blood)	☐ URINALYSIS
☐ COMPUTER INPUT	☐ INSTRUMENT STERILIZATION	☐ POSTING	☐ X-RAY
OFFICE EQUIPMENT USED: ☐ COMPUTER	☐ DICTATING EQUIPMENT	☐ WORD PROCESSOR	☐ OTHER:

| Other Kinds Of Tasks Performed Or Skills That May Be Applicable To Position: | Typing Speed | Shorthand Speed |

ORDER # **72-110** • © 1976 BIBBERO SYSTEMS, INC. • PETALUMA, CA. • (REV. 1/95)
TO REORDER CALL TOLL FREE: (800) BIBBERO (800-242-2376) OR FAX (800) 242-9330   MFG IN U.S.A.

(PLEASE COMPLETE OTHER SIDE)

Figure 15–1. Applicants for an open position in a medical office may be required to complete an employment application. (Form courtesy of Bibbero Systems, Inc., Petaluma, California, 800-242-2376. Fax 800-242-9330. www.bibbero.com.)

E. EMPLOYMENT RECORD

LIST MOST RECENT EMPLOYMENT FIRST	May We Contact Your Previous Employer(s) For A Reference? ☐ Yes ☐ No

1) Employer — Worked Performed. Be Specific:

Address	Street	City	State	Zip Code

Phone Number ( )

Type of Business	Dates	Mo.	Yr.		Mo.	Yr.
	From			To		

Your Position	Hourly Rate/Salary
	Starting Final

Supervisor©s Name

Reason For Leaving

2) Employer — Worked Performed. Be Specific:

Address	Street	City	State	Zip Code

Phone Number ( )

Type of Business	Dates	Mo.	Yr.		Mo.	Yr.
	From			To		

Your Position	Hourly Rate/Salary
	Starting Final

Supervisor©s Name

Reason For Leaving

3) Employer — Worked Performed. Be Specific:

Address	Street	City	State	Zip Code

Phone Number ( )

Type of Business	Dates	Mo.	Yr.		Mo.	Yr.
	From			To		

Your Position	Hourly Rate/Salary
	Starting Final

Supervisor©s Name

Reason For Leaving

F. REFERENCES — FRIENDS / ACQUAINTANCES NON-RELATED

(1)

Name	Address	Telephone Number	(☐ Work ☐ Home)	Occupation	Years Acquainted

(1)

Name	Address	Telephone Number	(☐ Work ☐ Home)	Occupation	Years Acquainted

Please Feel Free To Add Any Information Which You Feel Will Help Us Consider You For Employment

READ THE FOLLOWING CAREFULLY, THEN SIGN AND DATE THE APPLICATION

"I certify that all answers given by me on this application are true, correct and complete to the best of my knowledge. I acknowledge notice that the information contained in this application is subject to check. I agree that, if hired, my continued employment may be contingent upon the accuracy of that information. If employed, I further agree to comply with Company/Office rules and regulations."

Signature: _____   Date: _____

Figure 15–1. *Continued*

Taylor J. Reed

272 Meadowlawn Lane
Farmington, ND 58000
(012) 555-7717

Objective	To obtain a position as a medical administrative assistant in a family practice clinic.
Education	**1999–2001 Best Technical College** Farmington, ND • Medical Assisting, AAS. • Graduated with honors, GPA 3.92
	1996–1999 Southside High School Farmington, ND • Diploma • Member of National Honor Society
Experience	**1997–1999 Southside School Bookstore** Farmington, ND Sales Clerk • Worked in school store helping customers and stocking shelves. • Responsible for totaling daily receipts and making bank deposits.
	1999–2001 Green Valley Pharmacy Farmington, ND Sales Associate • Maintain computerized customer database. • Responsible for financial transactions (charges and cash payments). • Performed store opening and closing procedures. • Worked 30 hours per week while attending college.
Interests	Bike riding, team sports, reading, crossword puzzles
References	Mary K. Hanson, Faculty Advisor Best Technical College 308 Main Ave. Farmington, ND 58000 (555) 111-7899
	Christian Matthew, Store Manager Green Valley Pharmacy 709 Pine St. Farmington, ND 58000 (555) 111-3456

Figure 15–2. A professional-looking resumé that identifies an applicant's education and experience is essential when applying for a position in a medical office.

Professional Employment Services

There are two types of professional employment services: those that charge a fee and those that do not charge a fee. Of the services that charge a fee, the fee may be paid by the employer or the employee. A medical administrative assistant with the right job skills should **never** have to pay a fee to obtain a job.

Many employment agencies assist employers in finding the right people for jobs. Some agencies also place people in temporary positions to assist employers with short-term employment shortages. Sometimes, these temporary positions lead to permanent employment.

Some states have employment agencies (sometimes called *Job Service*) that provide services to employers looking to hire employees. A large practice may require that all entry-level positions be applied for through the state employment service in its city. Services are provided at no cost to the employer, and positions are available at no cost to the employee.

Classified Ads

One of the traditional spots to look for a job is in the classified section of a local newspaper. Sometimes, these ads can bring a flood of applicants to the office, and competition may be tough. Ads may also offer little information about the position, such as the job responsibilities or wages, so the assistant may not be able to discern whether the position is one he or she would like. When looking for openings, the best day for job listings is Sunday, but classified ads should be read every day to ensure that all openings are seen.

Box 15-1 Tips for a Great Resumé

- List the most important items first on the resumé. For example, if education in a medical office–related program has just been completed and the graduate has no experience working in a medical office, list the education first.
- If possible, keep a resumé to one page; employers may look only at the first page. A resumé should not be more than two pages.
- Use a font that is easy to read. A resumé is no place to experiment with elaborate font styles.
- Pay attention to format. Use a format that makes the resumé easy to read.
- Use high-quality paper with matching envelopes. Office supply stores carry a wide variety of papers. White or off-white papers look professional; avoid colors, especially vivid ones.
- Make the resumé unique. Incorporate a personal touch, if possible.
- Use a resumé template found in many popular office software packages or use specific software to develop a professional-looking resumé. Research approaches to preparing resumés.

PROCEDURE 15-1 *Prepare a Resumé*

Materials Needed

- Professional resumé paper (white or off-white)
- Computer with word processing software
- Education, work experience, and student portfolio information

1. Choose a format for the resumé. A resumé computer program or resumé template from a word processing program may be used.
2. List your full name, address, and telephone number at the top of the resumé. If available, an e-mail address can also be furnished.
3. Write a career objective specific to the position desired.
4. List your education, with the most recent first.
5. List your work experience, with the most recent first. Any volunteer experience or student internship experience can be listed under "work experience."
6. List your personal interests.
7. List your personal references. Instructors and work supervisors are good choices. Friends and relatives should not be listed as personal references. Be sure to ask each reference for permission before listing him or her as a reference.
8. Proofread the resumé for typos or grammatical errors. If possible, have another person read the resumé.*
9. Review the resumé to ensure that the format is easy to read. Make any necessary adjustments.
10. Print a copy of the resumé and retain a copy for yourself.

Denotes crucial step in procedure. Student must complete this step satisfactorily in order to complete the procedure satisfactorily.

Internet Job Search

The Internet can be a useful tool for recruiting employees. Several large health care institutions have established their own employment listings on their Web sites. Governmental agencies and large health care facilities such as the Mayo Clinic post open positions on the Internet. Assistants wishing to relocate may find the Internet a valuable resource for locating employment in the area desired.

Professional Associations

Students who belong to a professional organization during their education may find out about openings in the organization's newsletter or at membership meetings.

Cold Calls

If an assistant desires employment with a specific medical practice, the assistant should not wait for a position to be advertised. The assistant may choose to apply to an office by sending a cover letter and resumé expressing interest in working with the organization. The possibility always exists that an opening might be available. After all, what is there to lose?

Internship Opportunities

In preparation for entering the workforce, medical administrative assistants should take advantage of internship experiences that may be available to them (Fig. 15–4).

A part of many educational programs, an **internship** can provide an assistant with an opportunity to apply learned skills and behaviors and to experience the work environment of the medical office. Depending on the arrangements made, an internship experience may also be referred to as an *externship, clinical,* or *practicum.* In an internship, a student works under the supervision of a medical office employee and receives on-the-job experience in a medical office.

No matter what it is called, this experience can prove invaluable to the assistant when beginning the job hunt. An internship should be listed on the student's resumé under "work experience." Often, if the internship experience goes well and the medical office has an opening, the intern may have a good chance of securing employment at the internship site.

February 14, 2002

Ms. Taylor Hudson, Office Manager
Horizons Healthcare Center
123 Main Avenue
Farmington, ND 58000

Dear Ms. Hudson:

I have recently completed my education for Medical Administrative Assistant at Best Technical College in Farmington, ND. I am interested in staying in the local area to begin my career in the health care industry. I am applying for a customer service position in your insurance department and am enclosing my resume.

I am a hard-working, dedicated individual with customer service-related work experience over the past few years. I enjoy working with the public and have a particular interest in work related to the financial aspects of a business.

I would appreciate the opportunity to interview with you and appreciate your consideration of my qualifications for this position. I look forward to hearing from you.

Sincerely,

Taylor J. Reed

Taylor J. Reed

enclosure

Figure 15–3. A cover letter is used to introduce an applicant and is included along with a resumé.

AN APPLICATION FOR EMPLOYMENT

Sometimes, an application (see Fig. 15–1) is used in the medical office to gain specific information from each applicant. If the office needs specific expertise in a certain area, that area may be specifically listed on the application form. The application shown in Figure 15–1 asks specific questions about when the applicant is available for work. The use of an application form ensures that certain information is asked of each applicant that might not otherwise be included in a resume.

When filling out an application, an assistant should carefully complete all required blanks on the form and follow all instructions on the form. An employer will be negatively influenced if the assistant does not complete the application properly or if the application is incomplete. Procedure Box 15–3 outlines how to complete an employment application.

CHECKPOINT

You want to work in a large well-known facility that is located about 700 miles from your current home. What are some good strategies on locating and applying for a position there?

PREPARING FOR A GREAT INTERVIEW

Once the assistant has been selected to be interviewed for a position, there are many things he or she should consider that are part of a successful interview. Good preparation for an interview can help make it a successful experience.

● Know something about the organization. Research information on company operations. Know where any branch offices might be located and what medical specialties they have. Be ready to ask questions about the organization.
● Rehearse answers to questions that may be asked. Prepare answers to basic questions, such as "Tell me about your education at the technical college" or "What makes you the best person for the job?" Be prepared to answer tough questions, such as "Why are you leaving your present position?" or "What would you do if . . ."

PROCEDURE 15–2 *Prepare a Cover Letter*

Materials Needed

- Professional resumé paper (white or off-white)
- Computer with word processing software
- Completed resumé

1. Use a proper format for the letter (see Chapter 6).
2. Address the letter to the individual designated to receive applications.
3. Write the letter expressing your interest in a position and identifying some of your qualifications and strengths.
4. Close the letter with the appropriate salutation and your full name.
5. Proofread the letter for typos and grammatical errors. If possible, have another person also read the letter.*
6. Print a copy of the letter and retain a copy for yourself.
7. Sign the letter that will be included with your resumé.*
8. Place the letter appropriately in a business envelope along with the resumé (see Fig. 6–12).

Denotes crucial step in procedure. Student must complete this step satisfactorily in order to complete the procedure satisfactorily.

- Practice interviewing with a friend. Practicing or role-playing an interview can help relieve the anxiety often present during an interview.
- Arrive on time. Do not be late. Try to arrive 5 to 10 minutes early for the interview but not so early it may appear you are overanxious.

Box 15–2 Possible Employment Opportunities for a Medical Administrative Assistant

- Large multispecialty clinic.
- Private practice.
- Hospital.
- Nursing home.
- Insurance company.
- Home health agency.
- Hospice.
- Dental office.
- Law office specializing in medical-related cases.
- Medical school.
- Pharmaceutical company.
- Chiropractic office.

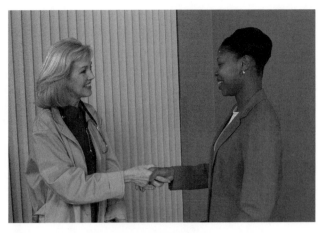

Figure 15–4. An applicant should shake the interviewer's hand both before and after an employment interview.

- Make sure to emphasize strong points. If you have outstanding or exceptional skills in a certain area, do not be afraid to "toot your own horn"—with a certain degree of modesty, of course.
- Dress appropriately. Remember that what is worn to an interview creates a first impression for others. Good grooming is expected. Do not smoke before the interview. An example of proper interview dress is included in Figure 15–5.
- Do not chew gum during the interview.
- Be prepared to ask questions about the position. Be ready with questions about the work hours, responsibilities, opportunity for advancement, and employee benefits.

The Interview

The anticipation of a job interview is often enough to make most people a little nervous. Rest assured; it is okay to be apprehensive—as a matter of fact, it is perfectly normal. It is very important to relax and trust that if you have the right qualifications, appear genuinely interested in working for the practice, and are sincere in your answers to interview questions, you will have a good chance of receiving a job offer.

The interview is an applicant's chance to support the qualifications presented in the resumé and an opportunity to display personal qualities. Some tips for a successful interview are as follows:

- Shake hands with the interviewer at the beginning of the interview. Practice a friendly greeting when preparing for the interview, such as "Good morning, my name is Jane Doe. I'm here for the 11:00 interview" or "Hello, my name is John Doe. It's a pleasure to meet you." Be sure to get the interviewer's name—you will need it later.
- Even if an application is required, give a resumé along with the application or bring one to the interview.
- Be positive. Do not spend time "bashing" a former employer. Present a positive attitude.
- Shake hands with the interviewer at the end of the interview. Use the person's name and thank him or her for the interview.

PROCEDURE 15–3 Complete an Employment Application

Materials Needed

Many employment applications are now available online over the Internet. The same steps would be followed, but the information would be entered electronically.

- Employment application
- Pen

1. Read the instructions on the form and follow them carefully. Provide the information requested here in addition to any other information requested on the application.
2. Identify your personal information.
3. List your educational history.
4. List your employment history.
5. List your personal references.
6. Review the application to make sure it is complete.*
7. Sign and date the application.*
8. Submit the application to the individual designated.

Denotes crucial step in procedure. Student must complete this step satisfactorily in order to complete the procedure satisfactorily.

- Send a follow-up letter (Fig. 15–6) thanking the interviewer for the interview. Be sure to address the letter to the interviewer personally.

Employee Benefit Packages

An important item of discussion during an interview is the types of benefits available for the position. Because of health care industry forecasts of continued employment growth, employers will likely need to provide incentives to attract and retain employees. Many employers offer substantial benefit packages that provide essential insurance coverages and some "perks" as well.

Individuals who are employed on a full-time basis usually have many benefits paid in full by the employer. Part-time employees in some facilities may have full benefits, but others may receive partial benefits or may need to pay a sum to obtain full benefits.

Not all benefits are available from every organization. Large organizations may be able to offer more benefits simply because of their size. Depending on the organization, it may be possible to negotiate some components of a benefit package.

Health Insurance. Health insurance varies widely in the types of incidents covered. Health insurance plans usually cover hospital and clinic charges related to illness or injury,

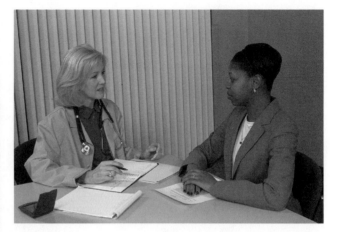

Figure 15–5. During an employment interview, proper posture, eye contact, and professional dress convey genuine interest in a job opening.

and some plans even provide coverage for preventive care, such as routine physicals and eye examinations. Employers may cover the entire cost of the insurance premium or may require employees to pay a portion of the premium. Many health insurance plans are quite comprehensive and provide many benefits, including reduced costs for prescriptions.

Life Insurance. Many employers provide a basic life insurance benefit that may be a set amount or may be proportionate to the employee's salary. The life insurance benefit is usually provided at no cost to the employee, but, occasionally, additional life insurance coverage for the employee or any member of the immediate family may be available for purchase at the employee's discretion.

Dental Insurance. Dental insurance coverage customarily covers illness or trauma related to the teeth as well as regular dental checkups. Dental procedures are usually covered, and many dental policies have an orthodontics benefit.

Disability Insurance. Disability insurance covers people who become disabled and are not able to work. Disability insurance is available in two forms: short-term and long-term. This type of insurance is designed to make up for income that might otherwise be lost if an employee were out of work for a brief or extended period of time.

Disability insurance is a type of insurance different from workers' compensation. Workers' compensation covers injuries that are job related; disability insurance provides coverage for time missed from work due to illness that may not be work related.

Sick Leave. Sick leave benefits provide paid time off when an employee is sick. Some employers allow employees to use sick leave if a family member is sick and needs to be cared for by the employee. Sick leave may be issued in terms of hours or days. It may be awarded at a set time each year or may be accrued during each pay period. Limits are sometimes set by employers on the amount of sick leave days or hours an employee may accumulate.

Vacation. Almost every health care employer offers some type of paid time off. Similar to sick leave, vacation

February 21, 2002

Ms. Taylor Hudson, Office Manager
Horizons Healthcare Center
123 Main Avenue
Farmington, ND 58000

Dear Ms. Hudson:

Thank you for the opportunity to interview yesterday for the customer service position in the insurance department at your facility. I appreciate the time you took to give me a tour of the facility as well as to discuss the responsibilities and expectations for the position.

If you have any additional questions for me, I can be reached after 3:00 weekdays at 555-7717. I look forward to receiving your decision regarding the position.

Sincerely,

Taylor J. Reed

Taylor J. Reed

Figure 15–6. A follow-up letter should be sent to thank an interviewer for the opportunity to interview.

leave may also be accumulated either by hours or per day and may be awarded at a specific time of the year or may accrue each pay period. A limit on vacation accumulation is common among most employers.

Holidays. Employers in facilities that are not open around the clock usually establish paid holidays. Common holidays recognized are religious holidays and many federal holidays.

Paid Time Off. For facilities that are open 24 hours a day, 365 days a year, employers may consolidate vacation, holiday pay, and sick leave in one pool for the employee. This pool is often referred to as paid time off (PTO). Employers will then allow employees to use the time as they choose, provided that adequate coverage is maintained throughout the facility's vital areas.

Pre-tax Plans. Employers may offer the chance for employees to set aside a specified amount for eligible expenses from each paycheck that is not taxed. Typical eligible expenses include child care and medical and dental expenses. The money that is set aside is deposited in an account with an outside agency. Participation in a pre-tax plan is totally voluntary. Participants in the plan submit proof of expenses to the outside agency and are reimbursed for their expenses up to the amount they have set aside.

Retirement. Many employers offer some type of retirement plan. Some plans allow employees to take additional money out of their paychecks to set aside for retirement. The additional money may even be matched by the employer. The thought of a retirement plan when you are just starting out in a career may seem strange, but the sooner an employee participates in a retirement plan, the more time the investment will have to grow.

Education Reimbursement. One of the less common benefits that is sometimes available is an educational reimbursement program provided by the employer. These programs encourage employees to continue their education and keep up with current technologies and trends. Educational reimbursement can pay some or all of the tuition associated with a course for credit. An employer may choose to fund only courses related to the individual's employment or may pay for any educational opportunity in which the employee has an interest. Some employers require proof of successful completion of the course before the tuition is reimbursed.

CHOOSING THE RIGHT POSITION

An assistant who is well suited to a position exemplifies that satisfaction when interacting with patients and coworkers. An assistant should take an honest look at the positions available and choose the one for which he or she is best suited. For instance, a talkative person may have difficulty in a transcription position that has little to no contact with people during the day, or a person who is relaxed and methodical may have difficulty in a fast-paced urgent care center. An assistant spends a good portion of each day at work, and the type of employment chosen will have an impact on his or her life. That impact will be a good one if an assistant is prepared for and interested in the job he or she chooses.

When a job offer is made, must the assistant give an answer right away? Of course not. Very few employers expect an answer immediately after an offer is made. Very often, an applicant will ask to "sleep on it" and get back to the employer the next day with an answer to the offer. This practice allows the applicant to think about what it would be like to work in that particular office.

How do you tell whether a position is right for you? Basically, you need to be satisfied with answers to questions such as the following:

- Is the job interesting?
- Does the practice appear to be an enjoyable place to work?
- Are the wages appropriate? (Information on wages in a local area can usually be obtained through state employment offices, school placement offices, or local libraries.)
- Are the benefits satisfactory?
- Does the work schedule meet with your expectations?

Once you have asked yourself questions such as these and have given yourself some time to think over a job offer, chances are good that you will make the right decision.

SUMMARY

Now that you have come to the end of this book, you may think that you have read and learned all you need to know to go out and get a job as a medical administrative assistant. However, recall what was mentioned in the very first chapter: in the medical field, learning never ends! Technologies used in health care change almost as quickly as we become aware of them.

Entering the world of work will bring many new challenges and opportunities. Working in a medical office will bring about many opportunities to apply the skills and techniques learned while in school. A career in medical administrative assisting is an exciting, interesting, and worthwhile occupation that a dedicated assistant will find continually rewarding. Best of luck to you in your career ahead!

Bibliography

U.S. Office of Personnel Management, Federal Employees Health Benefits.
U.S. Department of Labor.
U.S. Bureau of Labor and Statistics.

Exercise 15–1 TRUE OR FALSE

Read each statement and determine whether the statement is true or false. Record the answer in the blank provided. T = true; F = false

_____ 1. When applying for a position in a medical office, an assistant should bring along a resumé even if an employment application is completed.

_____ 2. Information on wages in your local area may be obtained through a state employment office or through other resources.

_____ 3. An applicant should review an application for completeness before it is handed in.

_____ 4. On a resumé, it is best to list "available on request" for personal references to save you the time of asking individuals for permission to list them as personal references.

_____ 5. Mistakes on an application can cost you a chance at an interview.

_____ 6. Medical and life insurance are typical employee benefits provided by employers.

_____ 7. If an employee is injured on the job, he or she must have disability insurance or compensation will not be received for time missed from work or injuries caused by work.

_____ 8. Retirement plans may allow additional contributions to be made by employees.

_____ 9. Employers may offer medical, dental, and life insurance to their employees at little or no additional cost.

_____ 10. A pre-tax plan allows employees to set aside part of their earnings tax-free to pay for medical and child care expenses.

Exercise 15–2 CHAPTER CONCEPTS

Read each statement and choose the answer that best completes the statement. Record the answer in the blank provided.

_____ 1. Which of the following is not true about seeking employment in a medical office?
(a) Some offices require an application to be completed.
(b) Courses in computer technology are of little value because technology changes too rapidly.
(c) Your personal strengths and interests should be considered when seeking employment.
(d) Continuing education will be necessary to keep pace with industry changes.

_____ 2. Which of the following is true about a cover letter?
(a) A cover letter contains detailed information regarding an applicant's education and work history.
(b) It is best to address the letter "To whom it may concern."
(c) A cover letter allows an applicant to emphasize chief qualifications for a position.
(d) A cover letter is sent separately from a resumé.

_____ 3. Which of the following is true about locating job openings?
(a) Fees are normally charged for using an academic placement service.
(b) Health care job openings are listed only in the Sunday newspaper.
(c) In order to find a job, an assistant should expect to use a professional employment service and should expect to pay a fee.
(d) Openings in another part of the country may be located using the Internet.

_____ 4. All of the following apply to a student internship except
(a) On an internship, a student experiences real-life situations.
(b) A student may be paid while on an internship.
(c) Internships often increase a student's chances of later being employed at the internship site.
(d) Every student wishing to work in a medical office must take an internship.

_____ 5. Benefits are an important consideration when accepting employment. Which of the following is not true in regard to employee benefits?
(a) An employee may be required to pay part of a health insurance premium.
(b) All employers are required to provide dental insurance for employees.
(c) PTO is an accumulation of vacation, holiday, and sick leave pay.
(d) Employers may limit the amount of vacation time that an employee can accumulate.

_____ 6. Which of the following is true about employee benefits?
(a) Employers may limit the amount of sick leave that an employee can accumulate.
(b) Education reimbursement benefits means an employer may pay for some educational courses or programs in which employees may enroll.
(c) An employee may be able to purchase additional life insurance coverage for himself or herself.
(d) All are correct.
(e) Only b and c are correct.

_____ 7. Which of the following does not belong?
(a) Reference
(b) Internship
(c) Practicum
(d) Clinical
(e) Externship

Exercise 15–3 INTERVIEW TECHNIQUES

Identify whether the following interview techniques are good or bad practice when applying for a position. Record the answer in the blank provided. G = good practice; B = bad practice.

_____ 1. Leave resumé at home until it is requested.

_____ 2. Be prepared to ask questions about the position and the organization.

_____ 3. Establish eye contact with the interviewer.

_____ 4. It is acceptable to chew gum during an interview.

_____ 5. Rehearse answers to potentially hard questions.

_____ 6. Ask the employer ahead of time for all questions that will be discussed during the interview.

_____ 7. Have a cigarette or alcoholic drink before the interview to relax.

_____ 8. Arrive on time or slightly late because doctors' offices usually are behind schedule.

_____ 9. Rehearse for the interview with a friend.

_____ 10. Focus on your needs and wants.

_____ 11. Shake hands with the interviewer before and after the interview.

_____ 12. Be interested in the position for which you are interviewing.

_____ 13. Ask current employees what they do not like about the office atmosphere.

_____ 14. Ask questions about the work schedule.

_____ 15. Send a follow-up letter thanking the interviewer for the opportunity to interview.

_____ 16. Use proper speech during the interview.

15
ACTIVITIES

ACTIVITY 15–1   Review the contents of your student portfolio begun in Activity 1–5 with the list here. Identify items that are included and items that should be added.
- Copy of school transcripts.
- Record of employment.
- Academic awards.
- Other achievement awards, personal accomplishments.
- Organization membership information.
- Committee membership/leadership information.
- Certifications or licensures.
- Examples of school projects.

ACTIVITY 15–2   Prepare a resumé using a professional resumé software or template from a word processing program. Follow the guidelines listed in Procedure Box 15–1.

ACTIVITY 15–3   Prepare a cover letter using a word processing program. Follow the guidelines in Procedure Box 15–2.

ACTIVITY 15–4   Prepare a list of questions that may be asked by an interviewer. Stay within the guidelines presented in Chapter 14, then participate in a mock interview with you acting as the interviewer.

ACTIVITY 15–5   Participate in a mock interview with another individual acting as the interviewer. Bring a prepared resumé to the interview and be prepared to answer interview questions.

ACTIVITY 15–6   Complete an employment application such as the one pictured in Figure 15–1 or use an application from a local health care facility. Follow the guidelines given in Procedure Box 15–3.

15
DISCUSSION

The following topics can be used for class discussion or for individual student essay.

DISCUSSION 15–1   Read the quotation at the beginning of the chapter. How might this quotation relate to your career plans and your life in the future?

DISCUSSION 15–2   Define professionalism and give examples of professional behavior.

DISCUSSION 15–3   Review your personal strengths and weaknesses. How would you discuss them with a potential employer?

DISCUSSION 15–4   Identify examples of how you could locate employment opportunities in your community using each of the following resources:
- Networking.
- Academic placement services.
- Professional employment services.
- Classified ads.
- Internet job search.
- Professional associations.
- Cold calls.
- Internship opportunities.

Appendices

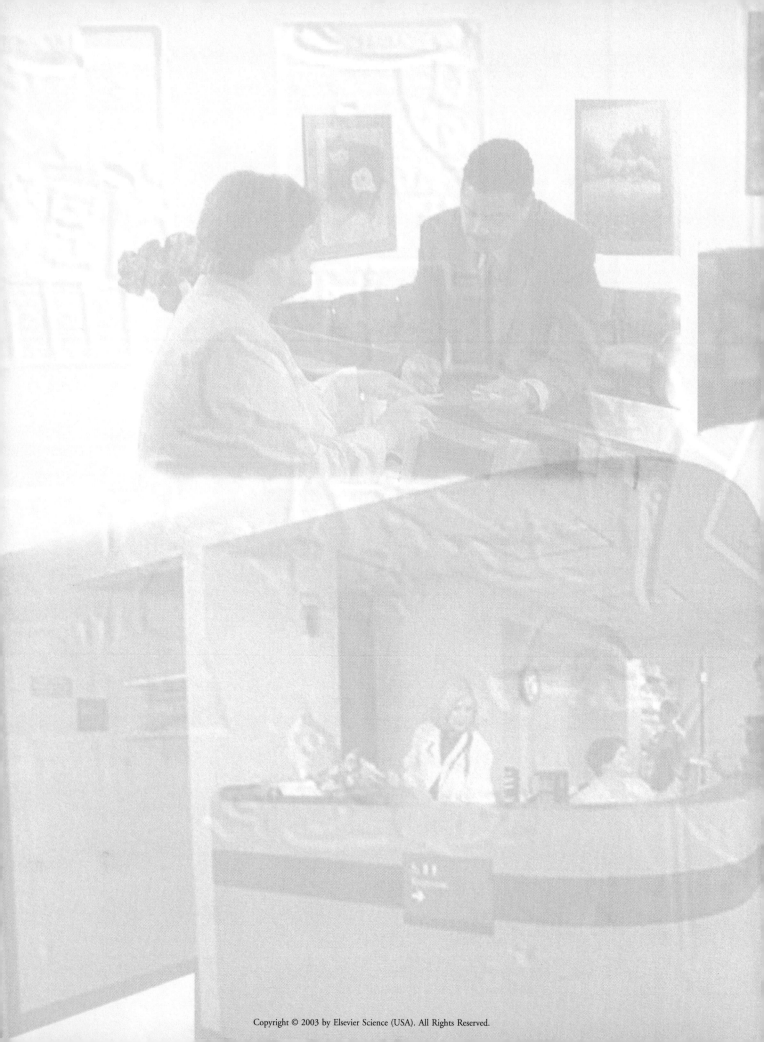

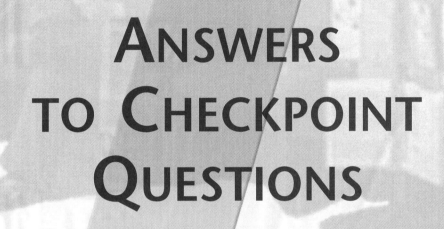

ANSWERS
TO CHECKPOINT
QUESTIONS

Chapter 1

Explain why education as a medical administrative assistant would be beneficial for employment in a dental office.

Students of medical administrative assistant programs take courses in office procedures, anatomy and physiology, medical terminology, and computer technology; the skills and knowledge acquired in such a program would be used frequently in a dental office setting.

Chapter 2

Explain why a group practice may want to employ more primary care physicians than specialists.

Primary care physicians provide comprehensive general health care for patients. These physicians are usually the first physician a patient with a health concern would consult, and patients are often required to obtain a referral from a primary care physician before seeing a specialist.

What advantage(s) would there be to a health care facility to hire health care providers other than physicians?

If there is a shortage of physicians in a particular area, a health care provider such as a nurse practitioner or physicians' assistant can help fulfill the need for additional health care providers. With regard to the financial aspect of using other health care providers, a salary for a nurse practitioner or physicians' assistant would be lower than a salary for a physician.

Nursing homes are required to have a certain number of RNs on duty at all times. A clinic may choose to hire LPNs to work with patients and may or may not have an RN present in the facility. Given what you know about the makeup of those facilities, explain why a clinic may not be required to hire RNs.

Because a physician does not continually work in a nursing home, a higher level of health care is required for care of the nursing home residents. The level of nursing care required in a clinic may not be as great as that required in a nursing home.

Chapter 3

Identify whether or not the following situations could be malpractice on the part of a health care professional:
1. A nurse gives the wrong dosage of a drug, and that dosage causes harm to the patient.
2. A patient phones the clinic with chest pain, and the nurse fails to inform the physician of the phone call. Later in the day, the patient suffers a massive heart attack while at home and dies.
3. A physician fails to notify a patient of normal laboratory results.
4. A physician fails to inform the patient of suspicious Pap smear results. The patient is not informed of the need for follow-up care, and 1 year later she is diagnosed with cervical cancer.

Referring to the information in the chapter regarding proving negligence in a malpractice suit, all cases except number 3

would probably be considered negligence. The patient in case number 3 would probably not be able to prove harm.

Could a patient with Alzheimer's disease enter into a contract?

No. If a patient has been diagnosed with Alzheimer's disease, the patient may no longer be of sound mind, and enforcing a contract signed by the patient (while suffering from the disease) would be difficult. Contracts made before the diagnosis may be valid but may be challenged if the contract was made close to the time of diagnosis.

Chapter 4

Physicians often provide treatment at no cost to their fellow physicians and their families. Is this in keeping with the Hippocratic Oath?

The Oath declares that a physician should "consider dear to me as my parents him who taught me this art; to live in common with him and if necessary to share my goods with him." This might be interpreted to support the practice of professional courtesy. (Professional courtesy is mentioned in the AMA's Current Opinions and is generally supported as ethical behavior.)

Examine the following examples of conduct, decide whether the conduct is in keeping with the information given about the AMA Principles of Medical Ethics, and state the reason for your answer:
1. Dr. Gonzalez is an obstetrician practicing in a large metropolitan city. Dr. Gonzalez has decided she will not accept any new obstetrics patients in her practice.

This practice is ethical because physicians are allowed to choose whom they will accept as patients (with the exception of emergency cases) (Principle VI).
2. Dr. Smith is an internist practicing in a state that has a law against physician-assisted suicide. Dr. Smith believes patients should have the right to choose physician-assisted suicide if they are terminally ill, so he helps a patient commit suicide.

Euthanasia is not supported by the AMA as ethical behavior. Physicians are dedicated to protecting life. A physician committing such an act would be practicing unethically and would likely face criminal charges if such an act was illegal (Principle III).
3. Dr. Anderson is aware of a physician in his health care facility that often bills Medicare for services that have not been performed. She does not report the physician's activity to the board of directors or to Medicare officials.

Physicians should report fraudulent activity of other physicians. If a physician has proof that fraudulent activity is occurring, the physician has an obligation to protect patients and the public (Principle II).
4. Dr. Kowalski has developed a new technique for suturing operative wounds. He demonstrates this new technique to colleagues at the AMA national convention.

Physicians are encouraged to develop new procedures and willingly share their discoveries with their colleagues (Principle IV).

A medical administrative assistant is confronted daily with situations to which she or he must decide how to respond.

The AAMA's code of medical ethics provides a framework for the assistant to determine appropriate behavior. Consider the following instances and determine whether or not the assistant's behavior is in keeping with the code of ethics:

1. An assistant volunteers for a local nonprofit health care organization.

   Yes. Participation in service activities is encouraged.

2. An assistant attends additional training to upgrade job skills.

   Yes. An assistant should continually seek to improve skills and knowledge.

3. An assistant unnecessarily discusses a patient's medical condition with a fellow employee.

   No. Such activity is a breach of confidentiality.

Consider the following case and determine the appropriate action that you as a medical administrative assistant should take:

Sue Adams, an unmarried pregnant patient of the office, cannot decide whether or not she should have an abortion. Sue asks Dr. Johnson what she thinks should be done. How would Dr. Johnson reply?

Dr. Johnson probably has a personal opinion about abortion, but she would likely present the facts (e.g., risks, alternatives) to the patient and leave it up to the patient to decide. Sue is the one who will have to live with her decision, not Dr. Johnson.

Is euthanasia a procedure that is consistent with the Hippocratic Oath? Why?

Not likely. The Hippocratic Oath, as given in the chapter, states, "to please no one will I prescribe a deadly drug, nor give advice which may cause his death."

Chapter 5

A physician specializing in family practice often sees patients who bring their young children to the office. Explain how and why the office staff might be expected to assist with the children in the office.

Although it is not the office staff's responsibility to take care of every child who accompanies a patient to the office, once in a while a child will not be able to be present in an examination room during an examination or procedure. At that time, an assistant should keep a watchful eye on the child until the procedure or examination is completed and the child can rejoin the parent.

Chapter 6

A few people in the office like to gossip about other staff members. How could this affect the medical office environment?

The more people who work in a medical office, the more likely there may be problems among some of the staff members. Office gossip can divide an office staff and create an unpleasant atmosphere in which to work. Gossip is negative and detrimental and should not be tolerated.

Explain why training in proper telephone technique is important for every staff member of the medical office.

Although the front desk staff may be chiefly responsible for answering the telephone, other staff members frequently use the telephone to talk with patients or other staff members. Training in proper telephone technique will help all personnel use the telephone more efficiently and effectively.

Explain the importance of deleting patient references from sample letters even though the letters remain in the office.

Although it is acceptable to keep samples of letters written in an office, anything that could potentially identify a patient should be obliterated from them. Names, chart numbers, addresses, account numbers—anything that could possibly be linked to a particular patient should be blacked out from a copy. Samples are usually kept near a transcriptionist's workstation and are not part of the medical records; thus, samples may not have the confidentiality protection (i.e., locked cabinets or rooms) that a medical record would have.

Chapter 7

The medical office where you are employed is evaluating two pieces of appointment scheduling software for implementation in the office. Software A is cheaper but only allows one user at a time to access the appointment system. Software B is twice as expensive but allows an unlimited number of users to access the appointment system at one time. There are three physicians, a nurse practitioner, three nurses, and three medical office assistants employed at the clinic. It is your job to recommend to the providers the appropriate software package for purchase. Which software package would you recommend? Defend your answer.

Of course, costs will be a factor, but if the office has sufficient funds to purchase software B, that should be the choice. Three assistants will be expected to schedule appointments for four health care providers. Software B allows more than one user at a time, so it is the better choice because assistants will need to schedule appointments and providers may need access to the system at the same time. Software B will enable the office staff to provide better service for patients.

Which of the following appointments could be scheduled as a double-booked appointment? (There may be more than one possible answer.)

Wart treatment	Headache	Depression
Lump	Sinus pain	Cough
Ear infection	Hearing check	Burn

Referring to Table 7–1, the following appointments could be double-booked: ear infection, sinus pain, cough. Double-booked appointments are usually appointments of an urgent-care nature. The three appointments identified are conditions that if left untreated could potentially become something more serious. Although the wart treatment is identified as a 15-minute appointment, wart treatment is usually not of an urgent nature.

Why is it important for the medical office assistant to have an excellent understanding of anatomy, physiology, and disease processes in order to appropriately schedule appointments in the medical office?

A basic understanding of the human body and conditions that affect a patient is absolutely essential for a medical administrative assistant. Although an assistant should never diagnose a patient, knowledge of the human body will enable an assistant to understand how extensive some health concerns could be. Also, it is usually an assistant who takes a patient's telephone call, screens the call, and decides how the call is handled (i.e., take a message, make an appointment, or transfer the call to a nurse or physician).

Chapter 8

An assistant who is new to the office likes to help make new patients feel more welcomed to the practice by sitting next to the patient in the lobby to answer any questions the patient has about completing the paperwork for registration. Is this a good idea?

No, this is not a good idea. Oftentimes on patient registration and history forms, personal questions may be listed, and the patient's confidentiality may be in jeopardy if questions are asked while the patient is seated in the lobby.

Explain why music or television, or both, is an important addition to a reception area.

Some type of entertainment that is appropriate for all ages will create a pleasant atmosphere and will help pass the time while patients and family members wait for appointments.

Explain why CPR training is a good idea for all medical office staff.

Whether an office is large or small, staff members never know whether they will be the first to encounter a patient who needs help. A staff member walking down a hallway or entering a restroom may be the first to encounter a patient who may need immediate attention.

Chapter 9

A medical office is using a terminal digit filing system in its records room. All chart numbers are composed of at least six digits. Charts will be marked with labels corresponding to the first unit used for filing. Should the medical office also use colored chart folders in addition to the colored labels, or will manila folders suffice?

Colored folders could also provide another check when filing charts. If a 10-color filing system such as the one pictured in Table 9–1 is implemented, the first digit in the secondary unit could signify the color. For example, the chart number 126342 would have labels identifying the 42, and the chart would have a green folder. Other charts—such as 126042, 126542, and 126842—would all be filed near 126342 and will all be the same color. If someone accidentally tries to file the chart numbered 123642 near those numbers, it would be recognized as a mistake because 123642 would be a white chart.

The credit department of the medical office has asked that an assistant place a colored label on the front of a patient's chart if the patient's account has a large balance that is grossly overdue. Is this a good idea? Why?

No, this is not a good idea. A patient's or guarantor's financial status or information regarding the balance of a patient's

or guarantor's account should not be included with the patient's medical record. A medical office would never want a patient to infer that treatment was not given because a large balance was owing on an account. Such activity might be an invitation to litigation.

Chapter 10

A patient telephones the office to report she has not yet received a bill for services performed a month ago. What do you do?

Take the patient's name and number and say that you will need to check the status of the bill. You may tell the patient that depending on the services that were rendered it sometimes takes a short time for charges to be posted to an account. You would then need to trace the bill to determine why it has not appeared on the patient's account. After finding the status of the bill, telephone the patient with the answer.

A minor telephones the office and wishes to see a physician for information on birth control. The minor does not want her parents to know about the visit. Based on what you learned in Chapter 3 and in this chapter, what might your answer be?

It is likely the physician will see the patient without the parents' consent. Before scheduling any type of appointment, confirm with the physician that the physician will see the patient for such a visit.

Your physician is contemplating switching from a pegboard system to a computerized system. What might be the advantages of a computerized system?

Although it may be costly up front, a computerized system will save the office time and money in the long run. Statements for patients' accounts will be generated easily, and a computerized system will provide tracking for all transactions related to patients' accounts.

Chapter 11

Which coverage could potentially be more costly for an insurance company to provide: a fee-for-service plan or a managed care plan?

A fee-for-service plan is usually more costly because a patient is usually not required to get approval to see a specialist. Under a managed care plan, patients are required to see a primary care physician in order to get approval to see a specialist. Oftentimes, the primary care physician will be able to treat the patient's condition, and the cost of a specialist will be avoided. With a fee-for-service plan, an insurance company will need to pay for every visit covered by the policy.

Chapter 12

A medical office employee trips and falls over some boxes in the medical records room. One of the staff physicians examines the employee, obtains x-rays of the employee's wrist, and determines that the x-rays are negative and that the employee has only sustained a wrist sprain. Because the worker is already employed by the clinic, the services are performed at no charge. Should anything else be done by the employee?

The employee must file a first report of injury form to document the case for workers' compensation reasons. In addition, the employee should make sure that the visit is documented in the employee's medical record. Regardless of whether or not anyone is billed, both the workers' compensation and medical record documentation must be done.

Chapter 13

At the end of many workdays, your coworkers comment that there is "too much to be done" to get ready for patients the next day and that the receipts of the day should be handled when the office atmosphere is less hectic—maybe at the end of the week or the next week. What is your response?

If assistants are having trouble meeting all responsibilities of a position because of their workload, something must be done. Receipts should not sit until they can be processed; because of lack of deposits, cash flow will be affected, which, in turn, will have an impact on the ability of the office to pay accounts payable. Letting receipts pile up also increases the chance that some payments will be lost or misplaced. Receipts must be handled on a timely basis. In this particular situation, taking action could mean overtime for office staff, additional office help, or reassignment of office duties, if necessary.

One of the assistants in the office proposes that receipts should no longer be written for payments received in person in the office, citing that patients who send checks in the mail do not get a receipt. What is your response?

Payments made in person in the office may occasionally be made in cash (e.g., small co-payments may be required by insurance companies). Without a receipt, persons paying cash would have no record of payment. In addition, receipts provide

an excellent tracking device for recording information regarding a payment. It is likely that checks received in the mail will be returned with a portion of the patient's statement, which will allow an assistant to identify which account will be credited with the payment. The receipt that accompanies a payment also identifies what account should be credited with the payment.

Chapter 14

You are responsible for hiring an additional medical assistant to work in the office. A physician in the practice has asked you to find an older woman whose children are grown so that she will be able to stay late if necessary. How do you reply?

*Such a question should never be asked. The question that could be asked of **any** applicant is whether the applicant would be able to stay late if necessary, and the question should be asked of all applicants.*

You are working for a pediatric practice. When hiring, the pediatricians have asked you to screen for an assistant who likes children. Would this be acceptable in an interview?

Most likely, this is an acceptable question. The question must be asked of all applicants, but because working with children is an essential part of the job, such a quality would be critical in an applicant.

Chapter 15

You want to work in a large well-known facility that is located about 700 miles from your current home. What are some good strategies on locating and applying for a position there?

The Internet is a good place to start. Because the facility is large and well known, chances are that information will be available from a Web site. In addition, a local library may carry a newspaper that may have employment listings from the facility.

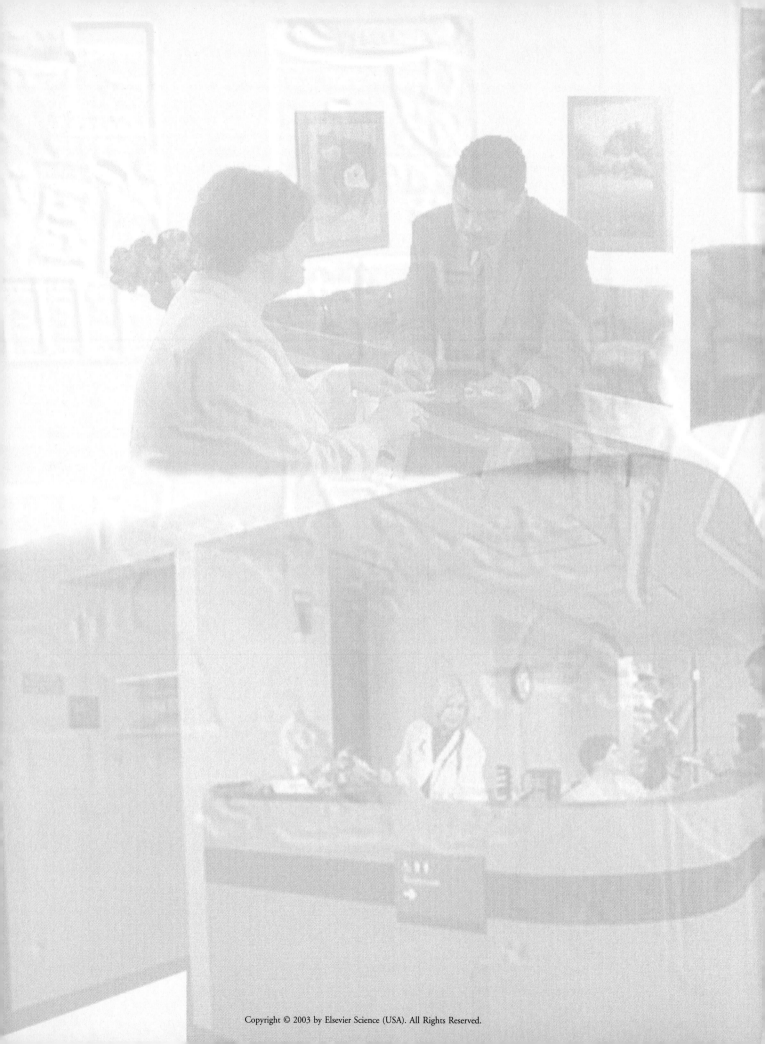

PROCEDURE COMPETENCY CHECKLISTS

Competency Assessment Checklist
Procedure 6–1: Demonstrate Telephone Techniques

Student name _____ Date _____

Learning Outcome: Demonstrate telephone techniques.

Performance Standards: 　　　　　Time allowed _____ min
　　　　　　　　　　　　　　　　Accuracy _____ %

Conditions: The student will follow the procedure outlined below to demonstrate telephone techniques within the standards identified using the following materials:
• Telephone set-up with two separate lines
• Pen or pencil

Evaluation Criterion	Performance Evaluation Checklist	Points Possible	Student's score 1st	2nd
■	1. Answer telephone using proper greeting: 　• welcome 　• identification of facility 　• identification of operator 　• offer to help			
●	2. Determine the reason for the call.			
■	3. Identity the caller.			
▲	4. Determine the appropriate action based on reason for the call.			
■	5. Confirm the call.			
■	6. Close the call.			
▲	*Optional* 7. Demonstrate holding.			
▲	8. Demonstrate transferring a call.			
	Total Points			

Minimum total points required for satisfactory score _____

Evaluation Criteria

Symbol	Category	point value
●	**crucial step**	_____
■	**essential step**	_____
▲	**theory**	_____

Evaluator's comments:

Evaluator's name _____ Date _____

● denotes crucial step in procedure. Student must complete this step satisfactorily in order to complete the procedure satisfactorily.

National curriculum competencies achieved:
• Demonstrate telephone techniques.
• Answer telephone calls employing proper etiquette.
• Manage telephone calls requiring special attention (including lab and x-ray reports, angry callers, and personal calls).

Competency Assessment Checklist
Procedure 6–2: Demonstrate Taking Telephone Messages

Student name _____ Date _____

Learning Outcome: Demonstrate taking telephone messages.

Performance Standards: Time allowed _____ min
                                      Accuracy _____ %

Conditions: The student will follow the procedure outlined below to demonstrate taking telephone messages within the standards identified using the following materials:
• Telephone set-up with two separate lines
• Message blanks
• Pen or pencil

Evaluation Criterion	Performance Evaluation Checklist	Points Possible	Student's score 1st	2nd
▲	1. Determine that a message is needed for an incoming telephnone call and obtain a message blank to record the message.			
■	2. Record date and time on message blank.			
■	3. Record caller's name on message blank.			
●	4. Record patient's name on message blank.			
■	5. Obtain patient's chart number. If chart number is not available, obtain patient's date of birth to help locate the chart number.			
■	6. Record name of individual to whom the call is directed–physician or another individual.			
■	7. Record message narrative including action requested on message blank.			
■	8. Record telephone number to return call.			
■	9. Sign the message with your name or initials.			
	Total Points			

Minimum total points required for satisfactory score _____

Evaluation Criteria

Symbol	Category	point value
●	crucial step	_____
■	essential step	_____
▲	theory	_____

Evaluator's comments:

Evaluator's name _____ Date _____

● denotes crucial step in procedure. Student must complete this step satisfactorily in order to complete the procedure satisfactorily.

National curriculum competencies achieved:
• Demonstrate telephone techniques.
• Manage telephone calls requiring special attention (including lab and x-ray reports, angry callers, and personal calls).

Competency Assessment Checklist
Procedure 6–3: Prepare a Patient Letter

Student name _____ Date _____

Learning Outcome: Prepare a patient letter.

Performance Standards: Time allowed _____ min
                                  Accuracy _____ %

Conditions: The student will follow the procedure outlined below to prepare a patient letter within standards identified using the following materials:
- Computer with word processing software
- Printer
- Letterhead stationery
- #10 business envelope
- Reference materials as necessary (dictionary, grammar reference)

Evaluation Criterion	Performance Evaluation Checklist	Points Possible	Student's score 1st	2nd
■	1. Prepare a letter to a patient using the proper format illustrated in Figures 6–8, 6–9 or 6–10.			
●	2. Proofread the letter for proper grammar and punctuation.			
■	3. Print enough copies of the letter.			
■	3. Address a business envelope using proper format for an OCR as shown in Figure 6–11.			
■	4. Fold and insert letter in an envelope as shown in Figure 6–12.			
	Total Points			

Minimum total points required for satisfactory score _____

Evaluation Criteria

Symbol	Category	point value
●	**crucial step**	_____
■	**essential step**	_____
▲	**theory**	_____

Evaluator's comments:

Evaluator's name _____ Date _____

● denotes crucial step in procedure. Student must complete this step satisfactorily in order to complete the procedure satisfactorily.

National curriculum competencies achieved:
- Respond to and initiate written communication.
- Compose correspondence according to acceptable business format.
- Employ effective written communication skills.
- Use computer for word processing.

Competency Assessment Checklist
Procedure 6–4: Prepare an Interoffice Memo

Student name _____ Date _____

Learning Outcome: Prepare an interoffice memo.

Performance Standards:　　　　　　　Time allowed _____ min
　　　　　　　　　　　　　　　　　　Accuracy _____ %

Conditions: The student will follow the procedure outlined below to prepare an interoffice memo within standards identified using the following materials:
• Computer with word processing software
• Printer
• Reference materials as necessary (dictionary, grammar reference)

Evaluation Criterion	Performance Evaluation Checklist	Points Possible	Student's score 1st	2nd
■	1. Prepare an interoffice memo using the proper format illustrated in Figure 6–13.			
●	2. Proofread the memo for proper grammar and punctuation.			
■	3. Print enough copies of the memo for distribution.			
	Total Points			

Minimum total points required for satisfactory score _____

Evaluation Criteria

Symbol	Category	point value
●	crucial step	_____
■	essential step	_____
▲	theory	_____

Evaluator's comments:

Evaluator's name _____ Date _____

● denotes crucial step in procedure. Student must complete this step satisfactorily in order to complete the procedure satisfactorily.

National curriculum competencies achieved:
• Respond to and initiate written communication.
• Compose correspondence according to acceptable business format.
• Employ effective written communication skills.
• Use computer for word processing.

Competency Assessment Checklist
Procedure 7–1: Prepare an Appointment Schedule for a Medical Office

Student name _____ Date _____

Learning Outcome: Prepare an appointment schedule for a medical office.

Performance Standards: Time allowed _____ min
                                    Accuracy _____ %

Conditions: The student will follow the procedure outlined below to prepare an appointment schedule for a medical office within standards identified using the following materials:
• Appointment scheduling software on a computer system
   or
• Appointment book and pencil

Evaluation Criterion	Performance Evaluation Checklist	Points Possible	Student's score 1st	2nd
■	1. Identify and mark off days the office is closed.			
■	2. Identify and mark off time of each day that the office is closed.			
■	3. Identify and mark off time of each day that each physician is unavailable.			
	Total Points			

Minimum total points required for satisfactory score _____

Evaluation Criteria

Symbol	Category	point value
●	crucial step	_____
■	essential step	_____
▲	theory	_____

Evaluator's comments:

Evaluator's name _____ Date _____

● denotes crucial step in procedure. Student must complete this step satisfactorily in order to complete the procedure satisfactorily.

National curriculum competencies achieved:
• Schedule and manage appointments.
• Utilize computer software to maintain office systems.
• Employ appointment scheduling system.
• Use computer for data entry and retrieval.

Competency Assessment Checklist
Procedure 7–2: Schedule Appointments

Student name _____ Date _____

Learning Outcome: Schedule appointments.

Performance Standards: Time allowed _____ min
                                  Accuracy _____ %

Conditions: The student will follow the procedure outlined below to schedule appointments within standards identified using the following materials:
- Appointment scheduling software on a computer system
    or
- Appointment book and pencil

Evaluation Criterion	Performance Evaluation Checklist	Points Possible	Student's score 1st	2nd
●	1. Determine the reason for the appointment.			
▲	2. Using scheduling guidelines, determine the length of the appointment.			
■	3. Identify the patient's name.			
■	4. Determine patient's preferences for desired appointment time.			
■	5. Identify date and time for appointment and obtain approval for date and time with patient (or patient's representative).			
■	6. Enter appointment on the schedule.			
■	7. Confirm appointment with patient (or patient's representative).			
■	*Optional*			
	8. If patient is in the office, give patient a written reminder for the appointment.			
	Total Points			

Minimum total points required for satisfactory score _____

Evaluation Criteria

Symbol	Category	point value
●	crucial step	_____
■	essential step	_____
▲	theory	_____

Evaluator's comments:

Evaluator's name _____ Date _____

● denotes crucial step in procedure. Student must complete this step satisfactorily in order to complete the procedure satisfactorily.

National curriculum competencies achieved:
- Schedule and manage appointments.
- Utilize computer software to maintain office systems.
- Employ appointment scheduling system.
- Use computer for data entry and retrieval.

Competency Assessment Checklist
Procedure 7–3: Document Appointment Changes

Student name _____ Date _____

Learning Outcome: Document appointment changes.

Performance Standards: Time allowed _____ min
Accuracy _____ %

Conditions: The student will follow the procedure outlined below to document appointment changes within standards identified using the following materials:
• Patient's medical record
• Black ink pen

Evaluation Criterion	Performance Evaluation Checklist	Points Possible	Student's score 1st	2nd
■	1. Identify appointment change (no-show, cancellation, reschedule, etc.)			
●	2. Obtain patient's medical record.			
●	3. In appropriate location in the patient's record, enter the date and document the appointment change.			
●	4. Sign the chart entry.			
	Total Points			

Minimum total points required for satisfactory score _____

Evaluation Criteria
Symbol	Category	point value
●	crucial step	_____
■	essential step	_____
▲	theory	_____

Evaluator's comments:

Evaluator's name _____ Date _____

● denotes crucial step in procedure. Student must complete this step satisfactorily in order to complete the procedure satisfactorily.

National curriculum competencies achieved:
• Schedule and manage appointments.
• Establish and maintain the medical record.
• Document appropriately.
• Employ procedures for handling cancellations and missed appointments.
• Use computer for data entry and retrieval.

Competency Assessment Checklist
Procedure 7–4: Reschedule Appointments

Student name _____ Date _____

Learning Outcome: Reschedule appointments.

Performance Standards:

Time allowed _____ min
Accuracy _____ %

Conditions: The student will follow the procedure outlined below to reschedule appointments within standards identified using the following materials:
• Appointment scheduling software on a computer system
  or
• Appointment book and pencil

Evaluation Criterion	Performance Evaluation Checklist	Points Possible	Student's score 1st	2nd
●	1. Obtain the patient's name.			
●	2. Locate the original appointment.			
▲	3. Verify the reason for the appointment. Using scheduling guidelines, determine if length of the appointment is correct.			
■	4. Determine preferences for desired appointment time.			
■	5. Identify date and time for appointment and obtain approval for date and time with patient (or patient's representative).			
■	6. Enter new appointment on the schedule.			
■	7. Confirm new appointment with patient (or patient's representative).			
	8. Delete original appointment.			
■	*Optional* 9. If patient is in the office, give patient a written reminder for the new appointment.			
	Total Points			

Minimum total points required for satisfactory score _____

Evaluation Criteria

Symbol	Category	point value
●	crucial step	_____
■	essential step	_____
▲	theory	_____

Evaluator's comments:

Evaluator's name _____ Date _____

● denotes crucial step in procedure. Student must complete this step satisfactorily in order to complete the procedure satisfactorily.

National curriculum competencies achieved:
• Schedule and manage appointments.
• Utilize computer software to maintain office systems.
• Employ appointment scheduling system.
• Use computer for data entry and retrieval.

Competency Assessment Checklist
Procedure 8–1: Update Existing Patient Registration Information

Student name _____ Date _____

Learning Outcome: Update existing patient registration information.

Performance Standards: Time allowed _____ min
                             Accuracy _____ %

Conditions: The student will follow the procedure outlined below to update existing patient registration information within standards identified using the following materials:
• Patient information
• Computer software for a medical office

Evaluation Criterion	Performance Evaluation Checklist	Points Possible	Student's score 1st	2nd
●	1. Ask patient for full legal name and locate patient information in patient database. Verify patient's date of birth to ensure that correct record is updated.			
■	2. Verify that the following information for the patient is current: • address • telephone number • employer • insurance company name, address, policy number and group number (copy insurance card if necessary) Record any changes given by the patient.			
■	3. Thank the patient for information and tell the patient to be seated in the lobby.			
■	4. Record any changes in registration information in patient's medical record (as applicable).			
	Total Points			

Minimum total points required for satisfactory score _____

Evaluation Criteria

Symbol	Category	point value
●	crucial step	_____
■	essential step	_____
▲	theory	_____

Evaluator's comments:

Evaluator's name _____ **Date** _____

● denotes crucial step in procedure. Student must complete this step satisfactorily in order to complete the procedure satisfactorily.

National curriculum competencies achieved:
• Establish and maintain the medical record.
• Obtain patient information.
• Use computer for data entry and retrieval.

Competency Assessment Checklist
Procedure 8–2: Obtain New Patient Registration Information

Student name _____ Date _____

Learning Outcome: Obtain new patient registration information.

Performance Standards: Time allowed _____min
                                         Accuracy _____%

Conditions: The student will follow the procedure outlined below to obtain registration information from a new patient within standards identified using the following materials:
• New patient registration form
• Patient medical history form
• Clipboard & pen or pencil
• Photocopier

Evaluation Criterion	Performance Evaluation Checklist	Points Possible	Student's score 1st	2nd
●	1. Ask patient for full legal name and check patient database to determine if patient is new to the medical office.			
■	2. Attach a registration form and patient history form to the clipboard and give to patient asking the patient to complete the forms and return to you when completed.			
■	3. After patient returns forms, review each form to determine if forms are complete. Ask patient for information if forms are incomplete.			
■	4. Ask patient for insurance card. Copy insurance card.			
■	5. Thank patient for information and tell patient to be seated in the lobby.			
	Total Points			

Minimum total points required for satisfactory score _____

Evaluation Criteria

Symbol	Category	point value
●	crucial step	_____
■	essential step	_____
▲	theory	_____

Evaluator's comments:

Evaluator's name _____ **Date** _____

● denotes crucial step in procedure. Student must complete this step satisfactorily in order to complete the procedure satisfactorily.

National curriculum competencies achieved:
• Establish and maintain the medical record.
• Obtain patient information.
• Use computer for data entry and retrieval.

Competency Assessment Checklist
Procedure 8–3: Record New Patient Registration Information

Student name _____ Date _____

Learning Outcome: Record new patient registration.

Performance Standards:

Time allowed _____ min
Accuracy _____ %

Conditions: The student will follow the procedure outlined below to record new patient registration within standards identified using the following materials:
- Computer software for a medical office
- Completed new patient registration form

Evaluation Criterion	Performance Evaluation Checklist	Points Possible	Student's score 1st	2nd
●	1. Check computer database to determine whether a record of the patient exists.			
■	2. Once patient has been verified as a new patient to the medical office, assign medical record number to the patient.			
■	3. Enter all pertinent data for the patient.			
■	4. Save the new record.			
	Total Points			

Minimum total points required for satisfactory score _____

Evaluation Criteria

Symbol	Category	point value
●	crucial step	_____
■	essential step	_____
▲	theory	_____

Evaluator's comments:

Evaluator's name _____ Date _____

● denotes crucial step in procedure. Student must complete this step satisfactorily in order to complete the procedure satisfactorily.

National curriculum competencies achieved:
- Establish and maintain the medical record.
- Obtain patient information.
- Use computer for data entry and retrieval.

Competency Assessment Checklist
Procedure 9–1: Document an Event in a Patient's Chart

Student name _____ Date _____

Learning Outcome: Document an event in a patient's chart.

Performance Standards: Time allowed _____ min
Accuracy _____ %

Conditions: The student will follow the procedure outlined below to document an event in a patient's chart within standards identified using the following materials:
• Patient's medical record
• Black ink pen

Evaluation Criterion	Performance Evaluation Checklist	Points Possible	Student's score 1st	2nd
●	1. Obtain patient's medical record. Locate next available place for documentation in the progress notes (continuation sheet).			
■	2. Determine information to be written in patient's chart. Be sure you are authorized to enter such information.			
●	3. With black ink, record date and information regarding the patient.			
●	4. Sign the chart entry.			
	Total Points			

Minimum total points required for satisfactory score _____

Evaluation Criteria

Symbol	Category	point value
●	crucial step	_____
■	essential step	_____
▲	theory	_____

Evaluator's comments:

Evaluator's name _____ Date _____

● denotes crucial step in procedure. Student must complete this step satisfactorily in order to complete the procedure satisfactorily.

National curriculum competencies achieved:
• Record laboratory results and patient communication in charts.
• Establish and maintain the medical record.
• Document appropriately.

Competency Assessment Checklist
Procedure 9–2: Transcribe a Medical Report

Student name _____ Date _____

Learning Outcome: Transcribe a medical report.

Performance Standards: Time allowed _____ min
 Accuracy _____ %

Conditions: The student will follow the procedure outlined below to transcribe a medical report within standards identified using the following materials:
• Dictated medical report
• Equipment to play report (digital or transcriber)
• Computer with word processing software
• Printer

Evaluation Criterion	Performance Evaluation Checklist	Points Possible	Student's score 1st	2nd
■	1. Locate beginning of report dictation.			
■	2. Adjust volume and speed of the dictation as necessary.			
▲	3. Choose appropriate report format.			
■	4. Type dictated report.			
●	5. Proofread report and make any necessary corrections.			
■	6. Print report for physician signature and insertion in patient's medical record.			
	Total Points			

Minimum total points required for satisfactory score _____

Evaluation Criteria

Symbol	Category	point value
●	crucial step	_____
■	essential step	_____
▲	theory	_____

Evaluator's comments:

Evaluator's name _____ Date _____

● denotes crucial step in procedure. Student must complete this step satisfactorily in order to complete the procedure satisfactorily.

National curriculum competencies achieved:
• Perform medical transcription.
• Utilize computer software to maintain office systems.
• Transcribe notes from a Dictaphone or tape recorder.
• Use computer for word processing.

Competency Assessment Checklist
Procedure 9 – 3: Organize a Patient's Medical Record

Student name _____ Date _____

Learning Outcome: Organize a patient's medical record.

Performance Standards:
Time allowed _____ min
Accuracy _____ %

Conditions: The student will follow the procedure outlined below to organize a patient's medical record within standards identified using the following materials:
• Patient's medical record
• Medical reports

Evaluation Criterion	Performance Evaluation Checklist	Points Possible	Student's score 1st	2nd
●	1. Verify patient's name on reports and on the medical record.			
■	2. Determine where the reports should be inserted in the medical record.			
■	3. Open fasteners holding chart documents together.			
■	4. Insert the reports in the appropriate location in the patient's medical record.			
■	5. Close fasteners to secure chart documents.			
	Total Points			

Minimum total points required for satisfactory score _____

Evaluation Criteria

Symbol	Category	point value
●	crucial step	_____
■	essential step	_____
▲	theory	_____

Evaluator's comments:

Evaluator's name _____ Date _____

● denotes crucial step in procedure. Student must complete this step satisfactorily in order to complete the procedure satisfactorily.

National curriculum competencies achieved:
• Organize a patient's medical record.
• Arrange contents of patient charts in appropriate order and perform audits for accuracy.

Competency Assessment Checklist
Procedure 9–4: Index and File Medical Records

Student name _____ Date _____

Learning Outcome: Index and file medical records.

Performance Standards: Time allowed _____ min
                                      Accuracy _____ %

Conditions: The student will follow the procedure outlined below to index and file medical records within standards identified using the following materials:
• Medical records

Evaluation Criterion	Performance Evaluation Checklist	Points Possible	Student's score 1st	2nd
■	1. Place medical records in indexing order following the guidelines for the filing system adopted by the medical office.			
●	2. Determine where the record will be filed.			
■	3. Verify that the filing location is correct by checking the record in front and in back of the record to be filed.			
■	4. Complete filing of each record by repeating steps 2 & 3 for each record.			
	Total Points			

Minimum total points required for satisfactory score _____

Evaluation Criteria

Symbol	Category	point value
●	crucial step	_____
■	essential step	_____
▲	theory	_____

Evaluator's comments:

Evaluator's name _____ Date _____

● denotes crucial step in procedure. Student must complete this step satisfactorily in order to complete the procedure satisfactorily.

National curriculum competencies achieved:
• File medical records.
• File records according to appropriate system.

Competency Assessment Checklist
Procedure 9–5: Color Code Medical Records

Student name _____ Date _____

Learning Outcome: Color code medical records.

Performance Standards:

Time allowed _____ min
Accuracy _____ %

Conditions: The student will follow the procedure outlined below to color code medical records within standards identified using the following materials:
- Medical records
- Color coding scheme
- Labels compatible with color coding scheme

Evaluation Criterion	Performance Evaluation Checklist	Points Possible	Student's score 1st	2nd
■	1. Obtain scheme for color coding medical records.			
●	2. Affix appropriate label to each medical record that corresponds to the filing system and associated color scheme. • Alphabetical filing—use label corresponding to first letter of patient's last name. • Consecutive number filing—use label corresponding to thousandths digit of chart number. • Terminal digit filing—use labels corresponding to the two digits in the primary indexing unit.			
■	3. Verify that color coding is correct by placing the records in order for filing, Colors will appear together.			
	Total Points			

Minimum total points required for satisfactory score _____

Evaluation Criteria

Symbol	Category	point value
●	crucial step	_____
■	essential step	_____
▲	theory	_____

Evaluator's comments:

Evaluator's name _____ Date _____

● denotes crucial step in procedure. Student must complete this step satisfactorily in order to complete the procedure satisfactorily.

National curriculum competencies achieved:

- File medical records.
- File records according to appropriate system.

Competency Assessment Checklist
Procedure 9–6: Process a Request to Release Medical Information

Student name _____ Date _____

Learning Outcome: Process a request to release medical information from the medical office.

Performance Standards: Time allowed _____ min

Accuracy _____ %

Conditions: The student will follow the procedure outlined below to process a request to release medical information from the medical office within standards identified using the following materials:
- Release of information form
- Black ink pen
- Patient's medical record

Evaluation Criterion	Performance Evaluation Checklist	Points Possible	Student's score 1st	2nd
■	1. If needed, help patient complete release request.			
▲	2. Verify that all necessary information is included on the release.			
●	3. Obtain patient's medical record and verify patient's name on release with name on medical record.			
■	4. Photocopy requested information to be released.			
■	5. Arrange information in logical order.			
■	6. Attach copy of release of information request on top of release.			
■	7. Place original release request in correspondence section of patient's medical record.			
●	8. Send information to the medical facility identified on the release.			
●	9. In a chart entry, document that the release was processed.			
	Total Points			

Minimum total points required for satisfactory score _____

Evaluation Criteria

Symbol	Category	point value
●	crucial step	_____
■	essential step	_____
▲	theory	_____

Evaluator's comments:

Evaluator's name _____ Date _____

● denotes crucial step in procedure. Student must complete this step satisfactorily in order to complete the procedure satisfactorily.

National curriculum competencies achieved:
- Identify and respond to issues of confidentiality.

Competency Assessment Checklist
Procedure 10–1: Assign Procedure Codes for a Patient's Encounter

Student name _____ Date _____

Learning Outcome: Assign procedure codes for a patient's encounter.

Performance Standards: Time allowed _____ min
                                    Accuracy _____ %

Conditions: The student will follow the procedure outlined below to assign procedure codes for a patient's encounter within standards identified using the following materials:
• Medical records
• CPT manual, current year's edition

Evaluation Criterion	Performance Evaluation Checklist	Points Possible	Student's score 1st	2nd
■	1. Identify all procedures treated during a patient's encounter.			
■	2. Locate the main term of each procedure code in the index by identifying the condition, anatomical site procedure or service provided.			
■	3. Look beneath in the main term for any additional modifiers. Identify all codes that may fit the procedure.			
■	4. Locate each of the codes from #3 in the appropriate section of CPT.			
●	5. Read the description for each code and choose the appropriate code for each procedure identified.			
	Total Points			

Minimum total points required for satisfactory score _____

Evaluation Criteria

Symbol	Category	point value
●	crucial step	_____
■	essential step	_____
▲	theory	_____

Evaluator's comments:

Evaluator's name _____ Date _____

● denotes crucial step in procedure. Student must complete this step satisfactorily in order to complete the procedure satisfactorily.

National curriculum competencies achieved:
• Perform procedural coding.
• Know coding systems used in insurance processing.
• Code diagnoses and procedures.

Competency Assessment Checklist
Procedure 10–2: Assign Diagnosis Codes for a Patient's Encounter

Student name _____ Date _____

Learning Outcome: Assign diagnosis codes for a patient's encounter.

Performance Standards:

Time allowed _____ min

Accuracy _____ %

Conditions: The student will follow the procedure outlined below to assign diagnosis codes for a patient's encounter within standards identified using the following materials:
• Medical records
• ICD-9-CM manual (current year)

Evaluation Criterion	Performance Evaluation Checklist	Points Possible	Student's score 1st	2nd
▲	1. Identify all diagnoses treated during a patient's encounter.			
▲	2. Determine the primary reason for the patient's office visit.			
■	3. Locate the main term of the diagnosis in the index (volume II).			
■	4. Locate any modifiers beneath the main term.			
■	5. Identify the numeric code referenced in volume II.			
■	6. Locate the code from volume II in the tabular (numerical) listing (volume I) in the manual.			
●	7. Read the description of the code. Determine if the code fits the diagnosis given for the patient.			
■	8. Code any additional diagnoses listed in the patient's encounter by repeating steps 3–7.			
	Total Points			

Minimum total points required for satisfactory score _____

Evaluation Criteria

Symbol	Category	point value
●	crucial step	_____
■	essential step	_____
▲	theory	_____

Evaluator's comments:

Evaluator's name _____ Date _____

● denotes crucial step in procedure. Student must complete this step satisfactorily in order to complete the procedure satisfactorily.

National curriculum competencies achieved:
• Perform diagnostic coding.
• Know coding systems used in insurance processing.
• Code diagnoses and procedures.

Competency Assessment Checklist
Procedure 10–3: Enter Patients' Charges into a Billing System

Student name _____ Date _____

Learning Outcome: Enter patients' charges into a billing system.

Performance Standards: Time allowed _____ min
                            Accuracy _____ %

Conditions: The student will follow the procedure outlined below to enter patients' charges into a billing system within standards identified using the following materials:
• Computer billing system or pegboard system
• Superbills from patients' encounters.

Evaluation Criterion	Performance Evaluation Checklist	Points Possible	Student's score 1st	2nd
▲	1. Gather superbills to be recorded.			
●	2. Assign correct procedure codes for each encounter.			
●	3. Assign correct diagnosis codes for each encounter.			
●	4. Record encounters in billing system. If using a pegboard system, use correct fee schedule for procedures. Enter correct information in each billing category.			
	Total Points			

Minimum total points required for satisfactory score _____

Evaluation Criteria

Symbol	Category	point value
●	crucial step	_____
■	essential step	_____
▲	theory	_____

Evaluator's comments:

Evaluator's name _____ Date _____

● denotes crucial step in procedure. Student must complete this step satisfactorily in order to complete the procedure satisfactorily.

National curriculum competencies achieved:
• Perform accounts receivable procedures.
• Perform billing and collection procedures.
• Use a physician's fee schedule.
• Know methods of billing.
• Employ appropriate accounting procedures.
• Know accounts payable/accounts receivable procedures.

Competency Assessment Checklist
Procedure 10–4: Produce Monthly Statements for Patient Accounts

Student name _____ Date _____

Learning Outcome: Produce monthly statements for patient accounts.

Performance Standards: Time allowed _____ min
                              Accuracy _____ %

Conditions: The student will follow the procedure outlined below to produce monthly statements for patients' accounts within standards identified using the following materials:
• Patients' account information (computer billing information or ledger cards)
• Outstanding charges and payments

Evaluation Criterion	Performance Evaluation Checklist	Points Possible	Student's score 1st	2nd
▲	1. Establish statement date.			
▲	2. Determine which accounts should have a statement generated. If using a cycle billing system, only certain statements may need to be generated.			
■	3. Post any outstanding charges to patients' accounts.			
■	4. Post any outstanding payments to patients' accounts.			
●	5. Print statements.			
	Total Points			

Minimum total points required for satisfactory score _____

Evaluation Criteria

Symbol	Category	point value
●	crucial step	_____
■	essential step	_____
▲	theory	_____

Evaluator's comments:

Evaluator's name _____ Date _____

● denotes crucial step in procedure. Student must complete this step satisfactorily in order to complete the procedure satisfactorily.

National curriculum competencies achieved:
• Perform accounts receivable procedures.
• Perform billing and collection procedures.
• Employ appropriate accounting procedures.
• Know accounts payable/accounts receivable procedures.

Competency Assessment Checklist
Procedure 11–1: Complete an Insurance Claim using the HCFA-1500

Student name _____ Date _____

Learning Outcome: Complete an insurance claim using the HCFA-1500.

Performance Standards: Time allowed _____ min
                                     Accuracy _____ %

Conditions: The student will follow the procedure outlined below to complete an insurance claim using the HCFA-1500 within standards identified using the following materials:
• Billing and insurance information for a patient
• Computer software or typewriter to complete form
• HCFA-1500 claim form

Evaluation Criterion	Performance Evaluation Checklist	Points Possible	Student's score 1st	2nd
▲	1. Obtain billing information for the claim.			
●	2. Code procedures and diagnoses for the claim.			
●	3. Obtain patient's insurance information for the claim.			
●	4. Complete HCFA-1500 claim form following guidelines established by the insurance plan.			
	Total Points			

Minimum total points required for satisfactory score _____

Evaluation Criteria

Symbol	Category	point value
●	crucial step	_____
■	essential step	_____
▲	theory	_____

Evaluator's comments:

Evaluator's name _____ Date _____

● denotes crucial step in procedure. Student must complete this step satisfactorily in order to complete the procedure satisfactorily.

National curriculum competencies achieved:
• Complete insurance claim forms.
• Utilize computer software to maintain office systems.
• Complete and file forms for insurance claims.
• Know billing requirements for insurance programs.

Competency Assessment Checklist
Procedure 12–1: Prepare a Meeting Agenda

Student name _____ Date _____

Learning Outcome: Prepare a meeting agenda.

Performance Standards:

Time allowed _____ min
Accuracy _____ %

Conditions: The student will follow the procedure outlined below to prepare a meeting agenda within standards identified using the following materials:
• Information about meeting
• Computer
• Printer

Evaluation Criterion	Performance Evaluation Checklist	Points Possible	Student's score 1st	2nd
■	1. Identify meeting date, time and place.			
■	2. Identify agenda items to be discussed and order of discussion.			
■	3. List agenda items in order of discussion.			
●	4. Proofread the agenda for typos and grammatical errors.			
■	5. Print a copy of the agenda.			
■	6. Make required number of copies of agenda and distribute to designated individuals.			
	Total Points			

Minimum total points required for satisfactory score _____

Evaluation Criteria

Symbol	Category	point value
●	crucial step	_____
■	essential step	_____
▲	theory	_____

Evaluator's comments:

Evaluator's name _____ Date _____

● denotes crucial step in procedure. Student must complete this step satisfactorily in order to complete the procedure satisfactorily.

National curriculum competencies achieved:
• Respond to and initiate written communication.
• Employ effective written communication skills.
• Use computer for word processing.

Competency Assessment Checklist
Procedure 12–2: Prepare Minutes of a Meeting

Student name _____ Date _____

Learning Outcome: Prepare minutes of a meeting.

Performance Standards: Time allowed _____ min
                                    Accuracy _____ %

Conditions: The student will follow the procedure outlined below to prepare minutes of a meeting within standards identified using the following materials:
• Meeting agenda
• Attendance at a meeting
• Computer and/or paper and pencil
• Printer

Evaluation Criterion	Performance Evaluation Checklist	Points Possible	Student's score 1st	2nd
■	1. Identify meeting date, time and place.			
■	2. Obtain copy of agenda.			
■	3. Attend meeting and list those present at the meeting.			
■	4. During the meeting, take notes regarding meeting discussion. Record the minutes in chronological order.			
■	5. Prepare minutes using the format provided in Chapter 12.			
●	6. Proofread the minutes for typos and grammatical errors.			
■	7. Print a copy of the minutes.			
■	8. Make required number of copies of minutes and distribute to designated individuals.			
	Total Points			

Minimum total points required for satisfactory score _____

Evaluation Criteria

Symbol	Category	point value
●	crucial step	_____
■	essential step	_____
▲	theory	_____

Evaluator's comments:

Evaluator's name _____ Date _____

● denotes crucial step in procedure. Student must complete this step satisfactorily in order to complete the procedure satisfactorily.

National curriculum competencies achieved:
• Respond to and initiate written communication.
• Employ effective written communication skills.
• Use computer for word processing.

Competency Assessment Checklist
Procedure 12–3: Prepare a Travel Itinerary

Student name _____ Date _____

Learning Outcome: Prepare a travel itinerary.

Performance Standards: Time allowed _____ min
                                    Accuracy _____ %

Conditions: The student will follow the procedure outlined below to prepare a travel itinerary within standards identified using the following materials:
• Information regarding travel plans
• Computer
• Printer

Evaluation Criterion	Performance Evaluation Checklist	Points Possible	Student's score 1st	2nd
■	1. Obtain information on air or ground transportation. Identify name of transportation provider, departure and arrival locations and travel confirmation numbers.			
■	2. Obtain information on hotel accommodations. Identify name, address, phone number and confirmation numbers.			
■	3. Obtain information on any meetings, conferences or other activities that will be attended. Identify name, address and phone numbers where possible.			
●	4. Prepare itinerary listing all information obtained above in chronological order.			
■	5. Distribute two copies of the itinerary to the traveler (one for traveler, one for traveler's family) and retain one copy for the office.			
	Total Points			

Minimum total points required for satisfactory score _____

Evaluation Criteria

Symbol	Category	point value
●	crucial step	_____
■	essential step	_____
▲	theory	_____

Evaluator's comments:

Evaluator's name _____ Date _____

● denotes crucial step in procedure. Student must complete this step satisfactorily in order to complete the procedure satisfactorily.

National curriculum competencies achieved:
• Respond to and initiate written communication.
• Employ effective written communication skills.
• Use computer for word processing.

Competency Assessment Checklist
Procedure 13–1: Prepare a Receipt for a Payment Received

Student name _____ Date _____

Learning Outcome: Prepare a receipt for a payment received.

Performance Standards: Time allowed _____ min
Accuracy _____ %

Conditions: The student will follow the procedure outlined below to prepare a receipt for a payment received within standards identified using the following materials:
• Receipts
• Payments received
• Pen

Evaluation Criterion	Performance Evaluation Checklist	Points Possible	Student's score 1st	2nd
■	1. Using the receipts in number order, enter the date payment is received.			
■	2. Enter the name of the payee.			
■	3. Specify the method of payment (check or cash).			
●	4. Enter the amount of payment numerically and in words in the spaces provided.			
●	5. Identify the account on which the payment should be applied.			
■	6. Enter the account balances if known.			
●	7. Sign the receipt.			
	Total Points			

Minimum total points required for satisfactory score _____

Evaluation Criteria
Symbol	Category	point value
●	crucial step	_____
■	essential step	_____
▲	theory	_____

Evaluator's comments:

Evaluator's name _____ Date _____

● denotes crucial step in procedure. Student must complete this step satisfactorily in order to complete the procedure satisfactorily.

National curriculum competencies achieved:
• Perform accounts receivable procedures.
• Collect and post payments; manage patient ledgers.
• Know accounts payable/accounts receivable procedures.

Competency Assessment Checklist
Procedure 13–2: Prepare a Bank Deposit

Student name _____ Date _____

Learning Outcome: Prepare a bank deposit.

Performance Standards: Time allowed _____ min
 Accuracy _____ %

Conditions: The student will follow the procedure outlined below to prepare a bank deposit within standards identified using the following materials:
• Checks and currency to be deposited
• Deposit slip
• Pen

Evaluation Criterion	Performance Evaluation Checklist	Points Possible	Student's score 1st	2nd
■	1. Enter date of deposit on deposit slip.			
■	2. Count currency to be deposited. Enter amount after currency on the deposit slip.			
■	3. Count coins to be deposited. Enter amount after coins on the deposit slip.			
■	4. Individually write the amount of each check to be deposited in the checks portion of the deposit slip.			
■	5. Calculate total of currency, coin, and checks to be deposited and enter amount under total.			
●	6. Verify deposit is correct by adding currency, coin, and the amount of each check.			
■	7. Record deposit in check register.			
	Total Points			

Minimum total points required for satisfactory score _____

Evaluation Criteria

Symbol	Category	point value
●	crucial step	_____
■	essential step	_____
▲	theory	_____

Evaluator's comments:

Evaluator's name _____ Date _____

● denotes crucial step in procedure. Student must complete this step satisfactorily in order to complete the procedure satisfactorily.

National curriculum competencies achieved:
• Prepare a bank deposit.

Competency Assessment Checklist
Procedure 13–3: Maintain a Petty Cash Fund

Student name _____ Date _____

Learning Outcome: Maintain a petty cash fund.

Performance Standards:

Time allowed _____ min
Accuracy _____ %

Conditions: The student will follow the procedure outlined below to maintain a petty cash fund within standards identified using the following materials:
• Petty cash record
• Receipts for expenditures
• Pen/pencil

Evaluation Criterion	Performance Evaluation Checklist	Points Possible	Student's score 1st	2nd
■	1. A cash fund of a pre-determined amount, possibly $100, is put in a secure location in a locked, zippered bank bag.			
■	2. When an approved purchase needs to be made, cash is removed from the bag that will cover the purchase and an employee makes the purchase.			
■	3. When the employee returns, a receipt for the item and change (if any) is placed in the bag. *The receipt and change should total the amount that was removed to make the purchase.*			
●	4. The item purchased is written in a petty cash log (Figure 13–5).			
■	5. When the fund becomes depleted, the expenses from the petty cash log are totaled and the log and receipts are kept as proof of expenses. A check is then written to Petty Cash for the amount of the expenses.			
■	6. The check is cashed by the employee responsible for the fund and the fund is replenished by placing the check proceeds in the bank bag. A new log sheet is started.			
●	7. After the fund is replenished, the cash in the bank bag should equal the original amount of the petty cash fund.			
	Total Points			

Minimum total points required for satisfactory score _____

Evaluation Criteria

Symbol	Category	point value
●	crucial step	_____
■	essential step	_____
▲	theory	_____

Evaluator's comments:

Evaluator's name _____ Date _____

● denotes crucial step in procedure. Student must complete this step satisfactorily in order to complete the procedure satisfactorily.

National curriculum competencies achieved:
• Establish and maintain a petty cash fund.
• Manage petty cash.

Competency Assessment Checklist
Procedure 13–4: Write a Check for Payment of an Invoice

Student name _____ Date _____

Learning Outcome: Write a check for payment of an invoice.

Performance Standards: Time allowed _____ min
                                     Accuracy _____ %

Conditions: The student will follow the procedure outlined below to write a check for payment of an invoice within standards identified using the following materials:
• Check register with checks
• Invoices to be paid
• Pen

Evaluation Criterion	Performance Evaluation Checklist	Points Possible	Student's score 1st	2nd
■	1. Complete the check stub, subtracting the amount of the check from the current balance of the account.			
●	2. Complete check using a pen. Use checks in numeric order.			
■	3. Enter current date on check.			
●	4. In the PAY TO THE ORDER OF line, enter the payee's name.			
●	5. Enter the amount of the check numerically in the blank provided after the $ sign. Begin entering the amount immediately after the $ sign to prevent anything from being added to the check amount.			
●	6. Enter the amount of the check in words in the line below the PAY TO THE ORDER OF line. If the entire line is not used, use dashes or a solid line to cross out the remainder of the line.			
●	7. The check is then signed by an individual who has been authorized to sign checks for the account. The check can then be placed in a window envelope for mailing to the payee if necessary.			
	Total Points			

Minimum total points required for satisfactory score _____

Evaluation Criteria

Symbol	Category	point value
●	crucial step	_____
■	essential step	_____
▲	theory	_____

Evaluator's comments:

Evaluator's name _____ Date _____

● denotes crucial step in procedure. Student must complete this step satisfactorily in order to complete the procedure satisfactorily.

National curriculum competencies achieved:
• Prepare a check.
• Perform accounts payable procedures.
• Use and process checks appropriately.
• Maintain checking account.
• Know accounts payable/accounts receivable procedures; process payables.

Competency Assessment Checklist
Procedure 13–5: Reconcile a Bank Statement

Student name _____ Date _____

Learning Outcome: Reconcile a bank statement.

Performance Standards: Time allowed _____ min
                              Accuracy _____ %

Conditions: The student will follow the procedure outlined below to reconcile a bank statement within standards identified using the following materials:
• Current month's bank statement
• Record of checks drawn or check register
• Calculator
• Pen or pencil

Evaluation Criterion	Performance Evaluation Checklist	Points Possible	Student's score 1st	2nd
■	1. All checks that have been paid by the bank should be checked on the Record of checks drawn or check register.			
■	2. Any charges applied to the account by the bank should be listed on the record/register and subtracted from the balance.			
■	3. Any interest deposits from the bank should be listed on the record/register and added to the balance.			
●	4. Take the ending monthly balance on the account and do the following. a. Add any deposits made by the practice that are not included on the statement. b. Subtract any checks written by the practice that have not been paid by the bank. c. The total should then equal the ending balance in the RECORD. If the total in 4C does not equal the balance in the RECORD, you should look for errors in addition and subtraction when figuring the ending balance, as well as any other errors that may be present in the record/register.			
	Total Points			

Minimum total points required for satisfactory score _____

Evaluation Criteria

Symbol	Category	point value
●	crucial step	_____
■	essential step	_____
▲	theory	_____

Evaluator's comments:

Evaluator's name _____ Date _____

● denotes crucial step in procedure. Student must complete this step satisfactorily in order to complete the procedure satisfactorily.

National curriculum competencies achieved:
• Reconcile a bank statement.

Competency Assessment Checklist
Procedure 14–1: Select Candidates for Interviewing

Student name _____ Date _____

Learning Outcome: Select candidates for interviewing.

Performance Standards:　　　　　　　Time allowed _____ min
　　　　　　　　　　　　　　　　　　　Accuracy _____ %

Conditions: The student will follow the procedure outlined below to select candidates for interviewing within standards identified using the following materials:
- Resumes or job applications
- Selection criteria
- Pen or pencil

Evaluation Criterion	Performance Evaluation Checklist	Points Possible	Student's score 1st	2nd
■	1. If at all possible, form a committee that will be involved in all aspects of the selection process. Using the committee selection process helps eliminate potential biases and future conflicts. (Sometimes this is not possible and the applicants will be interviewed by only one individual.) However, there should always be more than one interview. A second interview insures proper selection of the most qualified candidate.			
■	2. The committee or interviewer should establish a list of criteria necessary for the position and should assign points to each of those criteria.			
■	3. After all resumes are received, give copies of each resume to each member on the committee.			
●	4. Resumes are evaluated by each member and points are assigned for each candidate's qualifications.			
■	5. Point assignments are totaled and reviewed by the committee. The candidates with the most points are invited for an interview.			
	Total Points			

Minimum total points required for satisfactory score _____

Evaluation Criteria

Symbol	Category	point value
●	crucial step	_____
■	essential step	_____
▲	theory	_____

Evaluator's comments:

Evaluator's name _____ Date _____

● denotes crucial step in procedure. Student must complete this step satisfactorily in order to complete the procedure satisfactorily.

Competency Assessment Checklist
Procedure 14–2: Prepare Payroll

Student name _____ Date _____

Learning Outcome: Prepare payroll.

Performance Standards: Time allowed _____min
                                    Accuracy _____%

Conditions: The student will follow the procedure outlined below to prepare payroll within standards identified using the following materials:
• Timecards   • Calculator
• Tax tables or percentages

Evaluation Criterion	Performance Evaluation Checklist	Points Possible	Student's score 1st	2nd
●	1. Calculate wages earned by multiplying hours worked by hourly rate. If the employee has worked overtime, the overtime hours worked will be multiplied by $1\frac{1}{2}$ times the employee's hourly rate.			
●	2. Enter the total wages earned for the period in the gross (earnings) column.			
●	3. Enter FICA (Social Security and Medicare) tax in FICA column. Refer to employee's Form W-4 to obtain marital status and withholding allowances. Note any additional amount the employee wishes withheld.			
●	4. Using amount of employee's wages and withholding allowances, determine the amount of tax to be withheld. Enter federal income tax in FWT column.			
●	5. Using amount of employee's wages and withholding allowances, determine the amount of tax to be withheld. Enter state tax in SWT column.			
●	6. Enter total of other deductions in other column or columns on right.			
●	7. To figure employee's net earnings, subtract total deductions from gross earnings.			
●	8. Enter payroll amounts in employee compensation record.			
●	9. Prepare payroll check listing all payroll amounts on the check summary on the right.			
	Total Points			

Minimum total points required for satisfactory score _____

Evaluation Criteria

Symbol	Category	point value
●	crucial step	_____
■	essential step	_____
▲	theory	_____

Evaluator's comments:

Evaluator's name _____ Date _____

● denotes crucial step in procedure. Student must complete this step satisfactorily in order to complete the procedure satisfactorily.

National curriculum competencies achieved:
• Prepare employee payroll; know terminology pertaining to payroll and taxes.

Competency Assessment Checklist
Procedure 15–1: Prepare a Resumé

Student name _____ Date _____

Learning Outcome: Prepare a resumé.

Performance Standards: Time allowed _____ min
                             Accuracy _____ %

Conditions: The student will follow the procedure outlined below to prepare a resumé within standards identified using the following materials:
- Professional resumé paper (white or off-white)
- Computer with word processing software
- Education, work experience and student portfolio information

Evaluation Criterion	Performance Evaluation Checklist	Points Possible	Student's score 1st	2nd
■	1. Choose format for resumé. A resume computer program or resumé template from a word processing program may be used.			
■	2. List full name, address, and phone at the top of the resume. An e-mail address can also be furnished if available.			
	3. Write career objective specific to position desired.			
■	4. List education with most recent first.			
■	5. List work experience with most recent first. Any volunteer experience or student internship experience can be listed under work experience.			
■	6. List personal interests.			
■	7. List personal references. Instructors and work supervisors are good choices. Friends and relatives should not be listed as a personal reference. Be sure to ask each reference for permission before listing him or her as a reference.			
●	8. Proofread resumé for typos or grammatical errors. If possible, have another person read the resume for the same.			
■	9. Review resumé to assure that the format is easy to read. Make any adjustments necessary.			
■	10. Print a copy of the resumé and retain a copy for yourself.			
	Total Points			

Minimum total points required for satisfactory score _____

Evaluation Criteria

Symbol	Category	point value
●	crucial step	_____
■	essential step	_____
▲	theory	_____

Evaluator's comments:

Evaluator's name _____ Date _____

● denotes crucial step in procedure. Student must complete this step satisfactorily in order to complete the procedure satisfactorily.

Competency Assessment Checklist
Procedure 15–2: Prepare a Cover Letter

Student name _____ Date _____

Learning Outcome: Prepare a cover letter.

Performance Standards:　　　　　　　　Time allowed _____ min
　　　　　　　　　　　　　　　　　　　Accuracy _____ %

Conditions: The student will follow the procedure outlined below to prepare a cover letter within standards identified using the following materials:
• Professional resumé paper (white or off-white)
• Computer with word processing software
• Completed resumé

Evaluation Criterion	Performance Evaluation Checklist	Points Possible	Student's score 1st	2nd
▲	1. Use proper format for the letter. (Formats are located in Chapter 6.)			
■	2. Address the letter to the individual designated to receive applications.			
■	3. Write letter expressing your interest in a position and identifying some of your qualifications and strengths.			
▲	4. Close the letter with appropriate salutation and your full name.			
●	5. Proofread the letter for typos and grammatical errors. If possible, have another person also proof the letter.			
■	6. Print a copy of the letter and retain a copy for yourself.			
●	7. Sign the letter that will go with your resumé.			
■	8. Place the letter appropriately in a business envelope along with the resumé (Figure 6–12).			
	Total Points			

Minimum total points required for satisfactory score _____

Evaluation Criteria

Symbol	Category	point value
●	crucial step	_____
■	essential step	_____
▲	theory	_____

Evaluator's comments:

Evaluator's name _____ Date _____

● denotes crucial step in procedure. Student must complete this step satisfactorily in order to complete the procedure satisfactorily.

Competency Assessment Checklist
Procedure 15–3: Complete an Employment Application

Student name _____ Date _____

Learning Outcome: Complete an employment application.

Performance Standards: Time allowed _____ min
Accuracy _____ %

Conditions: The student will follow the procedure outlined below to complete an employment application within standards identified using the following materials:
- Employment application (Lately, many employment applications have been made available over the Internet. The same steps would be followed only the information would be entered electronically.)
- Pen

Evaluation Criterion	Performance Evaluation Checklist	Points Possible	Student's score 1st	2nd
■	1. Read instructions on the form and follow them carefully. Provide the information requested below in addition to any other information requested on the application.			
■	2. Identify personal information.			
■	3. List educational history.			
■	4. List history.			
■	5. List personal references.			
●	6. Review the application to make sure it is complete.			
●	7. Sign and date the application.			
■	8. Submit the application to the individual designated.			
	Total Points			

Minimum total points required for satisfactory score _____

Evaluation Criteria

Symbol	Category	point value
●	crucial step	_____
■	essential step	_____
▲	theory	_____

Evaluator's comments:

Evaluator's name _____ Date _____

● denotes crucial step in procedure. Student must complete this step satisfactorily in order to complete the procedure satisfactorily.

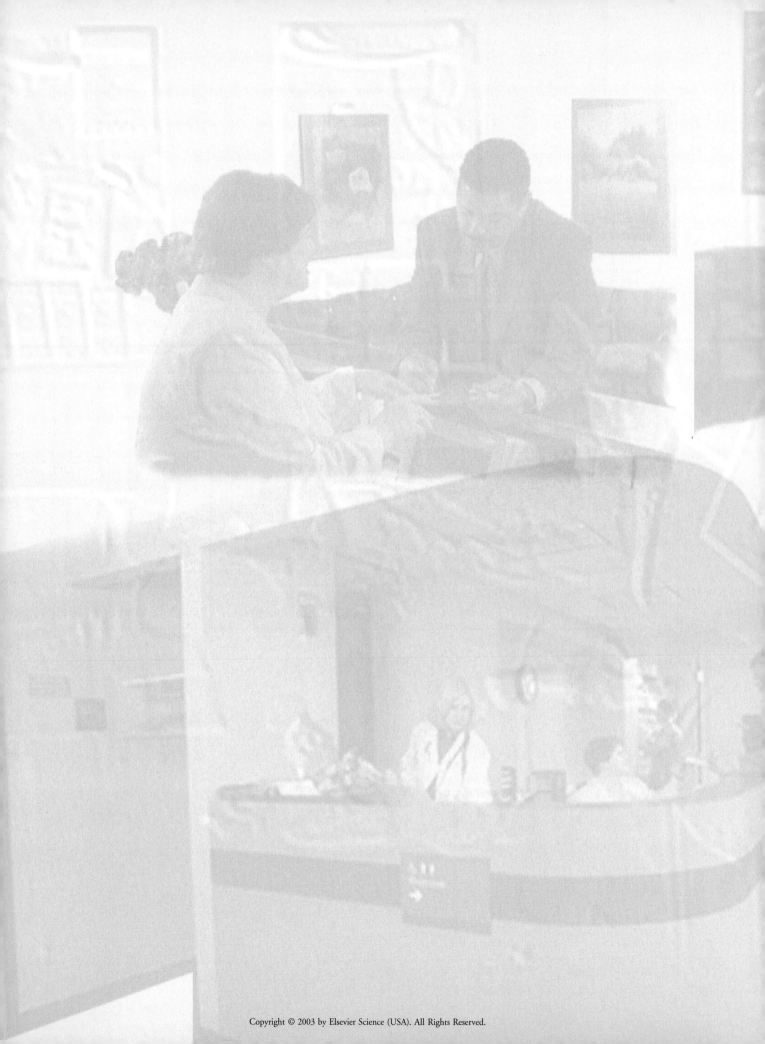

USING LYTEC MEDICAL 2001

The Lytec Medical 2001 computer program is included on the CD-ROM with the worktext *Medical Office Administration*. Lytec Medical 2001 is a Windows-based medical practice management program. In addition to workbook activities and activities on the CD-ROM, students have the opportunity to install and use this program to perform many administrative tasks of the medical office, such as

- Recording demographic and insurance information for patients.
- Scheduling appointments.
- Entering patient charges.
- Entering payments.
- Creating receipts, bills, and insurance billing.
- Submitting electronic claims.
- Creating reports such as day sheets and account aging reports.

INSTALLATION AND SETUP

To install Lytec Medical 2001, see the **Read-me** folder on the CD-ROM. Print out a copy of the installation instructions. Install the program from the CD-ROM. From **My Computer,** open the CD-ROM drive containing the "MOA_ALPHA1" application CD-ROM and double click on the "MOAsetup.EXE" icon. The application will launch upon loading.

CREATING YOUR OWN PRACTICE

You will need to make a copy of the practice files before beginning work on the Lytec 2001 computer projects. Under the *File* menu, click on *Open;* the *Open Practice* window will open. Right click on *Horizons Healthcare Center* and click on *copy.* Next, while still in the practice window, click in the blank space beneath the file names. Then, right click and choose *paste* to paste a copy of the practice information. The following should be displayed in the window: a Horizons Healthcare Center file and a copy of Horizons Healthcare Center file. Rename the copy file with your initials and HHCC and the extension .lpf, thereby creating your own personal "lpf" file to which you can save your own work. For example, if your name is Jane Doe, your file name should look like this: JDHHCC.lpf. **It is necessary to do this so you do not permanently alter the program and information supplied with the textbook.** This way, if you should need to reinstall the program and information, you will still have the original files. Also, if several people are sharing the same computer, each person will have a separate file to save changes. Do not make/save changes to the Horizons Healthcare Center file.

OPEN PRACTICE

Click on the *File* menu to view the options. Move your mouse to highlight and click on *Open Practice.* When the *Open Practice* window appears, select and open your personal "lpf" file. After you have opened your practice file, the practice name should appear on the title bar at the top of the window.

USING THE HELP FEATURE IN LYTEC

Lytec Medical 2001 has a help feature located under the *Help* menu. Click on *Help* on the menu bar and click on *Help Topics.* The content tab of the help feature allows you to locate information by clicking on the subject area. The index and search tabs allow you to enter keywords for which you may need some information. Both the index and search features give quick access to information on your keyword. When looking for information in the help feature, try your keyword under the index feature first. If no information is found, proceed to the search feature. The search feature provides a more comprehensive search of Lytec information. If you have questions when using Lytec 2001, the help feature provides a myriad of information about the program's operation.

FINDING A PATIENT

To determine which patients already have records in your practice, click on the *Lists* menu. Move your mouse to highlight and click on *Patients.* One of the patient records will be displayed. Click on the lookup button (magnifying glass) at the right of the *Patient Chart* box to see a list of patients. A list of patients with practice records will be displayed. Click on the patient whose record you wish to display and click *OK.*

ENTERING DATA FOR A NEW OR ESTABLISHED PATIENT

Every patient of the practice will require a Lytec patient record. If a patient is an established patient of the practice, click *Lists,* then *Patients,* and select the patient by clicking the magnifying glass to the right of the *Patient Chart* field.

To create a new patient record, open the patient list and click *New* on the right of the *Patients* window. Enter the patient's medical record (chart) number in the top field labeled *Patient Chart.* Below the chart number you will notice several tabs: *Patient Information* (the screen to which the dialog box opens automatically), *Primary Insurance, Secondary Insurance, Tertiary Insurance, Associations, Claim Information,* and *Diagnosis/Hold Codes.* Following is a summary of some of the tabs in the patient window:

Patient Information Tab

Fill in the following fields under the *Patient Information* tab with information from the text: Last Name, First Name, Middle Initial (if any), Street Address, City, State, Zip Code,

Home Phone, Work Phone, Birth Date, Social Security Number, Sex, and Marital Status. You will notice an arrow to the right of some fields, such as Sex or Marital Status). If you click on the arrow, a drop-down box will appear with the choices for that field. You can highlight and click on your choice. Leave the field labeled Recall Date blank. If the patient has a co-payment required for insurance, enter the amount of the co-payment in the Co-pay field, otherwise leave it blank. In the *Fee Schedule* field, select 1 for all patients. Leave the Patient Code and Patient Type fields blank.

Primary Insurance Tab

Select the *Primary Insurance* tab located beside the *Patient Information* tab. Click on the lookup button (magnifying glass) beside the Insurance Code field to identify the code for the patient's primary insurance company. In the Type field, click on the arrow and choose the type of insurance. If the patient has Medicare insurance, choose Medicare. Enter the patient's policy number in the ID Number field. For this exercise, leave the Policy Number field blank. Place a check next to Bill insurance automatically and Accept assignment for each patient in this exercise.

In the Relation to Insured field, *Self* is selected automatically. If the patient is not the insured, select the patient's relationship to the insured. Click the *Set Insured* button and identify whether the insured is another patient in the system or a guarantor who may have a file in the Lytec system. If the patient is NOT the insured, be sure to specify (under the *Set Insured* option) who is responsible for the bill.

Associations Tab

Select the *Associations* tab located in the row above the *Patient Information* tab to link the patient to his or her primary care physician. In the Provider field, click the magnifying glass on the right. Highlight the patient's primary physician and click *OK*.

ENTERING CHARGES AND PAYMENTS

On the main menu, click *billing*, then click *charges and payments*. The billing window will open. View patients by clicking the lookup button (magnifying glass) on the right side of the chart box. Find the patient to be billed on the patient list, highlight the patient's name, and click *OK*. The charges and payments window for the selected patient will be displayed. Enter the following information for the patient's encounter in the identified boxes. (To move from field to field in this window, simply press the *Enter* key.)

(a) *Billing #*—Accept the default number that appears in the box. (This box could also be used to record a superbill control number.)

(b) *Provider #*—The provider recorded under the patient's registration information will appear in this box.

(c) *Created*—Enter the billing correct date for the billing date.

(d) *Co-pay*—If the patient pays a co-payment with each office visit and the co-payment was entered in the patient's registration information, a co-payment will appear in this box. If a co-payment applies, a co-payment can also be entered manually. Accept the co-payment that appears for each patient.

(e) Under the *Bill to* portion of the window, a check mark should appear in the checkbox if the patient should receive a bill and the patient's insurance company should receive a claim form. If not, place a check in the *patient checkbox. (If a check is not placed in the patient checkbox, the patient's charges will not appear on a monthly statement.)* If an insurance company name appears on the primary insurance field, a check should be placed in the checkbox pertaining to that insurance. (To have the checkmark appear automatically in the charges and payments window, check the patient's registration data and be sure a checkmark appears in the *bill patient automatically* box.)

(f) Under *Detail items,* enter the following information (pressing the *Enter* key after information is entered will advance the cursor to the next box):

I. *Print*—A check should appear in the *Print checkbox*. This will print the transaction item on the patient's insurance claim.

II. *Payment*—When a payment is received on the patient's account, the payment may be applied to a specific item on the patient's account. If so, this field will be checked.

III. *Date from*—The current date appears in this box. Change the date to the patient's date of service.

IV. *Date to*—If a patient's charges apply to more than one day, the ending date should be entered in this box. Otherwise, leave the box blank.

V. *Provider*—The patient's assigned provider appears in this box. If the patient was seen by another provider, the provider can be selected by clicking the lookup button.

VI. *Diagnosis code*—Select a diagnosis code by clicking on the lookup button. If the diagnosis code is not listed, it may be manually entered or it may be added to the master list when the lookup button is clicked.

VII. *Procedure code*—Select a procedure code by clicking on the lookup button. If the procedure code is not listed, it may be manually entered or it may be added to the master list when the lookup button is clicked.

VIII. *Mod*—If a modifier applies to the procedure code listed, a two-digit modifier is entered in this box.

IX. *Place of service*—This field can be used to identify where a procedure was performed.

X. *Amount*—If a fee schedule has been assigned to the patient, the cost of the procedure will automatically appear in the amount box. An amount can be entered to override any automatic charge.

XI. *Units*—Enter the amount of times the procedure was done. The usual entry is 1.

XII. *Extended*—The number of units is multiplied by the amount to arrive at the extended amount. Once the *Enter* key is pressed after units, another line for billing will appear. If the patient has additional procedures to be entered, those procedures would be entered on the next line.

XIII. After all of the information for a patient's bill has been entered, click the *Save* button at the bottom of the window. A new billing screen will be displayed, and information for another patient may be entered (start with number III). When all bills have been entered, click *close* at the bottom of the window.

If a mistake is made after a line has been entered under detail items, click on the line and choose *Detail* at the bottom of the billing window. The *delete* option will delete the line currently in use. The *add* option will add a new blank line to the detail items portion of the billing window.

ENTERING PAYMENTS

Applying Payments to an Account Balance

1. Click *Billing,* then *Apply patient payment.*
2. Enter the appropriate information in the identified blanks.
   Patient or Guarantor: Identify who made the payment. Click on the button before patient or guarantor, then select the appropriate name from the patient and guarantor list.
   Payment date: Date payment was received.
   Reference: Number of check, if applicable.
   Payment amount: The amount of the payment.
   Codes—Patient payment: Identify the patient's method of payment (cash, check, or credit card.) ADJCREDIT should be listed in the *Write off* box.
3. Click *Next* to move to the next screen.
4. To apply payments to an account balance, enter payments in the section of the window entitled "To apply payments at the billing level." Enter the amount of the payment in the *apply* box. Press the *Enter* key after entering the payment amount. ***NOTE: At any time during this process, the back button can be clicked to revert to previous screens and wipe out any mistakes.***
5. Click *Post* to post the payment to the account.
6. To post a new payment from a patient, begin again at step 1.

Applying Payments Directly to a Specific Charge

1. Click *Billing,* then *Apply patient payment.*
2. Enter the appropriate information in the identified blanks.
   Patient or Guarantor: Identify who made the payment. Click on the button before patient or guarantor, then select the appropriate name from the patient and guarantor list.
   Payment date: Date payment was received.
   Reference: Check number.
   Payment amount: The amount of the payment.

Codes—Patient payment: Identify the patient's method of payment (cash, check, or credit card.) ADJCREDIT should be listed in the *Write off* box.
3. Click *Next* to move to the next screen.
4. To apply payments to a specific charge, enter payments in the section of the window entitled "To apply payments at the item level" and choose the specific charge that will be paid. Enter the amount of the payment to be applied in the *apply* box pertaining to the bill. Press the *Enter* key after entering the payment amount. If the patient is making a payment for more than one charge, enter the appropriate payment amount for each specific charge. Keep applying amounts until the entire payment has been applied. Note that the amount of the check appears in the upper portion of the window and the amount of the check that is unapplied also appears. ***NOTE: At any time during this process, the back button can be clicked to revert to previous screens and wipe out any mistakes.***
5. After all of the check has been applied, click *Post* to post the payment to the account.
6. To post a new payment from a patient, begin again at step 1.

Posting an Adjustment Credit to a Patient's Account

If an adjustment should be made to a patient's account, the adjustment can be entered at the same time the payment is made. To enter an adjustment, enter the amount of the adjustment in the *Write Off* column and press the *Enter* key. The amount of the write off should reduce the patient's balance.

Posting Payments and Adjustments when Charges Are Posted

Payments on account and adjustments can also be entered at the time a patient's account is charged for services. When in the charges and payment window, the procedure column can be used to specify the type of payment or adjustment that should be applied. This option would be used in such situations as a co-payment made by the patient on the date of a visit or a reduction in charges approved by the physician.

PRINTING REPORTS

A variety of report options is available under *Reports* on the Lytec 2001 menu bar. It is a good idea when printing reports to click the *preview* button before printing the reports to be sure the information requested is included in the report. Following is a list of instructions for some common reports:

Patient Account Balances

1. Click *reports,* then move down to *patient,* then click *patient balances.*

2. Click *total balance* and *greater than or equal to.*
3. In the *This amount* box, enter 0.01.
4. Click *sort by name* to display the results alphabetically.
5. Click *preview.* Patients with balances of greater than zero should be displayed.
6. Click the *print* icon in the preview window.

Day Sheet

1. Click *reports,* then click *Day sheet.*
2. Under the *Sort* option, click *patient name.*
3. Under the *Ranges* tab, specify the date(s) to be printed.
4. Click *preview.* Check to make sure the information requested is displayed.
5. Click the *print* icon in the preview window.

Monthly Summary Report

1. Click *reports,* then click *monthly summary.*
2. In the *Month* and *Year* boxes, enter October and 2002.
3. Click *preview.* The monthly summary for October 2002 should be displayed in the open window. If the display is correct, click the *print* icon.

Practice Analysis

1. Click *reports,* then click *practice analysis.*
2. The box before *Subtotal by provider* should be checked.
3. Click *preview.* The practice analysis should be displayed in the open window. If the display is correct, click the *print* icon.

Procedure Code Analysis

1. Click *reports,* then click *procedure code analysis.*
2. Remove the check in the box before *Subtotal by provider.*
3. Click *preview.* The procedure code analysis should be displayed in the open window. If the display is correct, click the *print* icon.

Patient Ledger Balances

1. Click *reports,* then move down to *patient,* then click *patient ledger.*
2. The following boxes should be checked: include paid billings; show paid detail; include transactions—active.

3. The following buttons should be selected: amounts—debit/credit; sort patients by—name; reference—do not print references.
4. Click *preview.*
5. If the preview display appears correct, click the *print* icon in the preview window.

PRINTING INSURANCE FORMS

To print the HCFA-1500 claim form, follow these steps:
1. On the main menu, click *billing,* then click *print insurance claims.* The *select custom form* window will open.
2. Highlight *HCFA Standard form* and click *open.* The *Print Insurance Claims* window will open.
3. The following selections should be made:
   - print claim types: primary
   - diagnoses per page: 4 (By leaving all other options blank, all outstanding claims will be generated.)
4. Click *Preview.* If the claims are correct, click the *printer* button in the preview window.

If claims do not appear, go back to the charges and payments window under the billing option. In the *Bill To* portion of the window, a check must appear next to the primary insurance company.

NOTE: To print an individual claim form for an existing billing, click *billing,* then *charges and payments.* Select the *patient name,* then click the lookup button after billing. Select the billing number for the claim and click *OK.* Then click *print,* then *primary insurance,* the *form name,* then *print.*

PRINTING A PATIENT STATEMENT

Patient statements are usually printed monthly for each account of a practice. To print statements, follow these steps:
1. On the main menu, click *Billing,* then click *Print Statements.* The select custom form window will then open.
2. Highlight *Standard Statement* and click *open.* The *Print Statements* window will open.
3. The following selections should be made:
   (a) Statement date: current date.
   (b) Statement messages: Standard and Dunning.
   (c) Sort Patients by: name.
4. Under the *Range* tab, ranges can be specified to print specific statements.
5. Click *Preview.* If the claims are correct, click the *printer* button in the preview window.

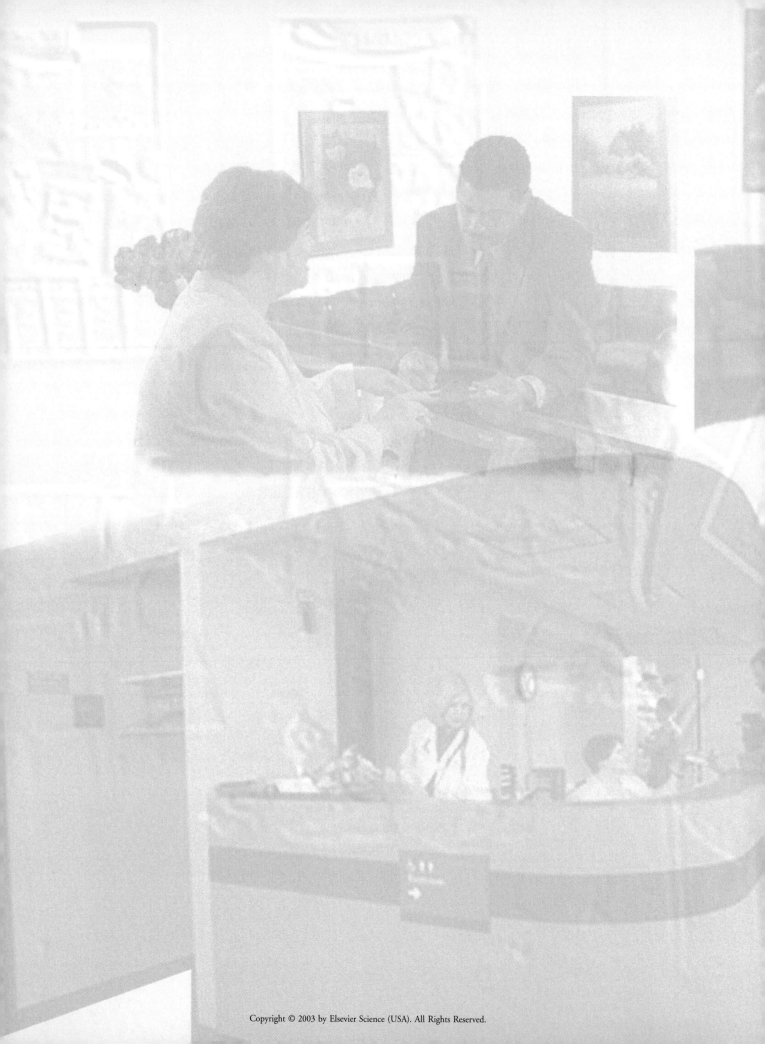

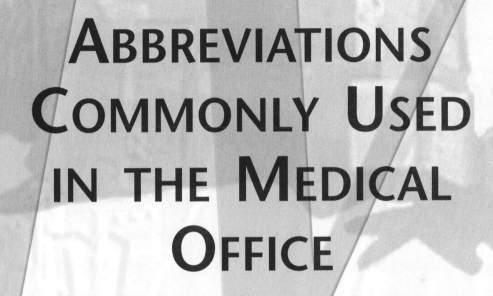

ABBREVIATIONS COMMONLY USED IN THE MEDICAL OFFICE

AAMA	American Association of Medical Assistants		DPM	Doctor of Podiatric Medicine
AAMT	American Association for Medical Transcription		DTR	deep tendon reflex
a.c.	*ante cibum* or before meals		DVT	deep vein thrombosis
AD	right ear		Dx	diagnosis
ADA	Americans with Disabilities Act		ECG, EKG	electrocardiogram
AHIMA	American Health Information Management Association		EDC	estimated date of confinement (due date of a pregnancy)
AMA	American Medical Association		EEG	electroencephalogram
AS	left ear		EENT	eyes, ears, nose, and throat
ASA	aspirin		EIN	employer identification number
AU	both ears		EMG	electromyogram
BC/BS	Blue Cross Blue Shield		ENT	ears, nose, and throat
b.i.d.	twice per day		EOB	explanation of benefits
BM	bowel movement		EPA	Environmental Protection Agency
BP	blood pressure		ESL	English as a second language
BUN	blood urea nitrogen		ESR	erythrocyte sedimentation rate
bx	biopsy		FB	foreign body
c̄	with		FBS	fasting blood sugar
C#	C followed by a number from 1–7 identifies a particular cervical vertebra (C1–C7)		FH	family history
			FICA	Federal Insurance Contributions Act
C&S	culture and sensitivity		FMLA	Family and Medical Leave Act
Ca	cancer		FUTA	Federal Unemployment Tax
CABG	coronary artery bypass graft		fx	fracture
cap	capsule		GI	gastrointestinal
CBC	complete blood count		GP	general practitioner
CC	chief complaint		gr	grain
cc	cubic centimeter		GTT	glucose tolerance test
CCU	Coronary Care Unit		gtt.	drops
CEU	continuing education unit		GU	genitourinary
CHF	congestive heart failure		gyn	gynecology
chol	cholesterol		H&H	hemoglobin and hematocrit
CLIA	Clinical Laboratory Improvement Amendments		H&P	history and physical
cm	centimeter		Hb, Hgb	hemoglobin
CMA	Certified Medical Assistant		HBV	hepatitis B virus
CMT	Certified Medical Transcriptionist		HCFA	Health Care Financing Administration
CNA	certified nursing assistant		HCT, Hct	hematocrit
CNM	Certified Nurse Midwife		HEENT	head, eyes, ears, nose, and throat
CNP	Certified Nurse Practitioner		HIV	human immunodeficiency virus
COB	coordination of benefits		HMO	health maintenance organization
COPD	chronic obstructive pulmonary disease		h.s.	at hour of sleep; bedtime
COTA	Certified Occupational Therapy Assistant		HTN	hypertension
CRTT	Certified Respiratory Therapist Technician		hx	history
CS	cesarean section		I&D	incision and drainage
CSA	Controlled Substances Act		ICU	Intensive Care Unit
CTS	carpal tunnel syndrome		IDDM	insulin-dependent diabetes mellitus
D&C	dilatation and curettage		IM	intramuscular
D.O.	Doctor of Osteopathy		Inj	injection
D/C	discontinued		IUD	intrauterine device
DC	Doctor of Chiropractic		IV	intravenous
DEA	Drug Enforcement Agency		IVP	intravenous pyelogram
DJD	degenerative joint disease		JCAHO	Joint Commission on Accreditation of Health Care Organizations
DM	diabetes mellitus			
DOB	date of birth		L	left, liter

L#	L followed by a number from 1–5 identifies a particular lumbar vertebra (L1–L5)	PTT	partial thromboplastin time
lat	lateral	px	physical examination
lb	pound	q	every
LBP	low back pain	q.d.	every day
LLQ	left lower quadrant	q.h.	every hour
LMP	last menstrual period	q.i.d.	four times per day
LPN	licensed practical nurse	q.o.d.	every other day
LUQ	left upper quadrant	R	right
LVN	licensed vocational nurse	R/O	rule out
M.D.	Doctor of Medicine	RA	rheumatoid arthritis
mcg	microgram	RBC	red blood (cell) count
MI	myocardial infarction	rbc	red blood cell
min	minute	RHIA	Registered Health Information Administrator
ml	milliliter	RHIT	Registered Health Information Technician
MRI	magnetic resonance imaging	RLQ	right lower quadrant
MS	multiple sclerosis	RMA	Registered Medical Assistant
MSD	musculoskeletal disorder	RN	registered nurse
MSDS	material safety data sheet	ROM	range of motion
MSN	Medicare Summary Notice	ROS	review of systems
Na	sodium	RRT	Registered Respiratory Therapist
NAD	no acute distress	RUQ	right upper quadrant
neg	negative	Rx	prescription, treatment, therapy
NIDDM	noninsulin-dependent diabetes mellitus	s̄	without
NKA	no known allergies	S#	S followed by a number from 1–5 identifies a particular sacral vertebra
NPO	nothing by mouth	s/p	status post
NSAID	nonsteroidal anti-inflammatory drug	sed rate	erythrocyte sedimentation rate
OB	obstetrics	SOB	shortness of breath
OB-GYN	obstetrics and gynecology	SSN	Social Security number
OD	Doctor of Optometry, right eye	stat	immediately
ORIF	open reduction internal fixation	STD	sexually transmitted disease
OS	left eye	Sx	symptoms
OSHA	Occupational Safety and Health Administration	T#	T followed by a number from 1–12 identifies a particular thoracic vertebra
OT	occupational therapy, occupational therapist	T&A	tonsillectomy and adenoidectomy
OTA	Occupational Therapy Assistant	t.i.d.	three times per day
OTC	over the counter	TAHBSO	total abdominal hysterectomy bilateral salpingo-oophorectomy
OU	both eyes	TB	tuberculosis
p̄	after	TEMP	temperature
p.c.	post cibum; after meals	tx	treatment
p.o.	by mouth	UA	urinalysis
p.r.n.	as needed	UCR	usual, customary, reasonable
PA	Physician Assistant	URI	upper respiratory infection
PE	physical examination	UTI	urinary tract infection
PH	past history	WBC	white blood (cell) count
Pharm.D.	Doctor of Pharmacy	wbc	white blood cell
PMH	past medical history	WNL	within normal limits
PMS	premenstrual syndrome	x	times
PO	purchase order		
PPO	preferred provider organization		
PT	physical therapy, physical therapist, prothrombin time		
PTA	Physical Therapy Assistant		

GLOSSARY

Abandonment   If a physician does not properly meet his or her obligation to treat a patient, *abandonment* has occurred.

Abortion   Termination of a pregnancy before the fetus is viable.

Accession ledger   Used to keep track of chart numbers assigned to patients.

Accounts payable   Functions of the practice include paying for items purchased for the sole use by the practice and expenses incurred by the practice.

Accounts receivable   Payment owed to the practice by patients, etc.

Administrative law   Regulations, or laws, established by government agencies to regulate activities within that agency's control.

Advance directive   Legal document that establishes a patient's wishes for medical care when the patient is no longer able to make those decisions.

Ambulatory care   Medical care provided for patients on an outpatient basis.

Ancillary appointments   Appointments that are made with departments such as laboratory or x-ray to have special diagnostic tests run.

Assessment   A part of the chart note in which a physician considers the subjective and the objective information gathered about the patient and comes to a conclusion; diagnosis; impression.

Assignment   Health care provider agrees to accept the Medicare (or other insurance program's) approved amount as payment in full.

Assignment of benefits   A patient's insurance claim benefits are sent directly from the insurance company to the physician's office.

Assisted living facility   A health care facility in which residents live in an apartment-type setting with services such as medication administration and meal preparation available.

Beneficiaries   Individuals who qualify for insurance benefits under a policy.

Birthday rule   Dependents are covered by the policy of the parent that has a birthday closest to the beginning of the year.

Board certified   A physician who has passed an examination in a specific specialty; once a physician successfully completes the examination, the physician is known as a *diplomate* and is *board certified*.

Breach of confidentiality   Release of medical information that should not be released.

Capitation   A prepaid plan (HMO) that provides all the care a patient needs for a flat fee or premium.

Case law   Common law; law established by judicial system.

Certified Coding Specialist (CCS)   One who has passed a coding proficiency examination.

Certified Medical Transcriptionist (CMT)   One who has passed a medical transcription proficiency examination.

Certified Professional Coder (CPC)   One who has passed a coding proficiency examination.

Certified Professional Secretary (CPS)   One who has passed an administrative professional proficiency examination.

Chart entries   Also known as chart notes.

Chart notes   Entries made in a patient's chart regarding the patient's visit to the doctor.

Chief complaint   The chief reason a patient visits the doctor; this is noted in the subjective portion of the chart note.

Civil law   The type of law that involves a relationship between individuals or groups (as opposed to criminal law).

Claim   Any request to the insurance company or government insurance program to receive benefits on the behalf of the insured.

Clinic   Facility in which a group of health care providers render medical treatment. A variety of medical specialties may be represented, or a clinic may consist of providers in one medical specialty, such as a family practice clinic or pediatric clinic.

Co-insurance   Percentage of a claim required to be paid by the patient.

Color coding   Involves assigning colors to represent letters and numbers to aid in record filing and retrieval.

Common law   Also known as case law; interpreted by the judicial branch or court system.

Communication   Conveying information from one person to another.

Compassion   Genuine caring and concern for people.

Compensatory damages   Monetary awards to compensate a plaintiff for damages such as physical injury, lost wages, emotional suffering, and loss of companionship.

Confidentiality   Keeping secret everything that is seen, heard, or performed in the medical office.

Consecutive number filing   Method of filing medical charts in the order of lowest to highest number.

Consent   To give approval.

Consideration   To complete a contractual agreement, something of value is exchanged between the two parties—this is *consideration*.

Consultation   A patient may be referred by a primary physician to a specialist; the meeting between the patient and the specialist is a *consultation*.

Continuation sheets   Also known as *progress notes*.

Contract   A legal agreement between two parties that creates an obligation.

Conventions   A symbol such as a set of parentheses or an abbreviation that alerts an assistant to any special notations or conditions of selecting a certain diagnosis code.

Co-payment   A set amount that must be paid by a patient or policy holder for each office visit regardless of the cost of the visit.

Corporation   A recognized separate entity operating independently of its employees and stockholders.

CPT   The numerical codes representing procedures for which a physician charges fees.

CPT-4 manual   A listing of codes assigned to medical procedures performed by physicians. *CPT* stands for *Current Procedural Terminology*.

Criminal law   The type of law that involves a relationship between an individual and the government.

Cross-referencing   A filing method that allows a patient's medical record to be easily located in the case of a name change. Therefore, a patient with a name change would be referenced under the old name and the new name in the master patient index.

Culture   Beliefs, behaviors, and attitudes shared by a particular group of people, passed from generation to generation.

Cycle billing   A billing method in which patients are billed at designated intervals throughout the month.

Damages   Monetary amounts requested by a plaintiff in consideration for injuries the plaintiff alleges to have received.

Database   Information containing health information about patients, their appointments, diagnoses, and procedures that will appear on insurance claims; results of diagnostic studies, laboratory tests, and x-rays can also be entered.

Deductible   A set amount of money that an insured person must pay each year before insurance benefits will be paid.

Defendant   Party or parties accused of wrongdoing.

Deposition   Sworn testimony given outside the courtroom.

Diagnosis   The physician's determination of a patient's illness or reason for the office visit.

Discharge summary   A synopsis of a patient's hospital treatment.

Double booking   The occurrence of overbooking a physician's appointment schedule.

Dunning message   Any type of message that makes a request for payment on an account.

Durable Power of Attorney for Health Care   A legal document giving authority to one person to make health care decisions for another person who is not able to make health care decisions.

Electronic mail (e-mail)   A message sent by means of a computer and telephone line.

Emancipated minor   A minor declared by the court to be capable of making adult decisions.

Emergency room   A department of a hospital that receives patients who are acutely, seriously, or critically ill or injured.

Empathy   The understanding of another person's feelings regarding his or her experiences.

Employee compensation record   Payroll data for each employee—amounts paid and deducted from each check as year-to-date totals. This information is used at the end of the year to produce W-2 forms.

Employer identification number (EIN)   A unique number assigned to each employer to use when reporting employment taxes or when giving tax statements to employees. This number identifies the tax account of the employer.

Empowerment   Employees are given some degree of responsibility (within their expertise) in achieving the mission of an organization.

Equal Credit Opportunity Act   Enacted in 1975; requires that once credit is extended to one individual, it must be extended to all others. Individuals cannot be denied credit on the basis of race, color, religion, national origin, sex, marital status, or age. Credit can be refused based only on the individual's inability to pay.

Ergonomics   Designing the work to fit the worker's physical capabilities.

Ethics   Rules or principles of right conduct.

Euthanasia   Taking an aggressive action that will hasten a patient's death.

Executive branch   The branch of government at both the state and federal level that is responsible for ensuring that laws within its jurisdiction are observed.

Explanation of Benefits (EOB)   Explanation of insurance benefits paid and what, if any, subtractions have been made from a claim. If the claim is rejected, the reason for the rejection is on the EOB.

Expressed consent   A statement from a patient that a physician should provide medical treatment for the patient.

Face sheet   Usually the first sheet in a patient's medical record; it includes patient's name, address, phone, employer and insurance information; also known as summary sheet or identification sheet.

Fair Debt Collection Practices Act   Legislation that protects debtors against debt collectors who use unfair practices when collecting a debt. Collectors cannot use threats of violence or offensive language, and they cannot misrepresent themselves.

Fee-for-service   An insurance plan that pays a physician a fee for his or her service. Patients do not have to see a primary care physician for referrals and are free to go anywhere they wish.

Fee schedule   A listing of every procedure done by a practice's physicians and the charge for each procedure.

Feedback   Information a receiver gives a sender about a message.

Fiscal intermediary   An insurance company that has contracted to process claims for Medicare.

Fraud   Knowingly and willingly billing an insurance company or individual for something that did not occur.

Group insurance   A group of people usually with the same employer who all have the same insurance policy and related benefits.

Group number   A number used to identify a group of people who all have the same insurance policy and related benefits.

Guarantor   The party responsible for payment of account.

HCFA Common Procedure Coding System (HCPCS)   CPT codes are part of a larger coding system established by the federal government. HCPCS consists of three levels of coding: level I codes are for physician procedures; level II codes are for nonphysician services, supplies, and procedures; level III codes are used at the local level for Medicare claims.

Health Care Financing Administration (HCFA)   An agency of the federal government that established a coding system. This agency is now called Centers for Medicare and Medicaid Services, or CMS.

Health information management   Directing and organizing all activities related to keeping and caring for information concerning health care provided for patients.

Health maintenance organization (HMO)   A prepaid plan that provides all the care a patient may need in exchange for a flat monthly fee or premium.

History and physical   Documents the patient's condition on admission to the hospital.

Home health care   Care given to a patient in his or her own home.

Hospital   A facility that provides inpatient care; health care that necessitates the patient staying overnight (usually more than a 24-hour period) and having the constant attention of the nursing staff.

Human resources   The department of a health care organization that provides services for the people who work for the organization.

ICD-9-CM   Diagnosis coding system of numerical codes; the *International Classification of Diseases, 9th Revision, Clinical Modification.* Coding consists of three parts: Volume 1, Tabular List of Diseases (in numerical order); Volume 2, Index of Diseases (in alphabetical order); Volume 3, Index and Tabular List of Procedures.

Identification sheet   A sheet in a patient's chart that identifies the patient and contains pertinent information, such as name, address, telephone number, and insurance.

Implied consent   Consent evidenced by a patient's actions; the very act of arriving at an appointment made with a physician.

Impression   Diagnosis or assessment.

Informed consent   Patient is given information about his/her medical condition, the treatment alternatives and why treatment is recommended.

Inpatient   Patient care given within a hospital setting, usually involving an overnight stay.

Insurance contract or policy   Specifies what types of health treatments are covered as well as the amount for which the treatments are covered.

Insured   Refers to the individual who holds an insurance policy; subscriber; policyholder.

Insurer   The insurance company.

Internship   A process whereby a student works under supervision of a medical office employee and receives on-the-job experience.

Interrogatories   A set of written questions asked of both the defendant and the plaintiff involved in a lawsuit.

Job description   Identifies what a person employed in a particular position will be required to do.

Judicial branch   The branch of government that establishes common law.

Laboratory report   A test report from a medical laboratory (e.g., results of urinalysis, complete blood cell count).

Law   Written rule established by society.

Legislative branch   The branch of government that consists of senators and representatives elected by the people.

Litigation   Legal action.

Living will   A legal document that communicates a patient's wishes with regard to life-sustaining treatment.

Malpractice   Professional misconduct, illegal or immoral, involving an unreasonable lack of skill or fidelity in the performance of professional duties.

Managed care   A type of insurance plan that often requires an insured to see a primary care physician initially for treatment. The primary care physician refers the patient to a specialist only if necessary. Managed care plans often require patients to obtain authorizations before beginning certain types of medical treatment.

Master patient index   An alphabetical system of filing medical records.

Material Safety Data Sheet (MSDS)   All facilities that have hazardous substances on site are required to keep a log that details the ingredients of the product as well as first aid measures to take in case of wrongful exposure. An MSDS is usually included with hazardous materials.

Mature minor   A minor recognized by some states as capable of making medical decisions without parental consent.

Medical administrative assistant   A multiskilled individual who performs administrative support services for the efficient operation of a medical office.

Medical assistant   An individual who is qualified to perform both administrative and clinical duties in a medical office.

Medical ethics   Values and guidelines governing decisions in medical practice.

Medical history   A questionnaire detailing a patient's past illnesses and treatment.

Medical transcription   Production of a typewritten medical report from a physician dictation for placement in a patient's file.

Minutes   A summary of information and discussion that occurred during a meeting.

Modifier   Used to communicate something different about a procedure or service (when coding).

MSDs   Musculoskeletal disorders.

Nursing home   A facility providing round-the-clock medical care for residents. Residents are often too ill to be cared for at home, but they are not sick enough to be hospitalized.

Objective   Portion of a chart note in which the results of the patient's physical examination are documented.

Offer and acceptance   The initial step in establishing a contract—an offer is made by one individual, and the other accepts the offer.

Operative report A detailed account of a patient's surgical procedure.

Outguide A plastic envelope with pockets; used to mark the place from which a medical record was removed.

Outpatient Medical care provided for patients outside a hospital setting.

Participating provider (PAR) Providers who accept assignment.

Participatory management Management style in which empowerment is present.

Partnership Two or more physicians who do not wish to incorporate can form a *partnership*. Partner physicians share all income and expenses of the practice. The disadvantage of a partnership is that each partner is liable for the other's actions.

Pathology report Analysis of diseased body tissue that has been sent for testing.

Performance review A review of an employee's performance over a period of 1 year; it is usually used to determine employee raises.

Plaintiff Initiator of a lawsuit.

Policy An agreement between an insurance company (otherwise known as an insurer) and an individual or group of individuals.

Policyholder The individual who holds an insurance policy; subscriber; insured.

Policy manual An office publication that details job descriptions and the practice's policies on various human resource–related topics.

Precertifications An insurance plan's approval for a health care provider to provide a health care service to a patient.

Preferred provider organization (PPO) A network of health care providers who agree to provide services at a discount for members of the PPO. A PPO may require patients to choose a primary care physician or a primary care clinic.

Premium A payment required for insurance coverage.

Primary care Health services focused on providing care for routine injury and illness. Common providers of primary care are family practice and internal medicine physicians, pediatricians, nurse practitioners, and physician assistants.

Primary care physician A physician designated by a patient to provide initial care for a medical condition.

Private practice A physician providing outpatient care from a private office in which the physician is the only provider.

Probationary period Specific amount of time, such as 90 days, when an employee is working under a temporary employment arrangement.

Problem-oriented medical record (POMR) Method of organizing a medical record in which all information pertaining to one specific problem is grouped together.

Procedure A service provided for a patient in the course of medical treatment.

Procedure manual A book or booklet that gives instruc-tions for procedures, guidelines, and protocols in a medical office.

Progress notes Information regarding a patient's visits to the doctor.

Protocol Instructions given to use in response to an event.

Provider The individuals who are chiefly responsible for coordinating and delivering health care services; such as physicians, nurses, and nurse practitioners.

Public health agency An agency that provides health care at little or no cost to lower-income individuals. These agencies often educate the community about healthy living, work to prevent or control epidemics, and track and report infectious and communicable diseases to state health departments.

Punitive damages Monetary awards designed to punish a defendant for wrongdoing.

Purchase order A request to purchase merchandise from an identified supplier.

Quantitative analysis The process in which a patient's record is reviewed to make sure that all necessary components are included in the chart; usually performed after the patient record has been returned to the record room.

Radiology report Results of a patient's radiologic study.

Reciprocity An agreement between states that allows an individual who has met the requirements in one state to meet requirements in another state; applies in the case of licensure of many medical professionals.

Reconciling Making sure that the bank statement and the bank balance are in agreement.

Referral Approval by the primary care physician for a patient to receive the services of a specialist.

Release of information A document that specifies what medical information regarding the patient is to be released. The release must be signed by the patient.

Residency A period of time in which a physician is educated in the specialty of his or her choice; the physician is known as a *resident*.

Resumé A document outlining an individual's qualifications for a position; allows one to highlight education, work experience, personal achievements, strengths, and qualities.

Restrictive endorsement Instructions allowing a check to be deposited only in the account of a particular business, practice, or physician. A check with a *restrictive endorsement* cannot be cashed if lost.

Risk management A means of minimizing the potential for legal action being taken against a practice.

Sexual harassment Unwelcome sexual behavior or innuendo.

Shingling Placing the oldest laboratory report near the back of the chart and laying new reports slightly above and overlapping the top of the previously placed report. This method is used to save space in a patient's chart.

SOAP method Method of documenting patient visits in a chart note. Each letter stands for the type of information in that section of the note: for example, S = Subjective, O = Objective, A = Assessment, P = Plan.

Sole proprietorship   A business arrangement that assumes all the liabilities for a practice and receives all income generated by the practice.

Sponsor   The veteran on whom CHAMPVA eligibility is based.

Source-oriented medical record   Like information grouped together in a patient's medical record.

SSN   Social Security number.

Standards of care   The level of acceptable care a health care provider is expected to give, usually reasonable and prudent.

Standard precautions   A protocol that treats all human blood and bodily fluids as potentially infectious for pathogens, such as the human immunodeficiency virus and hepatitis.

Statute   Laws established by legislative branch of government.

Statute of limitations   Time period in which a patient must file suit for medical malpractice.

Statutory adults   Minor who may consent to medical treatment at 14 years of age.

Student portfolio   A folder in which students have collected samples of projects and course work they have completed. Students should also keep track of accomplishments and special activities they participated in to present to prospective employers.

Subjective   Portion of the chart notes that documents information received from the patient.

Subpeona   An order to appear in court.

Subpeona duces tecum   An order to produce medical records for trial.

Subscriber   The individual who holds the insurance policy; policyholder.

Summary sheet   The top sheet in a medical file containing a patient's insurance information and address, telephone, employer, date of birth, and next of kin. May also include a brief summary of significant diagnoses, release information, and other necessary information.

Superbill   A documentation of a patient's office visit listing the charges incurred and patient's diagnosis; an invoice for a physician's services; also known as encounter form, fee slip, service record, or charge ticket.

Terminal digit filing   A filing method that involves breaking a chart number into a series of groups and filing within each group.

Tickler file   A system that reminds an assistant to perform a certain activity at a certain time.

Urgent care   Providing quick attention to a patient's health problem with immediate access to health care; urgent care centers usually operate on a walk-in basis.

Usual, customary, and reasonable (UCR) fee   Average amount charged by local physicians for services rendered. Insurers may not pay the portion of a fee that is higher than the UCR fee.

Vendor   Business or supplier from which merchandise is being purchased.

Voice mail   A telephone system that works like an answering machine: a message is recorded for the caller and the caller can leave a message.

Walk-in   A patient without an appointment. Some offices leave spots open for acutely ill patients who come in without a prior appointment.

Workers' compensation   Insurance coverage for employees who suffer from work-related injuries, diseases, illnesses, or even death.

INDEX

Note: Page numbers followed by the letter b refer to boxed material; those followed by the letter f refer to figures, and those followed by the letter t refer to tables.